Drug Delivery Nanosystems

Drug Delivery Nanosystems

From Bioinspiration and Biomimetics to Clinical Applications

edited by

Costas Demetzos
Stergios Pispas
Natassa Pippa

CRC Press
Taylor & Francis Group
Boca Raton London New York

CRC Press is an imprint of the
Taylor & Francis Group, an **informa** business

Drug Delivery Nanosystems: From Bioinspiration and Biomimetics to Clinical Applications

First published 2019 by Pan Stanford Publishing Pte. Ltd.

Published 2023 by CRC Press
Taylor & Francis Group
6000 Broken Sound Parkway NW, Suite 300
Boca Raton, FL 33487-2742

ISBN 978-981-4774-92-5 (hbk)
ISBN 978-0-429-49054-5 (ebk)

Visit the Taylor & Francis Web site at
http://www.taylorandfrancis.com

and the CRC Press Web site at
http://www.crcpress.com

British Library Cataloguing-in-Publication Data
A catalogue record for this book is available from the British Library.

Contents

Preface

Nanotechnology is the interdisciplinary field that deals with the development and utilization of materials that can be used to make devices and products with sizes equal to one-billionth of a meter. Nanotechnology is an emerging technology seeking to exploit distinct technological advances controlling the structure of nanoscale biomaterials at a nanodimensional scale approaching individual molecules and their aggregates or supramolecular structures. The term "nanomedicine" is used to describe the technologies under the umbrella of nanotechnology with therapeutic applications in human health.

Overall, this multiauthored book presents some recent trends and research achievements in the field of pharmaceutical nanotechnology and advanced drug delivery nanosystems. The applications of drug delivery nanosystems that are considered as carriers of active pharmaceutical ingredients (i.e., small molecules, proteins, peptides, and nucleic acids) will be analyzed on the basis of technology, preparation protocol, and biomedical applications. Liposomes, solid lipid nanoparticles, dendrimers, polymersomes, micelles, carbon nanotubes, nanoshells, hydrogels, etc., are presented in considerable depth, and special attention is given to the pharmaceutical technology and biomedical applications in terms of their design and development approaches. There is an extensive report on the principles and design protocols, as well as applications, of the nanosystems in drug delivery and targeting of active molecules with pharmaceutical interest. This multiauthored book summarizes several recent trends within the last five years in the field of drug delivery nanosystems, especially for theranostic purposes.

Pharmaceutical nanotechnology offers several solutions to resolve problems of water insolubility of active pharmaceutical ingredients. Production of drug nanocrystals is just one way to modify the intrinsic properties, like solubility, of the drug material. In Chapter 1 the characteristic properties of drug nanocrystals and the most important preparation techniques are presented. Furthermore, the benefits of the drug nanocrystals and examples of their applications in drug delivery and medical purposes are also reviewed in the chapter.

The scope of Chapter 2 is to define physicochemical properties and pharmaceutical applications of cyclodextrin-based nanosystems that have been investigated for utilization in diagnostics, therapeutics, and theranostics.

In line with the previous chapter, Chapter 3 discusses in depth the challenges associated with the development of hydrogels as delivery platforms and also issues that are related to their preparation process, their physicochemical properties, the drug release kinetics, and the conditions under which the therapeutic system is delivered to the human body. Special attention is given to stimuli-responsive nanogels.

The various nanotechnology formulation approaches in ocular drug delivery presented in the last few years are reviewed in Chapter 4, and their benefits, as well as limitations, are outlined.

Dendrimers and their biomedical applications are considered as emerging and exponentially growing technologies, with great potential in the development of novel therapeutic and preventive strategies against human immunodeficiency virus type 1 (HIV-1) infection because they are similar in size to biological structures. In particular, dendrimers are emerging as promising candidates for many applications in nanomedicine and deserve attention as they are used as solubility enhancers; anticancer, anti-inflammatory, and antiviral drugs; drug delivery carriers; and diagnosis and imaging agents. In this context, HIV-1 remains a growing and evolving epidemic, but new developments and enhanced models offer promising outcomes. This growing field is presented in Chapter 5.

Carbon nanotubes have attracted the attention of many researchers owing to their superior structural, mechanical, and electrical properties. In Chapter 6, the authors characterize albumin adsorption in terms of protein orientation, interacting residues, binding affinity, and protein conformational rearrangements due to albumin's interaction with carbon nanotubes.

The objective of Chapter 7 is to summarize recent research progress in the application of metal nanocrystals in biological systems, namely selective targeting of specific bio-oriented species and drug delivery, especially regarding cancer treatment. Moreover, a brief outlook regarding, current challenges in, and limitations in metal nanocluster research are also provided.

The series of examples of coupled experimental/modeling investigations in the field of self-assembled multivalent nanovectors for biological polyanion binding, illustrated and discussed in Chapter 8, emphasize both the fundamental role and the potentiality displayed by this approach in the pre- and postdevelopment of nanodevices for DNA and heparin binding and the hurdles that this field has to face before it can be translated into the clinical setting.

A novel 3D nucleic acid architecture, referred to as the spherical nucleic acid, is described in Chapter 9. A spherical nucleic acid (SNA) is typically a small (sub-100 nm) 3D structure composed of a gold core to which a shell of functionalized oligonucleotides is attached. These structures are characterized with a set of properties distinct from those of the linear forms of nucleic acids with the same sequence. They exhibit numerous advantages (colloidal stability, superior cellular uptake via scavenger receptor-mediated endocytosis, etc.). The capability of SNAs to interact with biological materials in unique ways, resulting from the arrangement of oligonucleotides into highly oriented, densely packed structures, provides us venues to use them in molecular diagnostics, gene regulation, and medicine.

Nanooncology is the application of nanobiotechnology in cancer, and it is the most important chapter of nanomedicine. Various applications in the diagnosis and therapy of cancer are discussed in Chapter 10, the aim being to show how nanotechnology is applied in the study of cancer and to discuss the various applications of nanotechnology in the diagnosis and treatment of this disease. Radiolabeled nanoparticles as diagnostic and therapeutic agents of cancer have been already designed and developed as useful weapons in the field of nanooncology.

In vivo imaging is an efficient noninvasive technique for testing innovative nanoparticles. Computed tomography, X-ray, scintigraphic, and single-photon emission tomography imaging techniques, as well as some other in vivo imaging techniques, are presented in Chapter 11. The basic principles and the instrumentation of them are discussed, and several examples from the recent literature are given.

Finally, nanotoxicology involves different aspects of science, from molecular biology to quantum physics and chemistry, and lays the foundations for eliminating all risks related to the manufacturing and applications of nanoparticles. All these very important issues are discussed in Chapter 12. According to the authors, the major obstacle associated with determining the hazardous impacts of nanoparticles is the variety of parameters that are probably responsible for their adverse effects. It is widely known that the dosage, size, composition, aggregation, surface charge, structure, and chemistry and even the route of administration of nanoparticles and the duration of exposure to them are the main characteristics upon which nanotoxicity depends.

We would like to express our gratitude to all authors for their complementary and important contributions. Their expertise in the fields of drug delivery, nanotechnology, and theranostics makes this book comprehensive and valuable for the scientists working in the area of nanomedicine.

Prof. Costas Demetzos
Dr. Stergios Pispas
Dr. Natassa Pippa
2018

Chapter 1

Nanocrystals in Medical Applications

Leena Peltonen and Jouni Hirvonen
Faculty of Pharmacy, University of Helsinki, P.O. Box 56,
Viikinkaari 5 E, 00014 University of Helsinki, Finland
leena.peltonen@helsinki.fi

Drug nanocrystals are solid drug nanoparticles covered by a stabilizer layer. Mostly they are utilized in order to improve solubility properties of poorly soluble drug materials, but they have also been used for controlled release purposes, for example, in implantable systems, where the drug release can last for months. Formation of drug nanocrystals is utilized in manipulating the physicochemical properties of compounds, like the solubility of drug materials, since many material-related properties are changed when going down into the nanorange. For drug administration purposes, the nanocrystals are further formulated to nanosuspensions, implants, tablets, capsules, etc. In this chapter the characteristic properties of drug nanocrystals, their production, and their potential biomedical applications are presented.

Drug Delivery Nanosystems: From Bioinspiration and Biomimetics to Clinical Applications
Edited by Costas Demetzos, Stergios Pispas, and Natassa Pippa

ISBN 978-981-4774-92-5 (Hardcover), 978-0-429-49054-5 (eBook)
www.panstanford.com

1.1 Introduction

Drug nanocrystals are solid, nanosized drug particles that are surrounded by a stabilizer layer. Stabilizers are needed due to the small particle size, because the nanosized particles are inherently unstable and tend to aggregate in order to minimize the total interfacial area of the system. Drug nanocrystals have been studied intensively since the beginning of the 1990s, and the first patent was issued in 1992 [1]. The first drug nanocrystals were formulated by a wet-milling technique, and since then the milling methods have been protected by numerous patents. This led to the invention of another industrially important production technique, namely high-pressure homogenization (HPH) [2]. Since the beginning of the 2010s the milling patents started to expire and there was more room for nanomilling formulations again. As of today, nanomilling is the most utilized technique for the production of drug nanocrystals [3].

Drug nanocrystals can be produced either by the so-called top-down or bottom-up techniques. In top-down methods the particle size of bulk material is decreased in a controlled way to the nanosized particle range, while in bottom-up techniques nanoparticles are built up molecule by molecule. In all these systems the final product is nanosized drug particles covered with a stabilizer layer, but depending on the formulation technique, particle properties like size, shape, level of crystallinity, morphology, etc., may differ.

Production of drug nanocrystals is just one way to modify the intrinsic properties, like solubility, of the drug material. Accordingly, for a final formulation, further process steps like drying of drug nanosuspensions, tableting, particle loading into a matrix system, etc., are needed. Drug nanocrystals are mostly utilized in improving the solubility properties of poorly soluble drug materials, but controlled release applications with over one-month drug release profiles also exist [4].

In this chapter the characteristic properties of drug nanocrystals and the most important preparation techniques are presented. Furthermore, the benefits of drug nanocrystals and examples on their applications in drug delivery and medical purposes are reviewed.

1.2 Characteristics of Drug Nanocrystals

Drug nanocrystals are solid drug particles, typically sized with some hundreds of nanometers, covered by a stabilizer layer (Fig. 1.1). Sometimes drug nanocrystals are referred to as solid micelles. The main role of the stabilizer is to stabilize the nanosized particles against aggregation. Typical stabilizers are either some kind of amphiphilic surfactants [5, 6] or polymers [7]; the stabilizers are discussed in more detail in Section 1.3.5.

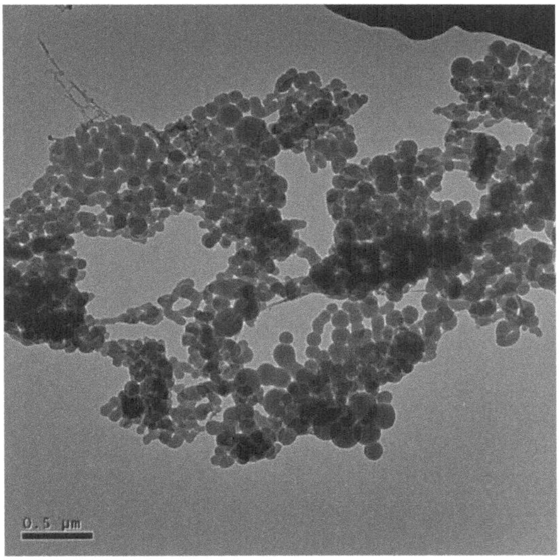

Figure 1.1 TEM images of hydrophobin protein–coated beclomethasone dipropionate nanocrystals. Reprinted with permission from [8]. Copyright (2008) American Chemical Society.

The most prominent benefits reached with nanocrystals are based on the increased surface area per mass solid, and they can be divided into three main classes: (i) fast dissolution, (ii) higher solubility, and (iii) increased adhesion to biological membranes. These benefits are presented more precisely next.

1.2.1 Improved Dissolution Rate

The most prominent effect reached with drug nanocrystals is the higher dissolution rate (Fig. 1.2).

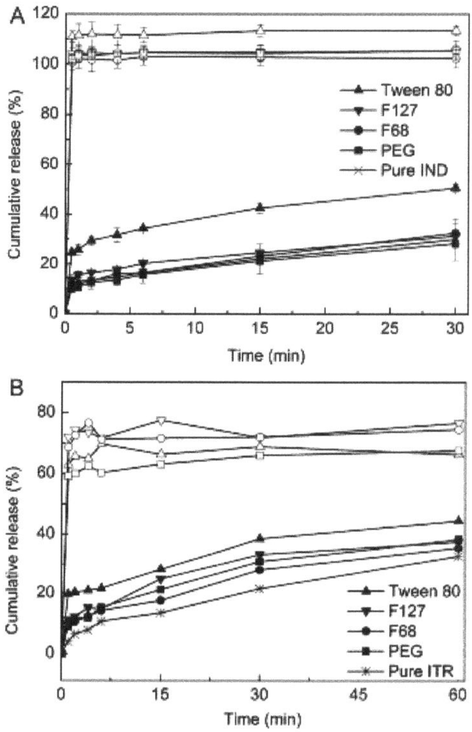

Figure 1.2 Dissolution profiles of (A) indomethacin and (B) itraconazole nanocrystals (open symbols) and corresponding dissolution curves of physical mixtures (solid symbols). Reprinted from [5], Copyright (2011), with permission from Elsevier.

Fast dissolution is based on increased interfacial area; when the particle size is decreased, the interfacial area per mass unit of drug for dissolution is increased. For example, for spherical particles, the surface area versus volume, $A/V = 3/r$; for example, if the particle size is reduced from 50 μm to 500 nm, the dissolution rate is increased a hundredfold. On the basis of Noyes–Whitney equation (Eq. 1.1)

$$\frac{dC}{dt} = \frac{DS}{Vh}(C_s - C), \tag{1.1}$$

where dC/dt is the dissolution rate (concentration change as a function of time), D is the diffusion coefficient, S is the surface area, V is the dissolution volume, h is the diffusion layer thickness, C_s is the saturation concentration, and C is the concentration at time t. For drug nanocrystals the increased dissolution rate is mainly due to the increased surface area (S) but also due to the higher saturation solubility (C_s). For particle sizes below approximately 50 μm the diffusion layer thickness is also decreased, which affects the total dissolution rate.

Dissolution of even very poorly soluble drug nanocrystals, when measured under sink conditions, is often very fast (Fig. 1.2) [5]. To find differences between different size fractions, higher separating conditions are required during dissolution testing, and thus, new techniques and methodologies have been developed for more precise and more discriminating dissolution testing [9]. On the basis of simulations, if the dissolution testing were performed exactly on the solubility limit of the drug (the volume of the medium in the dissolution test was exactly the same as that required for the total dissolution of all of the sample under test), the discriminating power was the highest [9]. This was further confirmed experimentally with a United States Pharmacopeia (USP) paddle method under nonsink conditions: differences in dissolution behavior were seen even between particle size fractions with mean sizes of 340 and 560 nm.

1.2.2 Increased Solubility

The solubility increase is based on Ostwald–Freundlich theory (Eq. 1.2). The theory was originally developed for liquid droplets in a gas phase, but later it was also considered valid for solid particles in liquids:

$$S_{\mathrm{NP}} = S_0 \left(\frac{2V_{\mathrm{m}}\gamma}{RTr} \right), \tag{1.2}$$

where S_{NP} is the solubility of nanoparticles with radius r, S_0 is the solubility of bulk material, V_{m} is the molar volume, γ is the interfacial tension, R is the gas constant, and T is the temperature.

Solubility of drug nanocrystals with different size fractions has been studied by measuring intrinsic dissolution rates in a flow-through dissolution equipment and by determining concentration profiles in a UV imaging system [10]. In the flow-through setup the measurements were performed from a constant surface area, and hence, the effect of increased dissolution area was ruled out. Results showed clearly that an increase in particle size led to a decreased dissolution rate. The highest differences, tenfold, were found when comparing the smallest nanocrystals (size 580 nm) to bulk drug. In the UV imaging tests it was shown that with nanocrystal samples a supersaturated state was reached: concentration levels reached with nanocrystal samples were even fivefold higher than the thermodynamic solubility value of the drug (Fig. 1.3).

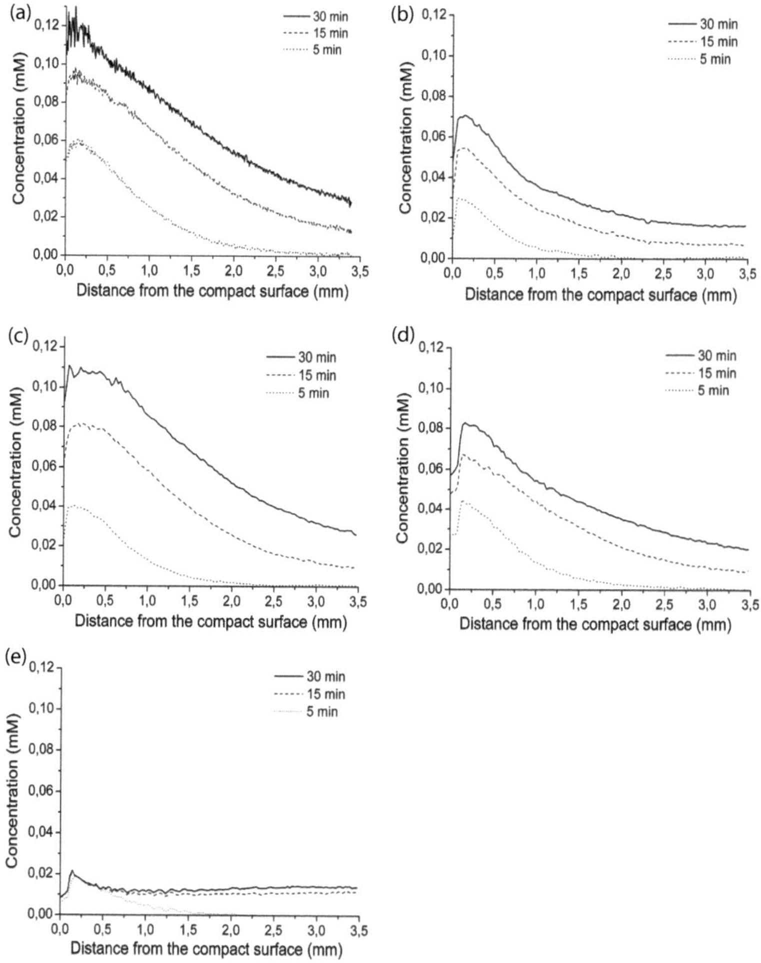

Figure 1.3 Apparent drug concentration values as a function of distance from compressed Poloxamer F68– or Poloxamer F127–stabilized indomethacin nanocrystal surfaces at time points 5, 15, and 30 min. (A) F68-stabilized 580 nm nanocrystals, (B) F68-stabilized microcrystals, (C) F127-stabilized 580 nm nanocrystals, (D) F127-stabilized microcrystals, and (E) bulk indomethacin. Reprinted from [10], Copyright (2013), with permission from Elsevier.

1.2.3 Improved Mucoadhesion

Mostly drug nanocrystals are utilized in order to improve the dissolution and/or solubility of poorly soluble drug materials, and in vivo the particles are dissolved almost immediately. However, when working with extremely poorly soluble materials, it may be the case that the nanocrystals remain in solid state for a longer time. Here the third benefit, increased adhesion of the nanocrystals on biological surfaces, may be a reality. Again, higher adhesion to surfaces is a consequence of the increased surface area as compared to the particle volume. Increased mucoadhesion leads to longer residence times in the body, and this can increase the drug bioavailability [11].

1.2.4 Possible Drug Candidates for Nanocrystallization

As already mentioned, drug nanocrystals are mostly utilized for improving the solubility of poorly soluble drug materials. New, efficient screening methods have led to increasing numbers of poorly soluble drug candidates, and it has been estimated that even 90% of the new chemical entities are poorly soluble, some 70% belonging to the Biopharmaceutics Classification System (BCS) class II and 20% to class IV [12, 13]. BCS class II drugs are poorly soluble but easily permeable, and those are obvious candidates for nanocrystallization [14].

BCS class II can still be divided into two subclasses, namely (i) class IIa, dissolution rate limited or so-called brick-dust molecules, and (ii) class IIb, solubility limited or so-called grease ball molecules. For grease ball molecules often the first choice of development is lipid formulations, although nanocrystal techniques have also been successfully used for these molecules [15]. For brick-dust molecules nanocrystallization is one of the first formulation options. Besides class II drugs, class IV drugs also may benefit from nanocrystallization. If the drug concentration, for example, in the gastrointestinal (GI) tract is higher due to the higher saturation solubility of drug nanocrystals, increased concentration gradient between the intestine and lumen may enhance permeation/absorption.

1.2.5 Cell Interactions of Drug Nanocrystals

Due to their small particle size, it is possible that drug nanocrystals are taken up by cells as solid undissolved particles. Chen and Li [16] studied the cellular uptake of sulforhodamine B–labeled paclitaxel nanocrystals with a KB cell line. They showed that nanocrystals could be taken up by the cells. The cell uptake mechanism was presumably via endocytosis, and higher intracellular drug concentrations were reached with a nanocrystal formulation as compared to the drug in solution. When the surface coatings (stabilizer layers on top of the nanocrystals) were changed, nanocrystal–cell interactions were altered.

Cellular interactions of paliperidone palmitate nano- and microcrystals were studied in macrophage cell cultures by coherent anti-Stokes Raman scattering (CARS) microscopy [17, 18], and the fate of nano- and microcrystals in vitro in macrophagial RAW cells as well as ex vivo in histological sections were imaged. It was shown that the nanocrystals were internalized into the cells in vitro and into the granulomatous tissue ex vivo (Fig. 1.4).

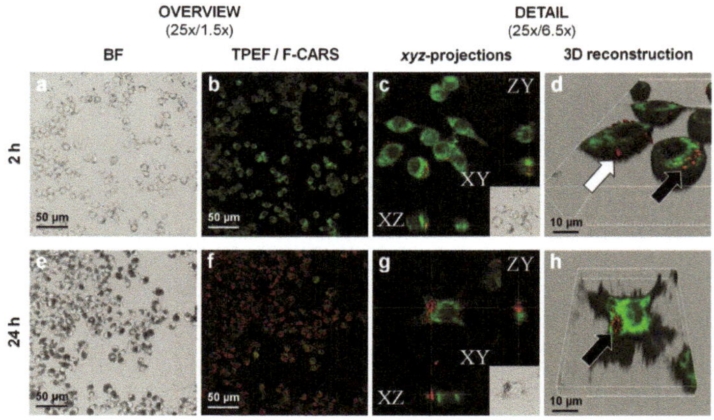

Figure 1.4 CARS imaging of paliperidone palmitate nano- and microcrystal interactions with RAW 264.7 macrophages. (a and e) Low- and high-magnification bright-field imaging. (b and f) Forward-detected CARS (F-CARS) (red)/two-photon excitation microscopy (TPEF) (green) merged micrographs of stained/fixed RAW 264.7 macrophages after incubation for 2 h (a–d) and 24 h (e–h). (c and g) Orthogonal projections of z-stacked F-CARS/TPEF overlays showing intracellular nano- and microcrystals. (d and h) Three-dimensional reconstructions of the z-stacked F-CARS/TPEF overlays. The white and black arrows indicate cell surface–adsorbed and phagocytosed nanocrystals, respectively. Reprinted from [17], Copyright (2015), with permission from Elsevier.

1.3 Preparation of Drug Nanocrystals

Drug nanocrystals can be produced by top-down or bottom-up methods. In top-down methods the nanosized particles are formed by decreasing the particle size of bulk material in a liquid dispersion, for example, by milling or homogenization techniques [2, 3, 19, 20]. On the other hand, in bottom-up techniques, the nanosized particles are formed by building up nanosized structures molecule by molecule with different kinds of precipitation-based methods [21–23]. It is also possible to combine the different methods for even more efficient particle size reduction. In the subsequent chapters different methods to produce drug nanocrystals are presented.

1.3.1 Top-Down Methods

Top-down methods are widely studied, and they utilize different kinds of media milling [5, 24, 25] and HPH [2] techniques. In these methods the scaling changes are considerably easy to perform and repeatability of processes is at a good level; almost all of the commercial nanocrystal products are produced by these techniques, most of them by different kinds of milling techniques [26].

Milling and homogenization are performed in suspension; mostly aqueous suspensions are used, although oil or polyethylene glycols (PEGs) can also be utilized. Thus, these techniques are water-based approaches without the use of organic solvents, which provides an environment-friendly approach [26, 27]. The presence of water increases molecular mobility and reduces the glass transition temperature of a compound, which hinders the formation of amorphous materials and stabilizes the crystalline form [28]. Accordingly, after milling, the drug typically remains in crystalline form, although polymorphic changes may take place [5, 29]. HPH can promote the formation of amorphous form, followed by possible subsequent recrystallization, but in this technique also, besides the other process variables, the presence of water stabilizes the crystalline form [28–31].

Particle size reduction is based on mechanical attrition (milling) or high-pressure collisions (HPH). The main drawbacks of these techniques are that the processes are considerably energy intensive, although today more efficient processes and reduced processing times have lowered the energy consumption. In the best cases, milling times for production of nanosized drug particles can be even a few minutes (Fig. 1.5) [5].

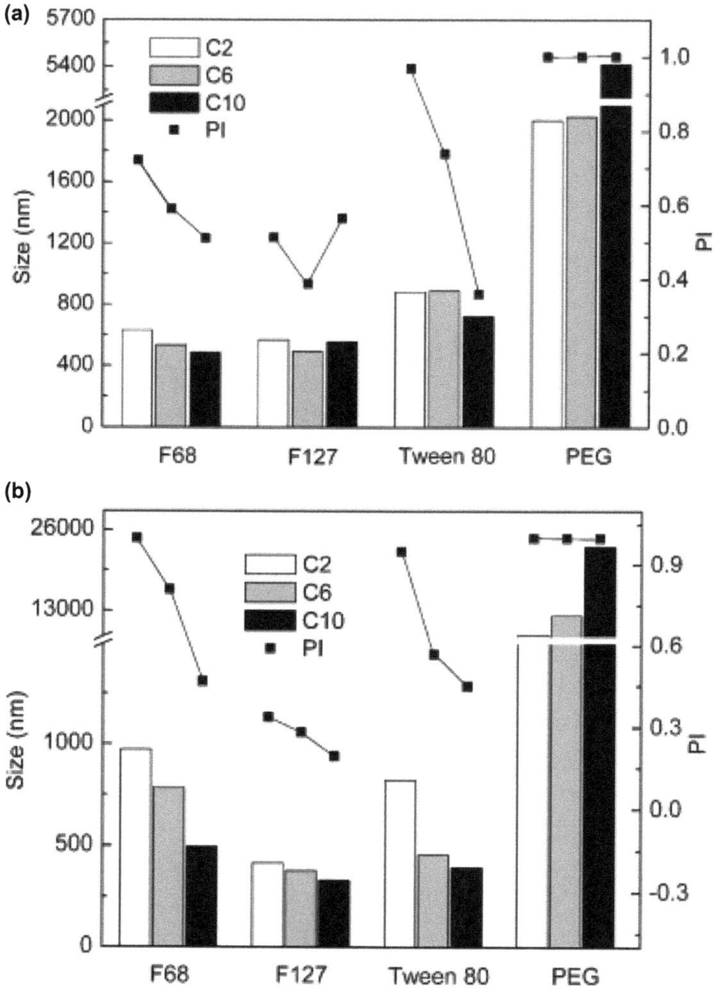

Figure 1.5 Mean particle size values and polydispersity indices (PIs) of (a) indomethacin and (b) itraconazole nanocrystals produced by wet milling with different stabilizers (poloxamer F68, poloxamer F127, Tween 80, and PEG) and after different milling times (C2, C6, and C10 in the figure mean after 6, 18, and 30 min. milling, correspondingly). Reprinted from [5], Copyright (2011), with permission from Elsevier.

The milling efficiency depends on, for example, hardness of the drug material, viscosity of the system (high viscosity can pose problems in milling or in HPH), energy input, and pearl size (smaller milling pearls typically produce smaller particle sizes) [14, 19, 20, 32]. Other drawbacks are possible wearing of equipment and contamination due to wearing, as well as hardness of the drug material, but this can be diminished by utilizing hard milling and vessel materials like ceramics (zirconium oxide) or coated milling pearls [33]. Milling media (pearls) and vessels should be made from the same material in order to avoid erosion.

HPH can be divided into three different approaches: (i) jet streaming (Microfluidizer, IDD-PTM, insoluble drug delivery microparticle technology), where high-energy suspension flows are collided in a microfluidizer system [2], and (ii) piston–gap homogenization, where particle size reduction is based on cavitation, shear forces and particle collision, when the drug suspension is forced through a small gap with high pressure (typically up to 1,500 bar) (iiia) in water (Dissocubes®) [34] or (iiib) in non-aqueous media (Nanopure®) [32, 35, 36].

1.3.2 Bottom-Up Methods

Bottom-up techniques are based on the precipitation of a drug from a supersaturated solution. Precipitation can be due to the addition of a nonsolvent, use of a supercritical fluid, solvent removal, or high-energy liquid atomization [21, 22, 37, 38]. These techniques are efficient at the laboratory scale, and often smaller particle sizes with high monodispersity can be reached with these techniques, but scaling up, controlled growth of particle size, laborious removal of solvents (often organic solvents are required due to the poor solubility of drug materials), and finding of a suitable nonsolvent/solvent combination, are often problematic. Most of the poorly soluble drug materials are also poorly soluble in many other solvents. Precipitation methods can produce amorphous materials [30, 31, 37]. This may cause stability problems, because the amorphous form tends to recrystallize and uncontrolled crystallization, for example, during storage can change the material and dosage form properties like solubility [31].

1.3.3 Combination Methods

To reach even smaller particle sizes, a combination of two different techniques can be used. In general, the combination techniques include a preprocess step followed by a high-energy top-down method. Besides a smaller particle size, combination techniques can be used to avoid, for example, clogging of the high-pressure homogenizer or shortening of milling times. The first combinatorial technique was nonsolvent precipitation followed by HPH (Nanoedge™ [3, 39]). Later it was mostly replaced by SmartCrystal® technology, where different preprocesses are combined with HPH [32]: Nanopure (no pretreatment step before HPH), H42 (spray-drying and HPH), H69 (precipitation and HPH), H96 (lyophilization and HPH), and combination technology (CT) (media milling and HPH). A quite novel combinatorial technique is nonsolvent precipitation followed by ultrasonication [31].

Although with combination techniques it is possible to reach even smaller particles or avoid some process-related problems, the fact is that extra process steps (preprocess) increase the overall complexity of the whole process and also the costs. Accordingly, combination techniques are not the first choice if the corresponding end product can be reached with a single process [3].

1.3.4 Comparison of Different Techniques

Independent of the selected technique, whether top-down, bottom-up, or combination, all the techniques mentioned produce solid drug cores coated with a stabilizer layer. However, for example, particle shape, porosity, size, or level of crystallinity may differ depending on the production method and the process parameters.

Milling, for example, typically produces edged particle shapes, while antisolvent precipitation or liquid atomization may result in almost spherical particles. But it is also important to note that not only the process but also the raw material have an impact on the formed particles (Fig. 1.6). In bottom-up techniques smaller particle sizes can be easily reached, even particles below 100 nm. For example, nonsolvent precipitation of hydrophobin-stabilized itraconazole [21] and beclomethasone dipropionate [8] nanocrystals with approximated particle sizes of 100 nm were reached. But top-down methods are also able to produce small particles: Bujnakova et al. produced arsenic sulfide nanocrystals by milling (rotational speed 4000 and milling time 2 h), and the final product had a mean particle size around 100 nm [33]. Accordingly, not only the technique itself but the equipment design, raw material properties, and process parameters affect the final product properties. Liquid atomization–based techniques generally produce more porous particles with a lower level of crystallinity [23]. All the above-mentioned particle properties affect dissolution and solubility [9, 10], as well as cellular interactions [40], and in that sense are important parameters to be controlled.

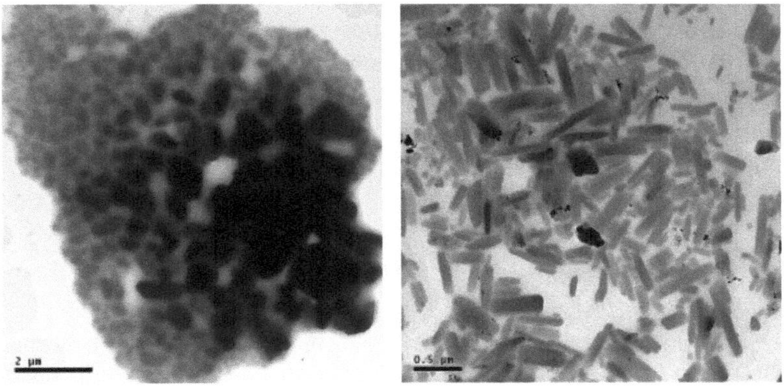

Figure 1.6 Transmission electron microscopy (TEM) images of indomethacin (left) and itraconazole (right) nanocrystals produced by nanomilling. Reprinted from [5], Copyright (2011), with permission from Elsevier.

1.3.5 Stabilizer

The selection and amount of stabilizer is often the crucial step for production of drug nanocrystals [5, 6]. In drug nanocrystals the main role of the stabilizer is to stabilize the inherently unstable nanosized particles against aggregation and Ostwald ripening. Typically the drug:stabilizer ratio is from 1:1 to 10:1. Normally all the stabilizer is added in the beginning of the process, but, for example, with high-viscosity polymers periodic addition may be beneficial.

Typical stabilizers of nanocrystals can be divided into the following groups: (i) semisynthetic nonionic polymers (e.g., celluloses like hydroxypropyl methylcellulose [HPMC], methyl cellulose [MC], hydroxyethyl cellulose [HEC], hydroxypropyl cellulose [HPC]) [7], (ii) semisynthetic ionic polymers (NaCMC, NaAlginate) [41], (iii) synthetic copolymers (poloxamers, polyvinyl alcohol–PEG graft copolymers) [42], (iv) ionic surfactants (sodium dodecyl sulfate [SDS], sodium docusate, sodium deoxycholate) [43], and (v) nonionic surfactants (polysorbates, sorbitan esters) [5]. Typically also mixtures of more than one stabilizer, like a polymer combined to a surfactant or nonionic and ionic stabilizer, have been used to increase the efficiency of the stabilization [43].

Many stabilizers can affect cells and cell layers and act as permeation enhancers (e.g., polysorbates, poloxamers) or as mucoadhesive materials and hence increase drug bioavailability even more [44, 45]. The permeation-enhancing effect can be due to the opening of the tight junctions, making the cell layers more leaky or having an impact on active transportation systems, like the permeability glycoprotein (P-gp) inhibiting factor. Via mucoadhesion the residence time in a certain body area is prolonged. The challenge in utilizing the transport activity/permeation-enhancing effect or mucoadhesion for higher bioavailability is that the drug and the excipient should be simultaneously available in the optimum absorption area.

When paclitaxel was formulated in solution together with vitamin E d-α-tocopheryl polyethylene glycol 1000 succinate (TPGS), a P-gp inhibitor, the drug was transported out from the cells by the P-gp because TPGS was not inside the cells at the same time than the drug [46]. However, when TPGS-stabilized paclitaxel nanocrystals were administered, no P-gp activity was detected because of successful TPGS inhibition [47].

1.3.6 Quality-by-Design Approach

Implementation of the quality-by-design (QbD) approach has increased in nanosuspension production during the past years [31, 48, 49]. In general, the QbD approach for nanosuspensions includes (i) selecting stabilizer(s) and processes on the basis of the quality target product profile (QTPP), (ii) defining critical quality attributes (CQAs) and critical process parameters (CPPs) on the basis of earlier experience, and (iii) with the aid of design of experiments (DoE) building a design space [50].

Depending on the target, factors like particle size, shape, solubility, and stability can be the CQAs [51]. The QbD approach comprehensively and systemically takes into account the impact of different variables in order to reach the optimal end product in terms of, for example, particle size or crystallinity. CPPs help in determining process-controlling tools during manufacturing. Proper design space ensures uniform product performance between different batches.

1.3.7 Scaling Up and Scaling Down

Some nanocrystal techniques offer flexibility of both up-scaling and down-scaling, depending on, for example, whether the process is a batch or a continuous process, but mostly studied are scaling changes with different milling processes [52, 53]. The HPH process forces suspension through a narrow gap, which can pose problems in miniaturization, but equipment with a volume of 3.5 mL has been described in the literature [29]. In HPH the equipment can be used in discontinuous mode at the laboratory scale [54].

In milling, the basic principle is agitation of devices containing the starting suspension with the drug and stabilizer and the milling medium, while scale-up or scale-down is considerably easy to perform. However, differences in product properties between small-scale experiments and large-scale production are possible due to the altered energy input and particle size reduction mechanisms [55, 56].

Small-scale milling tests have been performed with as low as 10 mg of drug per experiment: this amount is enough for a thorough physicochemical characterization of the product [57]. Seven different drugs were tested, and the milling was performed in a 96-well plate. Yttrium-stabilized milling pearls were used, and the suspension and milling pearls were put into the wells of the well plate on an orbital shaker. Another small-scale design is to put the suspension together with the milling medium in small glass vials, which are then put inside a milling vessel. Both of these settings were shown to be feasible for preclinical screening purposes, but wearing of the well plate/vials and contamination due to wearing limit the utilization of these techniques, because the vessel and milling media are from different materials (differences in hardness).

Scaling up of milling systems has been shown in many studies and also by an increasing number of marketed products [48, 56, 58]. Examples of successful scaling up of other methods are SmartCrystal combination technology scaled from laboratory to pilot scale [59], combination of static mixing and spray drying to large-scale continuous production of pharmaceutical nanocrystal formulations [60], and the precipitation–homogenization technique for large-scale nanocrystal production [61].

1.4 Applications of Drug Nanocrystals

The total number of nanocrystal drug product applications submitted to the Food and Drug Administration (FDA) during the years 1973–2015 was 82, and these applications formed 30% of all the drug product applications containing nanomaterials [62]. When divided on the basis of the route of administration, 65% were for oral administration, 20% for intravenous, 7% for intramuscular, 3% for ocular, 2% for inhalation, and 1% for both intraperitoneal and intratumoral drug delivery routes. If the therapeutic areas are taken into account, 26% were anti-infective, 24% anticancer, 11% anti-anorexia, 7% anti-emetic, 5% antipsychotic, 4% lipid lowering, 3% antihypertensive, and 3% antihyperthermic, while 2% each were for immunosuppression, pain relief, and other indications.

Administration of nanosuspensions and nanocrystals may take place via different drug delivery routes. The oral drug delivery route is the most popular and convenient, and oral solid dosage forms of nanocrystals are usually preferred for commercialization (Table 1.1). Sirolimus (Rapamune®) was the first nanocrystalline drug on the market in 2000, soon followed by other orally administered nanocrystalline formulations like megestrol acetate (Megace®, 2001), aprepitant (Emend®, 2003), and fenofibrate (Tricor®, 2004) [63].

Nanocrystals are often converted to dry powders, which are further formulated into dosage forms: tablets, capsules, pellets, or liquid nanosuspensions. Gao et al. [64] listed the benefits of nanocrystalline and nanoparticulate dosage forms in oral drug delivery: enhanced oral bioavailability (improved drug dissolution/solubility), reduced fasted-/fed-state variation, potentially improved transcellular uptake of the nanoparticles (or at least improved mucoadhesion of the nanoparticles), and improved safety profiles of the nanocrystal formulations. The mucoadhesive and gastroretentive properties of coated nanoparticles can be modified, for example, with hydrophobin proteins [11]. Upon entry of the nanoparticles from the stomach into the intestines, it was observed that the particles experienced a delay; hydrophobin-coated nanoparticles were retained in the rat stomach up to three hours after administration, whereas uncoated nanoparticles were released significantly faster in the same conditions.

Table 1.1 Nanocrystalline products on the market as approved by the US FDA [63]

Drug	Indication	Description
Aprepitant	Antiemetic	Faster absorption and increased bioavailability
Fenofibrate	Hyperlipidemia	Higher bioavailability, simplified administration
Sirolimus	Immunosupressant	Higher bioavailability
Megestrol acetate	Anti-anorectic	Reduced dosing
Morphine sulfate	Psychostimulant	Higher drug loading and improved bioavailability, extended release
Dexamethyl-phenidate HCl	Psychostimulant	Higher drug loading and improved bioavailability
Methylphyenidate HCl	Psychostimulant	Higher drug loading and improved bioavailability
Tizanidine HCl	Muscle relaxant	Higher drug loading and improved bioavailability
Calcium phosphate	Bone substitute	Mimicking bone structure; cell adhesive and allowing cell growth
Hydroxyapatite	Bone substitute	Mimicking bone structure; cell adhesive and allowing cell growth
Palperidone palmitate	Schizophrenia	Extended drug release
Dantrolene sodium	Malignant hypothermia	Faster administration with higher doses

Despite the benefits and ease of administration, nanocrystals provide special challenges in the design of oral solid drug formulations. Tuomela et al. [56] comprehensively screened powder and tablet compositions of indomethacin and itraconazole in order to find out optimal properties for the tableting of nanocrystalline formulations. As such, only the presence of nanocrystals in the composition improved the compressibility of tablets. The smaller the particle size was, the more contact surfaces there were providing potential interparticle bond formations and resulting in increased hardness/crushing strength of the tablets. When the nanocrystals were processed into granules before tableting, a further decrease in the required compression force was detected [56]. Disintegration testing results of the tablets revealed the fact that the less the amount of drug nanocrystals in the formulation, the more porous the structure formed; the disintegration times correlated well with the crushing strength values of the tablets. With at least indomethacin and itraconazole, the optimal amount of freeze-dried nanocrystals in the tablet composition was about 40% of the total mass, which was still able to maintain the improved dissolution profiles and disintegration times of the corresponding nanocrystal tablets.

Parenteral drug delivery (intravenous, intramuscular, and subcutaneous delivery routes) provides a quick (intravenous) or potentially retarded (intramuscular) onset of action, rapid targeting, and reduced dosage need of the drug. These routes are beneficial for drugs undergoing first-pass metabolism and drugs that are not absorbed or are degraded/irritating in the GI tract. Nanoparticles have potential as novel intravascular formulations for both diagnostic (imaging) and therapeutic purposes (drug delivery), or even a combination of these (theranostics). Successful parenteral nanoformulation delivery requests the drug to be able to target in specific tissues and cell types and escape from the reticuloendothelial system [65]. Parenteral administration of nanocrystals has advantages: administration of poorly soluble drugs without using high concentrations of toxic co-solvents, improved therapeutic effect of the drug, and targeted drug delivery to macrophages. Obvious drawbacks of this delivery route are the invasiveness of the mode of administration and the associated poor patient compliance.

Paliperidone palmitate nanocrystals as aqueous suspension formulations provide antipsychotic activity via monthly intramuscular injections (Table 1.1). The long-acting injection is effective in controlling the acute symptoms of schizophrenia, as well as in delaying the time to relapse. Factors influencing the drug release and absorption following the intramuscular injections are particle size (mean diameter 1.09 μm) and morphology [18]. Leng et al. [66] compared the pharmacokinetic behavior of two paliperidone palmitate nanosuspensions (prepared by wet media milling) with different particle sizes (1000 nm and 500 nm) after intramuscular administration. Also here the release of paliperidone lasted for almost one month after a single intramuscular dose. The area under the curve (AUC_{0-t}) and C_{max} (maximum concentration) values of the 1000 nm nanosuspensions were 2.0- and 1.8-fold higher, respectively, than the corresponding values of the 500 nm paliperidone nanosuspensions. However, the study demonstrated long-acting efficacy by both nanosuspensions.

Nanocrystal-covered implants provide a potential new strategy and extended therapeutic effect, especially in the development and utilization of orthopedic implants. Recently, titanium implant surfaces have been modified with calcium phosphate nanocrystals (Table 1.1), providing improved therapy for irradiated bone healing (osseointegration, development of structural and functional connection between the living bone and the surface of the implant) [67]. According to Bobo et al. [63], there exist no less than four different hydroxyapatite-containing nanocrystalline formulations on the market with the therapeutic indication of bone structure mimicking and enhancement of cellular adhesion and growth (Table 1.1).

Aqueous or dry powder nanosuspensions can be nebulized using mechanical or ultrasonic nebulizers for pulmonary drug delivery, reaching a uniform distribution of the drug in the lungs [24]. Nanocrystals may also increase the adhesiveness and prolong the pulmonary residence time of the drug. Müller and Jacobs [68] delivered budesonide drug nanoparticles with a nebulizer and the pharmacokinetic parameters showed a comparable AUC and higher C_{max} and lower T_{max} (time to reach maximum concentration) values compared to a control pulmonary dosage form.

Nanocrystal-based drug delivery systems also have important potential in the field of ocular drug delivery, especially when improving the poor bioavailability of poorly soluble drugs. Tuomela et al. [7] developed ophthalmic, intraocular pressure (IOP)-reducing nanocrystal suspensions from a poorly soluble drug, brinzolamide, by rapid wet milling. The elevated IOP values were reduced in vivo in rabbit eyes after nanocrystalline brinzolamide administration. The IOP-lowering effect was the most pronounced at pH 4.5, where the dissolved fraction of brinzolamide was the highest. Araújo et al. [69] have demonstrated that the poor bioavailability of drugs from ocular dosage forms is mainly due to precorneal loss factors, for example, tear dynamics, inefficient drug absorption, transient residence time in the cul-de-sac, and poor permeability of the corneal epithelial membrane. Thus, ocular nanocrystalline formulations are requested in order to improve drug penetration and maintain therapeutic drug levels with a reasonable application frequency and to reduce the unwanted local and systemic side effects.

1.5 Conclusions

When formulating raw materials to nanocrystals, not only the dissolution rate but also apparent solubility and mucoadhesive properties should be taken under consideration and research. On the basis of the above-mentioned physical properties of drug nanocrystals, they are mostly utilized in order to improve the solubility of poorly soluble drug materials, mainly BCS class II drugs, but are also used in applications for controlled release purposes, where the drug release lasts even for months. Numerous nanocrystalline drugs containing dosage forms have been commercialized since 2000, mostly delivered via oral or parenteral administration routes. It can be concluded that drug nanocrystals are a versatile option for improving and manipulation of the loading and release profiles of drug formulations.

References

1. Liversidge, G. G., Cundy, K. C., Bishop, J. F. and Czekai, D. A. (1992). Surface modified drug nanoparticles, USP patent 5145684.
2. Keck, C. M. and Müller, R. H. (2006). Drug nanocrystals of poorly soluble drugs produced by high pressure homogenization, *Eur. J. Pharm. Biopharm.*, **62**, pp. 3–16.

3. Möschwitzer, J. (2013). Drug nanocrystals in the commercial pharmaceutical development process, *Int. J. Pharm.*, **453**, pp. 142–156.

4. Wang, H., Zhang, G., Ma, X., Liu, Y., Feng, J., Park, K. and Wang, W. (2017). Enhanced encapsulation and bioavailability of breviscapine in PLGA microparticles by nanocystal and water-soluble polymer template techniques, *Eur. J. Pharm. Biopharm.*, **115**, pp. 177–185.

5. Liu, P., Rong, X., Laru, J., van Veen, B., Kiesvaara, J., Hirvonen, J., Laaksonen, T. and Peltonen, L. (2011). Nanosuspensions of poorly soluble drugs: preparation and development by wet milling, *Int. J. Pharm.*, **411**, pp. 215–222.

6. Liu, P., Viitala, T., Kartal-Hodzic, A., Liang, H., Laaksonen, T., Hirvonen, J. and Peltonen, L. (2015). Interaction studies between indomethacin nanocrystals and PEO/PPO copolymer stabilizers, *Pharm. Res.*, **32**, pp. 628–639.

7. Tuomela, A., Liu, P., Puranen, J., Rönkkö, S., Laaksonen, T., Kalesnykas, G., Oksala, O., Ilkka, J., Laru, J., Järvinen, K., Hirvonen, J. and Peltonen, L. (2014). Brinzolamide nanocrystal formulations for ophthalmic delivery: reduction of elevated intraocular pressure in vivo, *Int. J. Pharm.*, **467**, pp. 34–41.

8. Valo, H. K., Laaksonen, P. H., Peltonen, L. J., Linder, M. B., Hirvonen, J. T. and Laaksonen, T. J. (2010). Multifunctional hydrophobin: toward functional coatings for drug nanoparticles, *ACS Nano*, **4**, pp. 1750–1758.

9. Liu, P., De Wolf, O., Laru, J., Heikkilä, T., van Veen, B., Kiesvaara, J., Hirvonen, J., Peltonen, L. and Laaksonen, T. (2013). Dissolution studies of poorly soluble drug nanosuspensions in non-sink conditions, *AAPS PharmSciTech*, **14**, pp. 748–756.

10. Sarnes, A., Østergaard, J., Smedegaard Jensen, S., Aaltonen, J., Rantanen, J., Hirvonen, J. and Peltonen, L. (2013). Dissolution study of nanocrystal powders of a poorly soluble drug by UV imaging and channel flow methods, *Eur. J. Pharm. Sci.*, **50**, pp. 511–519.

11. Sarparanta, M. P., Bimbo, L. M., Mäkilä, E. M., Salonen, J. J., Laaksonen, P. H., Helariutta, K. A. M., Linder, M. B., Hirvonen, J. T., Laaksonen, T. J., Santos, H. A. and Airaksinen, A. J. (2012). The mucoadhesive and gastroretentive properties of hydrophobin-coated porous silicon nanoparticle oral drug delivery systems, *Biomaterials*, **33**, pp. 3353–3362.

12. Loftsson, T. and Brewster, M. E. (2010). Pharmaceutical applications of cyclodextrins: basic science and product development, *J. Pharm. Pharmacol.*, **62**, pp. 1607–1621.

13. Müller, R. H. and Keck, C. M. (2012). Twenty years of drug nanocrystals: where are we, and where do we go?, *Eur. J. Pharm. Biopharm.*, **80**, pp. 1–3.

14. Li, M., Alvarez, P. and Bilgili, E. (2017). A microhydrodynamic rationale for selection of bead size in preparation of drug nanosuspensions via wet stirred media milling, *Int. J. Pharm.*, **524**, pp. 178–192.

15. Rydberg, H. A., Arteta, M. Y., Berg, S., Lindfors, L. and Sigfridsson, K. (2016). Probing adsorption of DSPE-PEG2000 and DSPE-PEG5000 to the surface of felodipine and griseofulcin nanocrystals, *Int. J. Pharm.*, **510**, pp. 232–239.

16. Chen, Y. and Li, T. (2015). Cellular uptake mechanism of paclitaxel nanocrystals determined by confocal imaging and kinetic measurement, *AAPS J.*, **17**, pp. 1126–1134.

17. Darville, N., Saarinen, J., Isomäki, A., Khriachtchev, L., Cleeren, D., Sterkens, P., van Heerden, M., Annaert, P., Peltonen, L., Santos, H. A., Strachan, C. J. and van den Mooter, G. (2015). Multimodal non-linear optical imaging for the investigation of drug nano-/microcrystal-cell interactions, *Eur. J. Pharm. Biopharm.*, **96**, pp. 338–348.

18. Darville, N., van Heerden, M., Vynckie, A., DeMeuldeer, M., Sterkens, P., Annaert, P. and van den Mooter, G. (2014). Intramuscular administration of paliperidone palmitate extended-release injectable microsuspension induces a subclinical inflammatory reaction modulating the pharmacokinetics in rats, *J. Pharm. Sci.*, **103**, pp. 2072–2087.

19. Peltonen, L. and Hirvonen, J. (2010). Pharmaceutical nanocrystals by nanomilling: critical process parameters, particle fracturing and stabilization methods, *J. Pharm. Pharmacol.*, **62**, pp. 1569–1579.

20. Müller, R. H., Shegokar, R. and Keck, C. M. (2011). 20 years of lipid nanoparticles (SLN and NLC): present state of development and industrial applications, *Curr. Drug Discov. Technol.*, **8**, pp. 207–227.

21. Valo, H., Arola, S., Laaksonen, P., Torkkeli, M., Peltonen, L., Linder, M. B., Serimaa, R., Kuga, S., Hirvonen, J. and Laaksonen, T. (2013). Drug release from nanoparticles embedded in four different nanofibrillar cellulose aerogels, *Eur. J. Pharm. Sci.*, **50**, pp. 69–77.

22. Valo, H., Kovalainen, M., Laaksonen, P., Häkkinen, M., Auriola, S., Peltonen, L., Linder, M., Järvinen, K., Hirvonen, J. and Laaksonen, T. (2011). Immobilization of protein-coated drug nanoparticles in nanofibrillar cellulose matrices – enhanced stability and release, *J. Control. Release*, **156**, pp. 390–397.

23. Wang, M., Rutledge, G. C., Myerson, A. S. and Trout, B. L. (2012). Production and characterization of carbamazepine nanocrystals by electrospraying for continuous pharmaceutical manufacturing, *J. Pharm. Sci.*, **101**, pp. 1178–1188.

24. Laaksonen, T., Liu, P., Rahikkala, A., Peltonen, L., Kauppinen, E. I., Hirvonen, J., Järvinen, K. and Raula, J. (2011). Intact nanoparticulate indomethacin in fast-dissolving carrier particles by combined wet milling and aerosol flow reactor methods, *Pharm. Res.*, **28**, pp. 2403–2411.

25. Hou, Y., Shao, J., Fu, Q., Li, J., Sun, J. and He, Z. (2017). Spray-dried nanocrystals for a highly hydrophobic drug: increased drug loading, enhanced redispersity, and improved oral bioavailability, *Int. J. Pharm.*, **516**, pp. 372–279.

26. Chin, W. W. L., Parmentier, J., Widzinski, M., Tan, E. H. and Gokhale, R. (2014). A brief literature and patent review of nanosuspensions to a final drug product, *J. Pharm. Sci.*, **103**, pp. 2980–2999.

27. Peltonen, L., Hirvonen, J. and Laaksonen, J. T. (2014). Drug nanocrystals and nanosuspension in medicine, in *Handbook of Nanobiomedical Research, Fundamentals, Applications and Recent Developments, 1 Materials for Nanomedicine*, Vol. 3, ed. Torchilin, V., World Scientific, Singapore, pp. 169–197.

28. Sharma, P., Denny, W. A. and Garg, S. (2009). Effect of wet milling process on the solid state of indomethacin and simvastatin, *Int. J. Pharm.*, **380**, pp. 40–48.

29. Müller, R. H., Jacobs, C. and Kayser, O. (2001). Nanosuspensions as particulate drug formulations in therapy: rationale for development and what we can expect for the future, *Adv. Drug Deliv. Rev.*, **47**, pp. 3–19.

30. Homayouni, A., Sadeghi, F., Varshosaz, J., Garekani, H. A. and Nokhodchi, A. (2014). Comparing various techniques to produce micro/nanoparticles for enhancing the dissolution of celocoxib containing PVP, *Eur. J. Pharm. Biopharm.*, **88**, pp. 261–274.

31. Soliman, K. A., Ibrahim, H. K. and Ghorab, M. M. (2017). Effects of different combinations of nanocrystallization technologies on avanafil nanoparticles: *in vitro*, *in vivo* and stability evaluation, *Int. J. Pharm.*, **517**, pp. 148–156.

32. Shegokar, R. and Müller, R. H. (2010). Nanocrystals: industrially feasible multifunctional formulation technology for poorly soluble actives, *Int. J. Pharm.*, **399**, pp. 129–139.

33. Bujnakova, Z., Dutkova, E., Alaz, M., Turianicova, E. and Balaz, P. (2015). Stability studies of As4S4 nanosuspension prepared by wet milling in Poloxamer 407, *Int. J. Pharm.*, **478**, pp. 187–192.

34. Müller, R. H., Gohla, S. and Keck, C. M. (2011). State of the art of nanocrystals – special features, production, nanotoxicology aspects and intracellular delivery, *Eur. J. Pharm. Biopharm.*, **78**, pp. 1–9.

35. Radtke, M. and Müller, R. H. (2001). NanopureTM pure drug nanoparticles for the formulation of poorly soluble drugs, *New Drugs*, **3**, pp. 62–68.

36. Salazar, J., Müller, R. H. and Möschwitzer, J. P. (2014). Combinative particle size reduction technologies for the production of drug nanocrystals, *J. Pharm.*, **2014**, Article ID 265754 (14 pp.).

37. Sinha, B., Müller, R. H. and Möschwitzer, J. P. (2013). Bottom-up approaches for preparing drug nanocrystals: formulations and factors affecting particle size, *Int. J. Pharm.*, **453**, pp. 126–141.

38. Sahu, B. P. and Das, M. K. (2014). Preparation and in vitro/in vivo evaluation of felodipine nanosuspension, *Eur. J. Drug Metab. Pharmacokinet.*, **39**, pp. 183–193.

39. Kipp, J. E., Wong, J. C. T., Doty, M. J. and Rebbeck, C. L. (2003). Microprecipitation method for preparing submicron suspensions, United States Patent 6 607 784.

40. Shang, L., Nienhaus, K. and Nienhaus, G. U. (2014). Engineered nanoparticles interacting with cells: size matters, *J. Nanobiotechnol.*, **12**, pp. 1–11.

41. Rachmawati, H., Rahma, A., Al Shaal, L., Müller, R. H. and Keck, C. M. (2016). Destabilization mechanism of ionic surfactant on curcumin nanocrystal against electrolytes, *Sci. Pharm.*, **84**, pp. 685–693.

42. Sigfridsson, K., Skantze, P., Skantze, U., Svensson, L., Löfgren, L., Nordell, P., Michaëlsson, E., SmedsrØd, B., Fuglesteg, B., Elvevold, K. and Lindfors, L. (2017). Nanocrystal formulations of a poorly soluble drug. 2. Evaluation of nanocrystal liver uptake and distribution after intravenous administration to mice, *Int. J. Pharm.*, **524**, pp. 248–256.

43. Cerdeira, A. M., Mazzotti, M. and Gander, B. (2010). Miconazole nanosuspensions: influence of formulation variables on particle size reduction and physical stability, *Int. J. Pharm.*, **396**, pp. 210–218.

44. Soodvilai, S., Soodvilai, S., Chatsudthipong, V., Ngawhirunpat, T., Rojanarata, T. and Opanasopit, P. (2017). Interaction of pharmaceutical excipients with organic cation transporters, *Int. J. Pharm.*, **520**, pp. 14–20.

45. Chow, E. C. Y., Talattof, A., Tsakalozou, E., Fan, J., Zhao, L. and Zhang, X. (2016). Using physiologically based pharmacokinetic (PBPK) modeling to evaluate the impact of pharmaceutical excipients on oral drug absorption: sensitivity analyses, *AAPS J.*, **18**, pp. 1500–1511.

46. Varma, M. V. and Panchagnula, R. (2005). Enhanced oral paclitaxel absorption with vitamine E-TPGS: effect on solubility and permeability in vitro, in situ and in vivo, *Eur. J. Pharm. Sci.*, **25**, pp. 445–453.

47. Tang, X. J., Fu, Y. H., Meng, Q. H., Li, M., Ying, X. Y., Han, M., He, Q. J., Yang, B., Zeng, S., Hu, Y. Z., Sheng, X. X. and Gao, J. Q. (2013). Evaluation of pluronic nanosuspensions loading a novel insoluble anticancer drug both in vitro and in vivo, *Int. J. Pharm.*, **456**, pp. 243–250.

48. Ghosh, I., Schenck, D., Bose, S. and Ruegger, C. (2012). Optimization of formulation and process parameters for the production of nanosuspension by wet media milling technique: effect of vitamin E TPGS and nanocrystal particle size on oral absorption, *Eur. J. Pharm. Sci.*, **47**, pp. 718–728.

49. Kassem, M. A. A., ElMeshad, A. N. and Fares, A. R. (2017). Enhanced solubility and dissolution rate of lacidipine nanosuspension: formulation via antisolvent sonoprecipitation technique and optimization using Box-Behnken design, *AAPS PharmSciTech*, **18**, pp. 983–996.

50. Li, J., Qiao Y. and Wu, Z. (2017). Nanosystem trends in drug delivery using quality-by-design concept, *J. Control. Release*, **256**, pp. 9–18.

51. Peltonen, L. and Strachan, C. (2015). Understanding critical quality attributes for nanocrystals from preparation to delivery, *Molecules*, **20**, pp. 22286–22300.

52. Van Eerdenbrugh, B., Stuyven, B., Froyen, L., Van Humbeeck, J., Martens, J. A. and Augustijns, P., van den Mooter, G. (2009). Downscaling drug nanosuspension production: processing aspects and physicochemical characterization, *AAPS PharmSciTech*, **10**, pp. 44–53.

53. Singare, D. S., Marella, S., Gowthamrajan, K., Kulkarni, G. T., Vooturi, R. and Rao, P. S. (2010). Optimization of formulation and process variable of nanosuspension: an industrial perspective, *Int. J. Pharm.*, **402**, pp. 213–220.

54. Grau, M. J., Kayser, O. and Müller, R. H. (2000). Nanosuspensions of poorly soluble drugs – reproducibility of small scale production, *Int. J. Pharm.*, **196**, pp. 155–159.

55. Date, A. A. and Patravale, V. B. (2004). Current strategies for engineering drug nanoparticles, *Curr. Opin. Colloid Interface Sci.*, **9**, pp. 222–235.

56. Tuomela, A., Laaksonen, T., Laru, J., Antikainen, O., Kiesvaara, J., Ilkka, J., Oksala, O., Rönkkö, S., Järvinen, K., Hirvonen, J. and Peltonen, L. (2015). Solid formulations by a nanocrystal approach: critical process parameters regarding scale-ability of nanocrystals for tableting applications, *Int. J. Pharm.*, **485**, pp. 77–86.

57. van Eerdenbrugh, B., van den Mooter, G. and Augustijns, P. (2008). Top-down production of drug nanocrystals: nanosuspension stabilization, miniaturization and transformation into solid products, *Int. J. Pharm.*, **364**, pp. 64–75.

58. Niwa, T., Miura, S. and Danjo, K. (2011). Universal wet-milling technique to prepare oral nanosuspension focused on discovery and preclinical animal studies–development of particle design method, *Int. J. Pharm.*, **405**, pp. 218–227.

59. Shaal, A., Müller, R. and Shegokar, R. (2010). SmartCrystal combination technology–scale up from lab to pilot scale and long term starbility, *Pharmazie*, **65**, pp. 877–884.

60. Hu, J., Ng, W. K., Dong, Y., Shen, S. and Tan, R. B. H. (2011). Continuous and scalable process for water-redispersible nanoformulation of poorly aqueous soluble APIs by antisolvent precipitation and spray-drying, *Int. J. Pharm.*, **404**, pp. 198–204.

61. Quan, P., Xia, D., Piao, H., Piao, H., Shi, K., Jia, Y. and Cui, F. (2011). Nitrendipine nanocrystals: its preparation, characterization, and in vitro–in vivo evaluation, *AAPS PharmSciTech*, **12**, pp. 1136–1143.

62. Chen, M. L., John, M., Lee, S. L. and Tyner, K. M. (2017). Development considerations for nanocrystal drug products, *AAPS J.*, **19**, pp. 642–651.

63. Bobo, D., Robinson, K. J., Islam, J., Thurecht, K. J. and Corrie, S. R. (2016). Nanoparticle-based medicines: a review of FDA-approved materials and clinical trials to date, *Pharm. Res.*, **33**, pp. 2373–2387.

64. Gao, L., Liu, G., Ma, J., Wang, X., Zhou, L., Li, X. and Wang, F. (2013). Application of drug nanocrystal technologies on oral drug delivery of poorly soluble drugs, *Pharm. Res.*, **30**, pp. 307–324.

65. Åkerman, M. E., Chan, W. C. W., Laakkonen, P. and Bhatia, S. N. E. (2002). Nanocrystal targeting in vivo, *Proc. Natl. Acad. Sci. U.S.A.*, **99**, pp. 12617–12621.

66. Leng, D., Chen, H., Li, G., Guo, M., Zhu, Z., Xu, L. and Wang, Y. (2014). Development and comparison of intramuscularly long-acting paliperidone palmitate nanosuspensions with different particle size, *Int. J. Pharm.*, **472**, pp. 380–385.

67. Li, J. Y., Pow, E. H. N., Zheng, L. W., Ma, L., Kwong, D. L. W. and Cheung, L. K. (2015). Effects of calcium phosphate nanocrystals on osseointegration of titanium implant in irradiated bone, *BioMed Res. Int.*, Article ID 783894 (6 pp.).

68. Müller, R. H. and Jacobs, C. (2002). Production and characterization of budesonide nanosuspension for pulmonary administration, *Pharm. Res.*, **19**, pp. 189–194.

69. Araújo, J., Gonzalez, E., Egea, M. A., Garcia, M. L and Souto, E. B. (2009). Nanomedicines for ocular NSAIDs: safety on drug delivery, *Nanomedicine*, **5**, pp. 394–401.

Chapter 2

Cyclodextrin-Based Nanosystems: Current Status and Future Prospects

Cem Varan, Gamze Varan, Nazlı Erdoğar, and Erem Bilensoy
Department of Pharmaceutical Technology, Faculty of Pharmacy, Hacettepe University, Ankara, 06100, Turkey
eremino@hacettepe.edu.tr

Cyclodextrins have attracted the interest of scientists in various sectors since the day they were discovered. Cyclodextrins have been used in many different areas, thanks to their unique properties and chemical structures. Cyclodextrin derivatives can form inclusion complexes with very different molecules due to their different cavity diameters. In this context, there are a wide range of uses, especially in pharmacy. They are spherical oligosaccharides and are quite remarkable polymers in the preparation of nanosized systems. Cyclodextrins have many advantages; especially they encapsulate hydrophobic therapeutic molecules and imaging agents in their cavity and protect these molecules from the biological system and mask their bad taste or odor. Cyclodextrin-based systems can be prepared from different cyclodextrin derivatives according to the

Drug Delivery Nanosystems: From Bioinspiration and Biomimetics to Clinical Applications
Edited by Costas Demetzos, Stergios Pispas, and Natassa Pippa

ISBN 978-981-4774-92-5 (Hardcover), 978-0-429-49054-5 (eBook)
www.panstanford.com

molecule to be carried or the desired target site. In addition, the surfaces can be modified with the targeted site–specific agents. In this section, cyclodextrins and their derivatives are introduced and their use in nanoscale systems is explained. The scope of this chapter is to define physicochemical properties and pharmaceutical applications of cyclodextrin-based nanosystems that have been investigated for diagnostics, therapeutics, and theranostics.

2.1 Introduction

The scientific use of the term "nano" came from physicist Richard P. Feynman in 1959 [1]. Since then, the research, development, and use of nanotechnology has progressed rapidly in health, as well as in other fields. In healthcare, nanotechnology is used for diagnostic, therapeutic, and theranostic purposes and their combination [2]. Nanomedicine is a promising topic appearing in emerging therapeutics and diagnostics, especially in targeted and personalized medicine. In recent years, there has been enormous progress in nanotherapies and diagnostics in healthcare. The main objectives of the use of nanosized systems are as follows:

- Reduction in side effects by active targeting of cancer cells
- More effective treatment with less active substances
- Reduction of dosage frequency
- Development of systems containing imaging and therapeutic agents
- Increase in the stability of the drug and imaging agent
- Development of long-term imaging systems [3–5]

The process of replacing conventional medicines that have resulted in the spread of nanotechnology practices in healthcare has already begun. In the pharmaceutical industry cyclodextrins (CDs) are used to increase the water solubility, bioavailability, and stability of drugs. CDs are also used in masking bad taste and odor [6]. Currently, about 50 CD-based drugs are on the market [7]. Because CDs are frequently used in conventional drug systems as biocompatible polymers, it is preferred to prepare nanosized drug delivery systems [8–10]. Moreover, CDs can encapsulate imaging agents in their cavity, as well as drug molecules, or they can be used in the surface modification of nanosized imaging systems [11–13]. The development of smart and multifunctional systems in both diagnosis and treatment has been remarkable, taking advantage of the properties of nanoscale and CD chemistry.

2.2 Historical Perspective of Cyclodextrins

The CDs were discovered by French scientist Villiers in 1891. Villers isolated approximately 3 g of a crystalline product from 1000 g of starch and determined the product's composition as $C_6H_{10}O_5{\cdot}3H_2O$. This product, like cellulose, is acid-hydrolyzed because it is named "cellulosin." In 1903, Austrian microbiologist Franz Schardinger described two crystal compounds that formed as a result of bacterial breakage of potato starch during a study of bacteria causing food deterioration. He called them A and B and could isolate compound B in much greater amounts than compound A. In 1903, the name of the compound published by Schardinger was changed to the name "crystal dextrin" and the compounds A and B were named α-dextrin and β-dextrin. After eight years of work, he was able to isolate these compounds with different bacterial enzymes from different sources, such as potato, maize, and wheat. In a paper published in 1911, he explained the chemical structures of CDs. Although there was not much information available in those years, this work is considered to be the basis of CD chemistry. In 1935 Freudenberg discovered γ-CD, and in 1938 he showed the ring structure of CDs composed of α-(1-4)-dependent glucose units. Cramer then described the structures and resolutions and their physicochemical properties, such as complex forming abilities and internal cavity sizes of α-, β-, and γ-CDs [14–16] .

2.3 Chemistry and Properties of Cyclodextrins

2.3.1 Natural Cyclodextrins

Natural CDs are named according to the number of glucopyranose units present in the structures (Fig. 2.1). Among these, α-CD (six units), β-CD (seven units), and γ-CD (eight units) are important in terms of pharmaceutical interest [17]. There are no CDs with fewer than 6 glucopyranose units due to structural factors, but there are CDs containing 9–13 units and they are commonly referred to as δ-CDs [14].

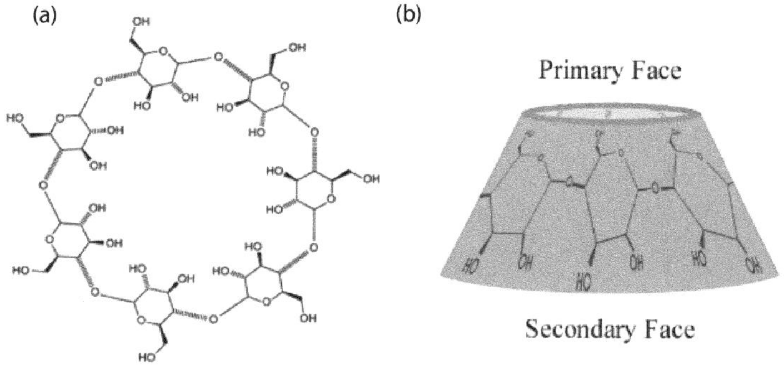

Figure 2.1 (a) The molecular structure and (b) the 3D structure of cyclodextrin.

The volume and diameter of the hydrophobic cavity vary depending on the number of glucopyranose units present in the constructions (Table 2.1).

Table 2.1 Physicochemical properties of natural CDs

Type of cyclodextrin	Cavity diameter (Å)	Outer diameter (Å)	Height of torus (Å)	Molecular weight (g/mol)	Solubility in water (mg/mL)
α- CD	4.7–5.3	14.6	7.9	972	145
β-CD	6–6.5	15.4	7.9	1135	18.5
γ-CD	7.5–8.3	17.5	7.9	1297	232

Natural CDs are crystalline, homogeneous, nonhygroscopic macrocyclic structures and have a $^4C_1$ chair conformation. They show a high electron density in the cavity because of the unpaired electron pairs of H atoms and the glycosidic O bridges in the hydrophobic cavity [18]. In aqueous media, water molecules inside the CD cavity can easily be replaced by apolar molecules, leading to an inclusion host–guest complex.

2.3.2 Modified Cyclodextrins

The water solubility of natural CDs is lower than that of linear dextrins due to the hydrogen bonds between the hydroxyl groups in the structures. It is also known that α-CD and β-CD cause nephrotoxicity [18, 19]. After parenteral administration, CDs are taken up by the renal tubule cells, resulting in impaired intracellular function. Natural CDs cause hemolysis in red blood cells and disruption of membrane components, such as cholesterol and phospholipids [20, 21]. CDs are modified by chemical methods in order to avoid these side effects, which are caused by natural CDs. The reasons for the modification of natural CDs can be summarized as follows:

- Increase the water solubility of natural CDs (especially β-CD)
- Remove nephrotoxicity, which is the most important side effect of natural CDs
- Increase the passage of CDs from biological membranes
- Increasing inclusion complex capacities of CDs
- Prevent hemolysis
- Establish a colloidal drug delivery system by giving self-organization properties to CDs [22, 23]

Within the modified natural CDs, up to three groups are used in the pharmaceutical field: methyl CD, hydroxypropyl (HP) CD, and sulfobutyl CD.

Methylated CD derivatives are obtained by the methylation of two or three hydroxyl groups to each glucopyranose unit. When there is methylation of two hydroxyl groups, dimethyl CD is formed and the methylation is selectively carried out on all C6 primary hydroxyl and all C2 secondary hydroxyl groups. When three hydroxyl groups are methylated, trimethyl CD is formed, and all C3 secondary hydroxyl groups are methylated. Methylated CD derivatives have a higher solubility than the CDs on which they are based [24, 25].

In the hydroxypropylated CD derivatives, selective substitution does not occur as in the methylated CD. HP CDs are highly soluble in water due to their amorphous structure. Their solubility is endothermic, and there is no decrease in solubility due to the increased temperature. Unlike methylated CDs, they are not hydrolyzed by gastrointestinal (GI) amylase. In parenteral administration, they exhibit less hemolytic activity than the baseline CD [26].

Sulfobutylether (SBE) CDs are anionic and water-soluble CD derivatives. Their ability to be superior to other CD derivatives is due to an increase in the degree of coupling due to the increase in the substitution level. This derivative increases drug stability and causes less hemolysis due to the polyanionic structure [27].

2.3.3 Amphiphilic Cyclodextrins

The greatest problem in the CD derivatives synthesized in order to increase the solubility of natural CDs is that the outer surface of the inner surface is also hydrophilic. This is because modification reduces the contact of the CDs with the biological membranes. In the last few years different amphiphilic CD derivatives have been synthesized to avoid this undesirable consequence. Other reasons for the synthesis of amphiphilic CDs are increasing the interaction with hydrophobic drugs by adding long aliphatic chains to the structure of CDs and allowing the formation of nanocapsules and nanospheres at physiological pH and spontaneous recovery in aqueous media [28, 29]. The first amphiphilic CD was synthesized by Kawabata in 1986 [30]. Kawabata made the primer surface of β-CD hydrophobic with alkylsulfinyl groups of various lengths.

2.3.3.1 Nonionic amphiphilic cyclodextrins

Nonionic amphiphilic CDs are obtained by attaching aliphatic chains of different lengths to the primary or secondary surface of glucopyranose units of CDs. There are different variants according to the structure (Fig. 2.2).

Lollipop CDs are amphiphilic CD derivatives obtained by the addition of only one aliphatic chain to the structure of 6-amino-β-CDs. In this CD derivative, the aliphatic chain can enter the cavity of the CD, preventing inclusion complex formation with the molecule [31]. A number of *tert*-butyl groups can be added to the end of the aliphatic chains to prevent this situation. This CD derivative is called "cup and ball CD". During, medusa-like CD synthesis, long chains containing 10–16 carbons are added to the primary hydroxyl groups of the β-CDs [32]. For skirt-shaped CDs, aliphatic esters containing 2–14 carbons are added to the secondary surfaces of α- and γ-CDs [33]. Bouquet-shaped CDs are synthesized by the addition of polymethylene chains on both surfaces with a total of 14 of 3-monomethyl-β-CDs [32].

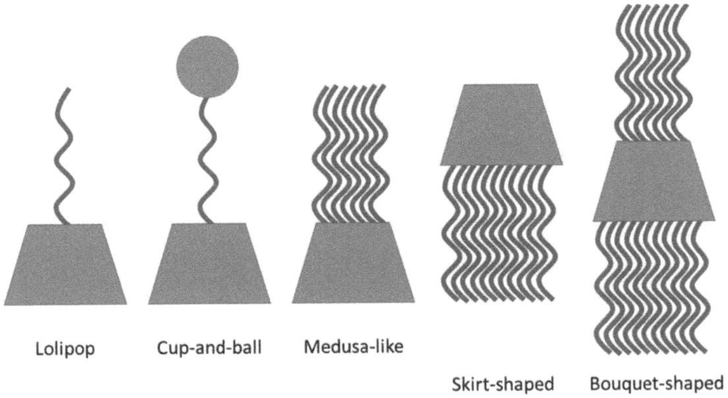

Figure 2.2 Different nonionic amphiphilic cyclodextrin derivatives presented in the literature.

2.3.3.2 Cationic amphiphilic cyclodextrins

Cationic amphiphilic CDs are CD derivatives garnering considerable interest in recent years. Amino groups are used as the ionic groups in the preparation of the cationic amphiphilic CD derivatives. It is believed that the formation of cationic amphiphilic CDs depends on the balance between the hydrophobic tail (thioalkyl chains) and the hydrophilic components (ethylene glycol oligomers) of the structure [34]. It is believed that the presence of ethylene glycol chains enhances the colloidal stability of multimolecular aggregates introduced by cationic CDs. In recent years, polyamino (polycationic) CDs have been used in medicine and especially gene delivery. Cationic polymers can easily bind to nucleic acids and nucleotides due to surface charges. The most important advantage of cationic/polycyclic CDs is their lower cytotoxicity to polymers, such as poly(amidine), as shown in in vitro and in vivo studies of gene transfer [35, 36]. Cationic CDs also tend to bind very strongly to nucleotides and enhance their transport acting as viral vectors. The greatest advantage of polycationic CDs and nanoparticles prepared therefrom is their ability to interact with nucleic acids, as well as their ability to organize themselves. Thus, they stand out as important components of polyplexes for use in gene therapy [37, 38].

2.3.3.3 Anionic amphiphilic cyclodextrins

In the preparation of anionic amphiphilic CD derivatives, anionic sulfate groups are used [22]. For the elimination of acyl-sulphated-β-

CDs, an efficient and specific synthetic pathway has been described in which sulphate groups are attached to the primary face of the CD and fatty acid esters are attached to the secondary face. These derivatives can form aggregates in aqueous media. Fluorine-containing anionic β-CDs were first obtained by Granger et al., through coupling of trifluoromethylthio groups [39]. They achieved an amphiphilic behavior in the air/water interface and considered it a good candidate for a new class of amphiphilic carriers.

2.4 Cyclodextrin-Based Nanosystems

CD-based nanosystems, as do all nanostructured systems, exhibit a wide variety with different features and structures. In this section, nanostructured systems prepared with CD as the main component, preparation methods of these systems, and literature examples are given.

2.4.1 Cyclodextrin-Based Nanoparticles

Polymeric-based CD nanoparticles are essentially separated into nanospheres and nanocapsules according to their structures. Nanospheres are carrier systems composed of a polymeric matrix (Fig. 2.3).

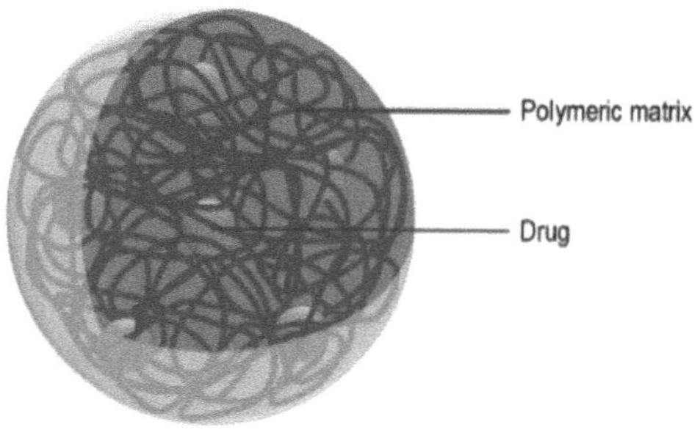

Figure 2.3 Nanospheres.

These systems can be likened to a ball of wool made of a polymeric thread. The therapeutic or diagnostic material may be dispersed within the polymeric sphere, adsorbed on the surface, or conjugated to the surface. Although the drug release rate is faster than that of nanocapsules, the particle size is usually smaller. In nanospheres, the therapeutic or diagnostic material may be diffused through the polymeric structure or released by the erosion of the polymeric structure or it may occur by the simultaneous occurrence of these two mechanisms. A nanocapsule is also a membrane-type system consisting of a polymeric envelope and an oily inner core. The therapeutic or diagnostic material is usually dissolved in the oily core and may be adsorbed on or conjugated to the surface (Fig. 2.4).

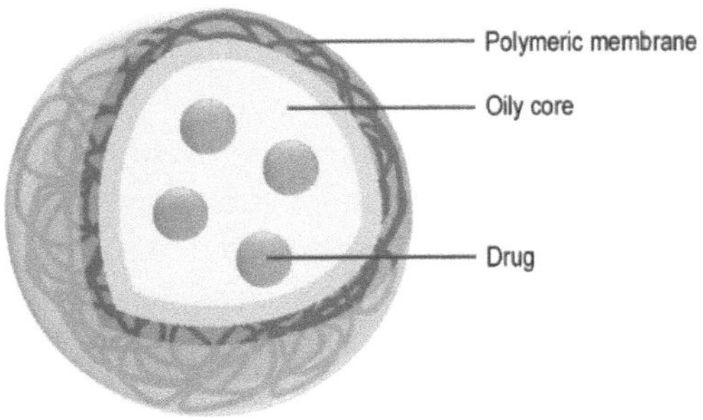

Figure 2.4 Nanocapsule.

The drug release rate is slower and the drug-loading capacity is higher for nanocapsules than for nanospheres due to their polymeric membrane structure. However, nanocapsules generally have larger particle sizes than nanospheres.

Although the nanoparticle preparation methods vary widely, there are two main approaches, polymerization of the monomers and dispersion of the polymers (Table 2.2).

Table 2.2 The classification of nanoparticle preparation method

Monomer polymerization	Polymer dispersion
Emulsion polymerization	Emulsion/Solvent evaporation
Dispersion polymerization	Nanoprecipitation
	Salting out
	Emulsion cross-linking
	Coacervation
	Spray-drying and spray-freezing
	Supercritical fluid technology
	Ionic gelation

The monomer polymerization technique works according to the bottom-up principle and allows the monomer units to be transformed into polymeric carrier systems by chemical reactions. Nanostructured systems consisting of synthetic polymers such as polyacrylamide are generally prepared by this method. With this technique, it is possible to obtain smaller and monodisperse particles.

The polymer dispersion technique does not contain any polymerization step, and it is based on the preparation of nanostructured systems directly from previously prepared or existing polymers. This method is quite suitable for preparing nanostructured systems from natural and biodegradable polymers, like CDs. Since there is no polymerization step in this technique, there is no need to purify toxic substances that may occur during polymerization. The nanosystems prepared by this technique have larger particle sizes and are more polydisperse [40, 41].

CD nanoparticles are prepared as both therapeutic and diagnostic systems in literature. Nanoprecipitation is a frequently used method in the literature for the preparation of CD nanoparticles because it is a simple and fast method. Bhattacharya et al. prepared piperolactam-A loaded HP-β-CD nanospheres by using the nanoprecipitation method for the treatment of leishmaniasis. With the drug-loaded stable nanoparticles 180 nm in size, they obtained macrophage initialization within 1 h. Thus, they demonstrated that the CD nanospheres are safe and affordable drug formulations for the treatment of leishmania infections [42]. By using the same preparation technique, Erdogar et al. prepared amphiphilic β-CD nanospheres loaded with the anticancer drug paclitaxel against breast cancer. In this study, folate receptors found in breast cancer cells were targeted with folate-conjugated CD nanoparticles and the active targeted drug formulation for the treatment of breast cancer was successfully prepared. The prepared anticancer drug-loaded nanosphere formulations were compared with paclitaxel in Cremophor®—which is used in clinics for the treatment of breast cancer—by in vivo animal studies. According to results, paclitaxel-loaded β-CD nanospheres have lower toxicity and are effective anticancer therapy for the treatment of breast cancer [43]. The emulsion solvent evaporation technique is another important method used in the preparation of CD nanoparticles. Quaglia et al.

[44] prepared docetaxel (DCX)-loaded CD nanoparticles by using the emulsion–solvent evaporation technique. With these prepared nanospheres, which have a particle size of 95 nm, they achieved an entrapment efficacy of 98% and a release profile of over eight weeks. According to the cell culture results from human Caucasian larynx carcinoma epidermoid cells (HEp-2) for a 48 h incubation period, DCX-loaded CD nanospheres were found to be more effective than free DCX on HEp-2 cells. With this study [44], they demonstrated that CD nanoparticles are promising in solid tumor therapy.

Studies demonstrate that nanoparticles prepared from some CD derivatives have anticancer efficacy. Varan et al. prepared different CD nanospheres from different CD derivatives. Interestingly, drug-free CD nanospheres have cytotoxic effects on cancer cell lines such as MCF-7, HeLa, HepG2, and MB49. Moreover, Varan et al. could not detect any cytotoxic effect when they incubated these nanospheres with healthy cell lines such as L929 and G/G. They examined this effect of CD nanospheres on cancer cell lines and showed that this apoptotic effect in cancer cells may be related to the cholesterol affinity of the CDs. Thus, they demonstrated that CD nanoparticles may be effective systems without anticancer drug in the treatment of cancer [45].

Besides the CD nanospheres, there are also CD nanocapsules as drug delivery systems in the literature. Unal et al. prepared core-shell CD nanocapsules in order to increase the oral bioavailability of camptothecin. The particle size of the prepared CD nanocapsules was determined to be 187 nm, and the zeta potential was found to be –11 mV. They also showed that the particle size increased by 17 nm and the zeta potential increased from –11 mV to +10 mV when CD nanocapsules were coated with chitosan to improve the cellular uptake. According to the in vitro cell culture studies drug-loaded nanocapsules have a more cytotoxic effect than the free drug solution on the MCF-7 cell line and the permeation of the drug across Caco-2 cells was threefold higher than the free drug solution. Consequently, it can be said that CD nanocapsules are a good candidate for increasing the oral bioavailability of camptothecin [46, 47]. CDs are used as the supporting or coating material for nanoparticles prepared from different polymers as well as the main polymer in the preparation of nanospheres or nanocapsules. Zhang et al. prepared SBE-CD chitosan nanoparticles by using an ionic gelation technique.

With this technique, they obtained naringenin-loaded spherical nanoparticles with a size of 446 nm and +22 mV zeta potential for ocular drug delivery. In vivo experiments on rabbits showed that prepared systems increased the bioavailability of naringenin. They also suggested that this system may be an alternative for the ocular administration of poorly soluble drugs [48]. Varan et al. used CD as the coating material in DCX-loaded poly(ε-caprolactone) (PCL) nanoparticles for the treatment of solid tumor [8]. CD-coated nanoparticles were found to have a higher drug-loading efficiency when they were coated compared to uncoated. On the other hand, the drug release profiles were said to be unaffected by the coating and close to each other for all formulations. In addition, the cytotoxic effect was enhanced when the DCX-loaded PCL nanoparticles were coated with CD in in vitro experiments on the MCF-7 cell line. Consequently, CD-coated PCL nanoparticles can be a suitable carrier for DCX in the treatment of solid tumors

In addition to drug delivery systems, CD nanoparticles are also used for gene therapy in the literature. Evans et al. prepared anisamide-targeted CD nanoparticles having particle sizes smaller than 200 nm and cationic surface charge to promote therapeutic gene silencing for prostate cancer. Cellular uptake of anisamide-targeted and untargeted nanoparticles were compared with each in the light of 2D and 3D cell culture studies. Anisamide-targeted CD nanoparticles were found to be more effective than untargeted nanoparticles in gene silencing. In addition to these targeted CD nanoparticles, it was predicted that the need for in vivo animal studies would be reduced by the developed 3D cell culture model of bone cancer metastasis [49]. Another study by Evan et al. on CD nanoparticles showed that polyethylene glycol (PEG)-conjugated folate–targeted amphiphilic CD nanoparticles increased the circulation time of small interfering RNA (siRNA) by eight times [50]. Likewise, Bruno et al. used PEGylated amphiphilic CD nanoparticles for the delivery of siRNA. When they examined the pharmacokinetic properties and stability of the system they prepared, they found that PEGylation length and density increase stability. Moreover, they showed that siRNA in CD nanoparticles increase systemic exposure and reduce clearance when compared with naked siRNA [51]. All these studies show that CD nanoparticles are promising and good alternatives to viral vectors.

2.4.2 Cyclodextrin-Based Nanosponges

Nanosponges, which are the colloidal structures of hyper-cross-linked polymers, have been especially developed in recent years, and interest in these structures is increasing. Nanosponges have several advantages, especially increasing the solubility of drugs with low solubility, having higher encapsulation efficacy, and prolonging drug release. In addition, nanosponges can be designed in different dosage forms, such as oral, parenteral, topical, and inhalation. Methods such as simple thermal desorption, extraction with solvents, microwave use, and ultrasonic techniques can be used to prepare CD nanosponges. CD nanosponges are prepared to eliminate problems of drugs such as solubility, permeability, and sensitivity; ensure effective and safe dosage forms, enhance drug-loading capacity; and prolong drug release [52].

Dora et al. prepared erlotinib-loaded CD nanosponges to increase the solubility and bioavailability of erlotinib. After determining the optimal drug formulations, they have done various in vitro characterization and cell culture studies. According to their results, the developed CD nanosponges increased the solubility, dissolution, and oral bioavailability of erlotinib. This system allows the drug to be used at lower doses, thus preventing dose-related side effects [53]. In another study, Roa et al. improved the CD nanosponge structure to improve the bioavailability and controlled release of gabapentin, which has a short biological half-life and low bioavailability. In addition, since this drug has a bitter taste, a pediatric drug formulation has been prepared by masking the taste of the drug in these CD nanosponges. As a result of the characterization studies, they found that the developed CD nanosponges were quite successful in masking the taste, increasing the bioavailability of the drug, and providing controlled release [54]. Shende et al. used CD nanosponges for the delivery of calcium in hyperphosphatemia. Characterization studies showed that CD nanosponges can successfully encapsulate, store, and release calcium carbonate for a prolonged period. This system shows promise in the treatment of hyperthermia by providing calcium carbonate stability and controlled release [55]. The work done with CD nanosponges is very new and limited, but the number of studies in this area is increasing day by day. In addition to the examples given above, there are several CD nanosponge formulations for the treatment of diseases such as cancer [56, 57], ocular diseases [58], and Parkinson's disease [59] in the literature.

2.4.3 Cyclodextrin-Based Liposomes

As a result of modern drug research studies, a large number of novel active substances with low solubility have been discovered [18, 60]. Due to low oral absorption, these compounds fail to get through advanced stages of development in spite of their pharmacological activity. Hence it is a great challenge for pharmaceutical researchers to formulate low-molecular-weight soluble molecules in oral administration [61].

One of the important approaches for improving poor solubility and low oral bioavailability is the application of CDs, which can form water-soluble inclusion complexes with hydrophobic molecules. Due to better biocompatibility, low toxicity, and nonimmune responses to humans, CDs have been widely applied in oral delivery systems for hydrophobic molecules in many studies [62]. Novel CD-based drug delivery systems provide increased drug solubility, cellular uptake, and intestinal permeation in the GI tract. Among these systems, drug-CD-liposome complexes have been widely studied for increasing drug solubility and bioavailability. A hydrophobic drug–CD complex is loaded in liposomes within the lipid bilayer, which potentially prevents a rapid leakage of the drug from the liposome [63, 64]. Major problems of liposomes (poor stability, etc.) and CDs (renal toxicity, etc.) were resolved by combining liposomes and CDs. Encapsulation of drug-CD complexes into liposomes increases the encapsulation efficiency of the hydrophobic drug and decreases its release from the carrier [65].

Zhu et al. developed Pluronic F127-modified liposome including a CD inclusion complex (FLIC) to improve solubility, cellular uptake, and intestinal permeation of tacrolimus in GI way. A drug-CD-liposome complex was prepared with the lipid film hydration technique. The drug uptake of the FLIC was two times higher against conventional liposomes using the Caco-2 cell line. After the oral administration of the FLIC in rats, high-intensity fluorescence could be detected in the basolateral of the intestinal mucus membrane. These results indicate that surface modification with Pluronic F127 could effectively enhance the intestinal penetration of the drug [66].

In another study, Zhang et al. investigated different flurbiprofen-loaded CD liposomes using β-CD, HP-β-CD, and SBE-β-CD in vitro and in vivo. Especially flurbiprofen-loaded HP-β-CD liposomes, prepared by coevaporation, give promising results with a higher encapsulation efficiency, size in the nanorange, and slow drug release. In addition to this, entrapment of HP-β-CD into the liposomes change the T_{max} (time taken to reach the maximum concentration) and improve the C_{max} (maximum concentration) and bioavailability [67] .

Maestrelli et al. developed HP-β-CD liposomes for the topical delivery of local anesthetics benzocaine and butamben. Double-loaded liposomes were prepared by adding the drug–HP-β-CD complex at its maximum aqueous solubility in the vesicles' hydrophilic phase and the remaining amount of up to 1% as free drug in the lipophilic phase. The formation of an inclusion complex was proved with differential scanning calorimetry, Fourier-transform infrared (FTIR), and X-ray analysis. The presence of HP-β-CD improves the dissolution rate of a drug in liposomes. For two drugs, double-loaded liposomes, benefiting from favorable effects of drug–CD complexation, allowed a significant increase in the intensity and duration of anesthetic effect compared to single-loaded ones in in vivo studies [68]. In another study, novel itraconazole-loaded deformable liposomes were developed in the presence of HP-β-CD in order to enhance antifungal efficacy using a *Candida albicans* model. The efficiency of these systems was compared with conventional liposomes and drug solution. Characterization studies showed that the presence of HP-β-CD played an important role in reducing the size to the nanorange. Moreover, deformable liposomes enhanced the drug amount in the stratum corneum and the deeper skin layers compared to conventional liposomes. The antifungal activity of itraconazole-loaded deformable liposomes remained intact compared to drug solution. It can be concluded that deformable liposomes in the presence of HP-β-CD may be a promising carrier for effective cutaneous delivery of itraconazole [69].

Different nanosized drug delivery systems have been studied that improved chemotherapeutic efficacy [70]. On the other hand, nanosized systems can control the release of active molecules and enhance intracellular concentration in tumor. For this reason, PEGylated liposomes prefer to incorporate a large range of hydrophilic and hydrophobic compounds with high drug-loading capacity within the aqueous core and lipid bilayer. Nevertheless, a burst release of molecules from liposomes is the major problem. To overcome this drawback, CDs were employed to load the anticancer drugs in the liposomes. Sun et al. evaluated DCX- and gemcitabine (GEM)-loaded PEGylated liposomes (DCX/GEM-L) to enhance the therapeutic efficacy in osteosarcoma (OS). A 2-HP-γ-CD/DCX inclusion complex was prepared to enhance DCX's poor aqueous solubility. An in vitro release study showed a sustained release profile for both drugs. These nanosystems significantly increased the cytotoxic effect compared to the free drug solution at the same concentration. The antitumor efficacy was performed in a human bone OS cell–bearing in vivo mice model. The results indicated that DCX/GEM-L significantly reduced the tumor burden compared to the free drug combination. PEGylated CD liposomes successfully delivered anticancer drugs in OS tumor interstitial spaces via an enhanced permeability and retention effect. DCX/GEM-L showed an excellent safety profile along with the remarkable tumor suppression ability [71].

2.4.4 Cyclodextrin-Based Hydrogels

Hydrogels are of great import for the delivery of active agents like proteins because of their biocompatibility and high water content. Recently, CD-based hydrogels have emerged as a new approach suitable for controlled drug delivery [72]. The combination of CDs and hydrogels leads to synergistic properties: increased biocompatibility and stability of inclusion complexes; also CDs set the mechanical properties and enable affinity-based drug loading and release. Otherwise, CDs might play a significant role in notably improving the capability of hydrogels to load active molecules and to control their release by communicating the ability of forming inclusion complexes [73]. Many researchers focused on hydrogels formed by CDs and polypseudorotaxane polymer (PPRX) for their potential use as injectable drug delivery systems, due to their thixotropic nature and biocompatibility [74]. In a study, insulin/α-CD PPRX and insulin/γ-CD PPRX hydrogels were prepared with inclusion complexation between PEG and CDs for protein and peptide delivery. In vitro release studies showed that the release rate of insulin from hydrogels decreased in the order of γ-CD PPRX hydrogel > α-CD

PPRX hydrogel. The serum insulin level after s.c. administration of γ-CD PPRX hydrogel to rats was significantly prolonged, which was obviously reflected in the prolonged hypoglycemic effect. As a result, these findings represented the potential use of the γ-CD PPRX hydrogel as an injectable sustained release system for insulin [75].

In another study, Machín et al. investigated the possibility of applying novel β-CD polymers as drug carriers for different model drugs (naproxen, nabumetone, naftifine, and terbinafine) release. The interaction of drugs with the β-CD polymers was proved by X-ray diffraction, FTIR spectroscopy, and differential thermal analysis. Drug release followed a simple Fickian diffusion mechanism for all model drugs. These results suggested that these hydrogel matrices are potentially suitable as sustained release systems [76]. Soft contact lenses (SCL) and hydrogels that contain conjugated CD units emerged as drug delivery systems to deliver high drug concentrations into the eye or other mucosal surfaces. Glisoni et al. investigated two different hydrophilic networks with conjugated β-CD for the localized release of a novel 1-indanone thiosemicarbazone (TSC) derivative in the eye and its potential application in ophthalmic diseases. Poly(2-hydroxyethyl methacrylate) (pHEMA) SCLs displaying β-CD functionality, namely pHEMA-*co*-β-CD, and superhydrophilic hydrogels of directly cross-linked HP-β-CD, were synthesized and characterized in terms of drug-loading capacity, swelling, and in vitro release in artificial lacrimal fluid. Controlled release was observed for at least two weeks, drug concentrations being within an optimal therapeutic window for the antimicrobial ocular treatment. Microbiological tests against *Pseudomonas aeruginosa* and *Staphylococcus aureus* verified the ability of the TSC-loaded pHEMA-*co*-β-CD network to inhibit bacterial growth [77].

2.4.5 Cyclodextrin-Based Nanofibers

Nanofibers are promising systems for many drug applications due to their large surface areas and surface functionalities. Among many approaches used for preparing nanofibers, electrospinning is a cost-efficient preparation technique for multifunctional nanofibers from a large number of molecules such as polymers and composites (Fig. 2.5). Electrospun nanofibers have many magnificent properties, like a very high surface-to-volume ratio, a nanoporous structure, and multifunctionality. Additionally, the major advantages of nanofibers are better stability, low toxicity, a high drug-loading capacity, encapsulation of a wide range of drugs, and suitability for thermolabile drugs [78]. It has been shown that these excellent properties of electrospun nanofibers make them applicable in various areas, including drug delivery, wound dressing, and tissue engineering [79–82].

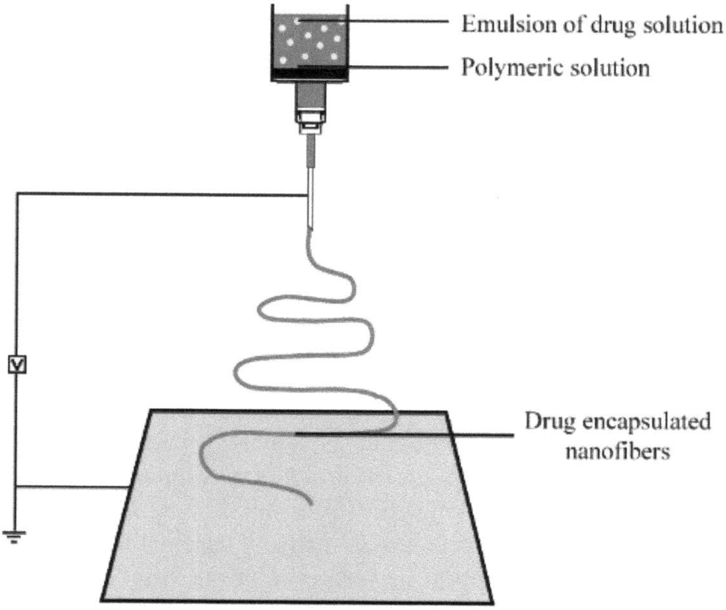

Figure 2.5 Electrospinning of polymer fibers.

Recently, CD electrospun nanofibers have received much attention due to their specific properties. Celebioglu and Uyar reported that due to the presence of a large number of aggregates and intermolecular interactions between CD molecules, CD-inclusion-complexed nanofibers could be obtained by electrospinning without using a polymeric matrix at a high concentration [83]. In another study, Vigh et al. investigated the dissolution enhancement of a drug with a polymer-free electrospun solid dosage form. The fast release could be successfully prevented by HP-β-CD. Polymer-free HP-β-CD nanofibers induce a dramatic release rate enhancement and dissolution improvement in the case of poorly water soluble drugs

[84]. On the contrary, many studies showed that the dissolution rate was enhanced on using CD-polymer nanofibers. The pharmaceutical dosage form may be prepared or modified depending on the polymer used to form the nanofibers. Canbolat et al. first prepared the inclusion complex with naproxen sodium and β-CD, and then the inclusion complex was incorporated into PCL nanofibers via electrospinning. The release profiles of the drug from CD-free PCL and CD-PCL nanofibers were compared. The release study clarified that CD-PCL nanofibers have a higher release amount of drug than the PCL nanofibers because the inclusion complex enhances the solubility of naproxen [85].

2.4.6 Cyclodextrin Molecular Imprints

Molecular imprinting technology is a research area attracting considerable interest as a synthetic method of developing molecular affinity systems that are able to recognize, form complexes with, and control the delivery of small drugs. This technology includes the design of a polymer matrix that has specific and complementary recognition sites for an active drug molecule [86]. By binding the interacting group of the functional monomers, the molecular structure of the polymer matrix is specifically adapted to the template of interest, leading to a higher drug-loading efficacy [87]. Oral drug delivery using molecular-imprinted polymers (MIPs) involves the protection of the template from GI degradation and the control of drug release and pharmacokinetic profile. A functional response to an external stimulus like pH or temperature and the opportunity to ensure both drug recognition and delivery properties continue to render MIPs attractive for oral drug delivery [88].

The application of CDs is useful to imprint biologically active molecules because templates have complex conformations, low solubility in organic monomer solutions, and slow diffusion rates and suffer from interference by other components in imprint systems [89]. The main drawbacks associated with imprinting are low mass-transfer kinetics, flexible structure of macrotemplates, and the attempt to generate molecular recognition in water. Additionally, macromolecules have different biological activity when redissolved in an aqueous medium. This is a conformational change in the protein due to refolding in the different media [90]. Here is the main strategy for utilizing CDs in this field: When several CD molecules are associated around the template, each CD molecule is provided with a portion of the template. Thus, the CD molecules are brought together so that the pattern is fully recognized [91].

Cerchiara et al. developed a CD-MIP network with the CD molecules spatially arranged to fit designated portions of a nanosized template, an antibiotic glycopeptide vancomycin with a limited oral administration [92]. Compared to the polymer matrix without recognition capacity, CD-MIP systems showed a twofold increase in drug loading. Besides, a 2.6-fold increase in the apparent stability constant showed that the CD-MIP is able to carry out a sustained release of the drug [93]. Recently, MIPs of CD nanosponges were developed by Trotta and colleagues for the oral delivery of L-DOPA [(S)-2-amino-3-(3,4-dihydroxyphenyl) propanoic acid] in the treatment of neurodegenerative diseases. The synthesis of CD-NS in the presence of the template alters its structural arrangement, molecular recognition ability, and in vivo behavior compared to drug-loaded CD-NS. The prolonged rate of L-DOPA release from MIP-CD-NS compared to that from nonimprinted CD-NS showed a stronger, molecular imprinting–mediated L-DOPA-CD-NS interaction [59].

2.4.7 Cyclodextrin Polymers

Another carrier system made with CDs is polyrotaxane. This system, also called "molecular necklace," is a polymer in which the CDs are threaded on a PEG chain [94]. CD polyrotaxanes are multifunctional and biocompatible as a drug carrier system. They have potential for pharmaceutical applications due to their low toxicity, controllable size, and unique properties, such as biodegradability, aqueous compatibility, targeting, and stimuli responsiveness [95, 96]. The drug may be covalently attached to the CD rings of a polyrotaxane. while the polyrotaxanes are used as the drug delivery system. The polymer formed in this manner dissolves in water [97].

These polyrotaxanes can be classified as follows:

- Directly formed polyrotaxanes with linear drug molecules
- Conjugates of polyrotaxanes with drugs
- Hydrogels including drugs
- Drug complexes with polyrotaxanes

CRLX101 is in Phase-2 development, which has camptothecin as an active molecule. CRLX101 is a self-assembled system that has been developed by covalently conjugating camptothecin to the β-CD-PEG copolymer. According to results of preclinical and clinical data, CRLX101 removes the solubility problem of camptothecin and reduces the pharmacokinetic drawbacks [98].

Jiang et. al reported that polyrotaxane-containing β-CDs have a higher drug-loading capacity due to the hydrogen bonding between amphotericin B (antifungal drug) and β-CD. Following this study, folic acid–conjugated amphiphilic polyrotaxane–based polymers were synthesized using β-CD and PEG methyl ether methacrylate. It was reported that the conjugated copolymers are able to self-assemble in an aqueous solution and encapsulate doxorubicin (anticancer drug) into the hydrophobic core. It was emphasized that the loaded drug content increased due to the hydrogen bond interaction between doxorubicin and polyrotaxane. In addition, these active-targeted polyrotaxane have a slower and sustained drug release. According to results of cell culture studies, anticancer drug–loaded polyrotaxanes were internalized in MDA-MB-231 cells via folic acid receptor–mediated endocytosis [99]. In another study, novel pH-labile micelles containing a polyrotaxane-based triblock copolymer with doxorubicin were studied. In vitro imaging data with a transmission electron microscope showed that drug-polyrotaxane conjugates form self-assembled micelles 70 nm in diameter in an aqueous solution. Moreover, in vitro release of doxorubicin from polyrotaxane was 37% over 72 h at acidic pH [100].

2.5 Future Perspectives

CD-based nanosized systems are described in this chapter, accompanied by studies made in recent years. As can be understood from the examples and ongoing studies, the number of studies carried out in the field of CD-based nanosystems is increasing every year. Studies using the unique properties of CDs are continuing at a rapid pace in the biomedical field, and especially in the pharmaceutical field. Their ability to be modified as desired, their high loading capacity, and their biocompatibility are the main reasons for their preference for drug/gene delivery. CDs are used not only to develop drug formulations but also to determine cellular interactions and uptake in the pharmaceutical field. The development of drug-CD conjugate systems such as CRLX101 is an inevitable consequence. The CDs specifically synthesized in the particular system make the system unique.

References

1. Satyanarayana, T. S. V. and Rai, R. (2011). Nanotechnology: the future, *J. Interdiscip. Dentistry*, **1**, pp. 93–100.
2. Parveen, S., Misra, R. and Sahoo, S. K. (2012). Nanoparticles: a boon to drug delivery, therapeutics, diagnostics and imaging, *Nanomedicine*, **8**, pp. 147–166.
3. Blanco, E., Hsiao, A., Mann, A. P., Landry, M. G., Meric-Bernstam, F. and Ferrari, M. (2011). Nanomedicine in cancer therapy: innovative trends and prospects, *Cancer Sci.*, **102**, pp. 1247–1252.
4. Sumer, B. and Gao, J. (2008). Theranostic nanomedicine for cancer, *Nanomedicine (Lond)*, **3**, pp. 137–140.
5. Wicki, A., Witzigmann, D., Balasubramanian, V. and Huwyler, J. (2015). Nanomedicine in cancer therapy: challenges, opportunities, and clinical applications, *J. Control. Release*, **200**, pp. 138–157.
6. Tiwari, G., Tiwari, R. and Rai, A. K. (2010). Cyclodextrins in delivery systems: applications, *J. Pharm. Bioallied Sci.*, **2**, pp. 72–79.
7. Fenyvesi, E. (2013). Approved pharmaceutical products containing cyclodextrins, *Cyclodextrin News*, **26**, pp. 2–4.
8. Varan, C. and Bilensoy, E. (2014). Development of implantable hydroxypropyl-beta-cyclodextrin coated polycaprolactone nanoparticles for the controlled delivery of docetaxel to solid tumors, *J. Incl. Phenom. Macrocycl. Chem.*, **80**, pp. 9–15.
9. Bilensoy, E., Gurkaynak, O., Ertan, M., Sen, M. and Hincal, A. A. (2008). Development of nonsurfactant cyclodextrin nanoparticles loaded with anticancer drug paclitaxel, *J. Pharm. Sci.*, **97**, pp. 1519–1529.
10. Nahaei, M., Valizadeh, H., Baradaran, B., Nahaei, M. R., Asgari, D., Hallaj-Nezhadi, S., Dastmalchi, S. and Lotfipour, F. (2013). Preparation and characterization of chitosan/beta-cyclodextrin nanoparticles containing plasmid DNA encoding interleukin-12, *Drug Res. (Stuttg)*, **63**, pp. 7–12.
11. Trapani, A., Tricarico, D., Mele, A., Maqoud, F., Mandracchia, D., Vitale, P., Capriati, V., Trapani, G., Dimiccoli, V., Tolomeo, A. and Scilimati, A. (2017). A novel injectable formulation of 6-fluoro-l-DOPA imaging

agent for diagnosis of neuroendocrine tumors and Parkinson's disease, *Int. J. Pharm.*, **519**, pp. 304–313.

12. Wang, H., Sun, D., Liao, H., Wang, Y., Zhao, S., Zhang, Y., Lv, G., Ma, X., Liu, Y. and Sun, G. (2017). Synthesis and characterization of a bimodal nanoparticle based on the host-guest self-assembly for targeted cellular imaging, *Talanta*, **171**, pp. 8–15.
13. Lin, W., Yao, N., Qian, L., Zhang, X., Chen, Q., Wang, J. and Zhang, L. (2017). pH-responsive unimolecular micelle-gold nanoparticles-drug nanohybrid system for cancer theranostics, *Acta Biomater.*, **58**, pp. 455–465.
14. Laza-Knoerr, A. L., Gref, R. and Couvreur, P. (2010). Cyclodextrins for drug delivery, *J. Drug Target.*, **18**, pp. 645–656.
15. Crini, G. (2014). Review: a history of cyclodextrins, *Chem. Rev.*, **114**, pp. 10940–10975.
16. Kurkov, S. V. and Loftsson, T. (2013). Cyclodextrins, *Int. J. Pharm.*, **453**, pp. 167–180.
17. Del Valle, E. M. M. (2004). Cyclodextrins and their uses: a review, *Process Biochem.*, **39**, pp. 1033–1046.
18. Loftsson, T. and Brewster, M. E. (2010). Pharmaceutical applications of cyclodextrins: basic science and product development, *J. Pharm. Pharmacol.*, **62**, pp. 1607–1621.
19. Wang, H., Xie, X., Zhang, F., Zhou, Q., Tao, Q., Zou, Y., Chen, C., Zhou, C. and Yu, S. (2011). Evaluation of cholesterol depletion as a marker of nephrotoxicity in vitro for novel β-cyclodextrin derivatives, *Food Chem. Toxicol.*, **49**, pp. 1387–1393.
20. Szejtli, J., Cserháti, T. and Szögyi, M. (1986). Interactions between cyclodextrins and cell-membrane phospholipids, *Carbohydr. Polym.*, **6**, pp. 35–49.
21. Steck, T. L., Ye, J. and Lange, Y. (2002). Probing red cell membrane cholesterol movement with cyclodextrin, *Biophys. J.*, **83**, pp. 2118–2125.
22. Zhang, J. and Ma, P. X. (2013). Cyclodextrin-based supramolecular systems for drug delivery: recent progress and future perspective, *Adv. Drug Deliv. Rev.*, **65**, pp. 1215–1233.
23. Brewster, M. E. and Loftsson, T. (2007). Cyclodextrins as pharmaceutical solubilizers, *Adv. Drug Deliv. Rev.*, **59**, pp. 645–666.
24. Casu, B., Reggiani, M. and Sanderson, G. R. (1979). Methylated cycloamyloses (cyclodextrins) and their inclusion properties, *Carbohydr. Res.*, **76**, pp. 59–66.

25. Loftsson, T. and Brewster, M. E. (1996). Pharmaceutical applications of cyclodextrins. 1. Drug solubilization and stabilization, *J. Pharm. Sci.*, **85**, pp. 1017–1025.

26. Pitha, J., Milecki, J., Fales, H., Pannell, L. and Uekama, K. (1986). Hydroxypropyl-β-cyclodextrin: preparation and characterization; effects on solubility of drugs, *Int. J. Pharm.*, **29**, pp. 73–82.

27. Duchêne, D., Ponchel, G. and Wouessidjewe, D. (1999). Cyclodextrins in targeting, *Adv. Drug Deliv. Rev.*, **36**, pp. 29–40.

28. Varan, G., Varan, C., Erdoğar, N., Hıncal, A. A. and Bilensoy, E. (2017). Amphiphilic cyclodextrin nanoparticles, *Int. J. Pharm.*, **531**(2), pp. 457–469.

29. Erdogar, N., Varan, G. and Bilensoy, E. (2017). Amphiphilic cyclodextrin derivatives for targeted drug delivery to tumors, *Curr. Top. Med. Chem.*, **17**, pp. 1521–1528.

30. Jabbari, A. and Sadeghian, H. (2012). Amphiphilic cyclodextrins, synthesis, utilities and application of molecular modeling in their design, in *Recent Advances in Novel Drug Carrier Systems*, ed. Sezer, A. D., InTech, Rijeka, pp. 331–354.

31. Bellanger, N. and Perly, B. (1992). NMR investigations of the conformation of new cyclodextrin-based amphiphilic transporters for hydrophobic drugs: molecular lollipops, *J. Mol. Struct.*, **273**, pp. 215–226.

32. Roux, M., Perly, B. and Djedaini-Pilard, F. (2007). Self-assemblies of amphiphilic cyclodextrins, *Eur. Biophys. J.*, **36**, pp. 861–867.

33. Lesieur, S., Charon, D., Lesieur, P., Ringard-Lefebvre, C., Muguet, V., Duchêne, D. and Wouessidjewe, D. (2000). Phase behavior of fully hydrated DMPC-amphiphilic cyclodextrin systems, *Chem. Phys. Lipids*, **106**, pp. 127–144.

34. Duchěne, D. and Wouessidjewe, D. (1990). Pharmaceutical uses of cyclodextrins and derivatives, *Drug Dev. Ind. Pharm.*, **16**, pp. 2487–2499.

35. Diaz-Moscoso, A., Balbuena, P., Gomez-Garcia, M., Ortiz Mellet, C., Benito, J. M., Le Gourrierec, L., Di Giorgio, C., Vierling, P., Mazzaglia, A., Micali, N., Defaye, J. and Garcia Fernandez, J. M. (2008). Rational design of cationic cyclooligosaccharides as efficient gene delivery systems, *Chem. Commun.*, pp. 2001–2003.

36. Díaz-Moscoso, A., Le Gourriérec, L., Gómez-García, M., Benito, J. M., Balbuena, P., Ortega-Caballero, F., Guilloteau, N., Di Giorgio, C., Vierling, P., Defaye, J., Ortiz Mellet, C. and García Fernández, J. M. (2009).

Polycationic amphiphilic cyclodextrins for gene delivery: synthesis and effect of structural modifications on plasmid DNA complex stability, cytotoxicity, and gene expression, *Chem. Eur. J.*, **15**, pp. 12871–12888.

37. Mendez-Ardoy, A., Urbiola, K., Aranda, C., Ortiz-Mellet, C., Garcia-Fernandez, J. M. and de Ilarduya, C. T. (2011). Polycationic amphiphilic cyclodextrin-based nanoparticles for therapeutic gene delivery, *Nanomedicine*, **6**, pp. 1697–1707.

38. Cryan, S. A., Holohan, A., Donohue, R., Darcy, R. and O'Driscoll, C. M. (2004). Cell transfection with polycationic cyclodextrin vectors, *Eur. J. Pharm. Sci.*, **21**, pp. 625–633.

39. Granger, C. E., Félix, C. P., Parrot-Lopez, H. P. and Langlois, B. R. (2000). Fluorine containing β-cyclodextrin: a new class of amphiphilic carriers, *Tetrahedron Lett.*, **41**, pp. 9257–9260.

40. Alonso, M. J. (1996). Nanoparticulate drug carrier technology, *Drugs Pharm. Sci.*, **77**, pp. 203–242.

41. Soppimath, K. S., Aminabhavi, T. M., Kulkarni, A. R. and Rudzinski, W. E. (2001). Biodegradable polymeric nanoparticles as drug delivery devices, *J. Control. Release*, **70**, pp. 1–20.

42. Bhattacharya, P., Mondal, S., Basak, S., Das, P., Saha, A. and Bera, T. (2016). In Vitro susceptibilities of wild and drug resistant *Leishmania donovani amastigotes* to piperolactam A loaded hydroxypropyl-beta-cyclodextrin nanoparticles, *Acta Trop.*, **158**, pp. 97–106.

43. Erdogar, N., Esendagli, G., Nielsen, T. T., Esendagli-Yilmaz, G., Yoyen-Ermis, D., Erdogdu, B., Sargon, M. F., Eroglu, H. and Bilensoy, E. (2017). Therapeutic efficacy of folate receptor-targeted amphiphilic cyclodextrin nanoparticles as a novel vehicle for paclitaxel delivery in breast cancer, *J. Drug Target.*, pp. 1–9.

44. Quaglia, F., Ostacolo, L., Mazzaglia, A., Villari, V, Zaccaria, D. and Sciortino, M. T. (2009). The intracellular effects of non-ionic amphiphilic cyclodextrin nanoparticles in the delivery of anticancer drugs, *Biomaterials*, **30**, pp. 374–382.

45. Varan, G., Oncul, S., Ercan, A., Benito, J. M., Ortiz Mellet, C. and Bilensoy, E. (2016). Cholesterol-targeted anticancer and apoptotic effects of anionic and polycationic amphiphilic cyclodextrin nanoparticles, *J. Pharm. Sci.*, **105**, pp. 3172–3182.

46. Unal, H., d'Angelo, I., Pagano, E., Borrelli, F., Izzo, A., Ungaro, F., Quaglia, F. and Bilensoy, E. (2015). Core-shell hybrid nanocapsules for oral delivery of camptothecin: formulation development, in vitro and in vivo evaluation, *J. Nanopart. Res.*, **17**, p. 42.

47. Unal, H., Ozturk, N. and Bilensoy, E. (2015). Formulation development, stability and anticancer efficacy of core-shell cyclodextrin nanocapsules for oral chemotherapy with camptothecin, *Beilstein J. Org. Chem.*, **11**, pp. 204–212.

48. Zhang, P., Liu, X., Hu, W., Bai, Y. and Zhang, L. (2016). Preparation and evaluation of naringenin-loaded sulfobutylether-beta-cyclodextrin/chitosan nanoparticles for ocular drug delivery, *Carbohydr. Polym.*, **149**, pp. 224–230.

49. Evans, J. C., Malhotra, M., Fitzgerald, K. A., Guo, J., Cronin, M. F., Curtin, C. M., O'Brien, F. J., Darcy, R. and O'Driscoll, C. M. (2017). Formulation and evaluation of anisamide-targeted amphiphilic cyclodextrin nanoparticles to promote therapeutic gene silencing in a 3D prostate cancer bone metastases model, *Mol. Pharmaceutics*, **14**, pp. 42–52.

50. Evans, J. C., Malhotra, M., Guo, J., O'Shea, J. P., Hanrahan, K., O'Neill, A., Landry, W. D., Griffin, B. T., Darcy, R., Watson, R. W. and O'Driscoll, C. M. (2016). Folate-targeted amphiphilic cyclodextrin.siRNA nanoparticles for prostate cancer therapy exhibit PSMA mediated uptake, therapeutic gene silencing in vitro and prolonged circulation in vivo, *Nanomedicine*, **12**, pp. 2341–2351.

51. Godinho, B. M., Ogier, J. R., Quinlan, A., Darcy, R., Griffin, B. T., Cryan, J. F. and O'Driscoll, C. M. (2014). PEGylated cyclodextrins as novel siRNA nanosystems: correlations between polyethylene glycol length and nanoparticle stability, *Int. J. Pharm.*, **473**, pp. 105–112.

52. Tejashri, G., Amrita, B. and Darshana, J. (2013). Cyclodextrin based nanosponges for pharmaceutical use: a review, *Acta Pharm.*, **63**, pp. 335–358.

53. Dora, C. P., Trotta, F., Kushwah, V., Devasari, N., Singh, C., Suresh, S. and Jain, S. (2016). Potential of erlotinib cyclodextrin nanosponge complex to enhance solubility, dissolution rate, in vitro cytotoxicity and oral bioavailability, *Carbohydr. Polym.*, **137**, pp. 339–349.

54. Rao, M. R. and Bhingole, R. C. (2015). Nanosponge-based pediatric-controlled release dry suspension of Gabapentin for reconstitution, *Drug Dev. Ind. Pharm.*, **41**, pp. 2029–2036.

55. Shende, P., Deshmukh, K., Trotta, F. and Caldera, F. (2013). Novel cyclodextrin nanosponges for delivery of calcium in hyperphosphatemia, *Int. J. Pharm.*, **456**, pp. 95–100.

56. Torne, S., Darandale, S., Vavia, P., Trotta, F. and Cavalli, R. (2013). Cyclodextrin-based nanosponges: effective nanocarrier for tamoxifen delivery, *Pharm. Dev. Technol.*, **18**, pp. 619–625.

57. Minelli, R., Cavalli, R., Ellis, L., Pettazzoni, P., Trotta, F., Ciamporcero, E., Barrera, G., Fantozzi, R., Dianzani, C. and Pili, R. (2012). Nanosponge-encapsulated camptothecin exerts anti-tumor activity in human prostate cancer cells, *Eur. J. Pharm. Sci.*, **47**, pp. 686–694.

58. Hayiyana, Z., Choonara, Y. E., Makgotloe, A., du Toit, L. C., Kumar, P. and Pillay, V. (2016). Ester-based hydrophilic cyclodextrin nanosponges for topical ocular drug delivery, *Curr. Pharm. Des.*, **22**, pp. 6988–6997.

59. Trotta, F., Caldera, F., Cavalli, R., Soster, M., Riedo, C., Biasizzo, M., Uccello Barretta, G., Balzano, F. and Brunella, V. (2016). Molecularly imprinted cyclodextrin nanosponges for the controlled delivery of L-DOPA: perspectives for the treatment of Parkinson's disease, *Expert Opin. Drug Deliv.*, **13**, pp. 1671–1680.

60. Davis, M. E. and Brewster, M. E. (2004). Cyclodextrin-based pharmaceutics: past, present and future, *Nat. Rev. Drug Discov.*, **3**, pp. 1023–1035.

61. Dahan, A. and Hoffman, A. (2008). Rationalizing the selection of oral lipid based drug delivery systems by an in vitro dynamic lipolysis model for improved oral bioavailability of poorly water soluble drugs, *J. Control. Release*, **129**, pp. 1–10.

62. Carrier, R. L., Miller, L. A. and Ahmed, I. (2007). The utility of cyclodextrins for enhancing oral bioavailability, *J. Control. Release*, **123**, pp. 78–99.

63. Gillet, A., Grammenos, A., Compere, P., Evrard, B. and Piel, G. (2009). Development of a new topical system: drug-in-cyclodextrin-in-deformable liposome, *Int. J. Pharm.*, **380**, pp. 174–180.

64. Hatzi, P., Mourtas, S., Klepetsanis, P. G. and Antimisiaris, S. G. (2007). Integrity of liposomes in presence of cyclodextrins: effect of liposome type and lipid composition, *Int. J. Pharm.*, **333**, pp. 167–176.

65. Chen, J., Lu, W. L., Gu, W., Lu, S. S., Chen, Z. P., Cai, B. C. and Yang, X. X. (2014). Drug-in-cyclodextrin-in-liposomes: a promising delivery system for hydrophobic drugs, *Expert Opin. Drug Deliv.*, **11**, pp. 565–577.

66. Zhu, Q., Guo, T., Xia, D., Li, X., Zhu, C., Li, H., Ouyang, D., Zhang, J. and Gan, Y. (2013). Pluronic F127-modified liposome-containing tacrolimus-cyclodextrin inclusion complexes: improved solubility, cellular uptake and intestinal penetration, *J. Pharm. Pharmacol.*, **65**, pp. 1107–1117.

67. Zhang, L., Zhang, Q., Wang, X., Zhang, W., Lin, C., Chen, F., Yang, X. and Pan, W. (2015). Drug-in-cyclodextrin-in-liposomes: a novel drug delivery system for flurbiprofen, *Int. J. Pharm.*, **492**, pp. 40–45.

68. Maestrelli, F., Gonzalez-Rodriguez, M. L., Rabasco, A. M., Ghelardini, C. and Mura, P. (2010). New "drug-in cyclodextrin-in deformable liposomes" formulations to improve the therapeutic efficacy of local anaesthetics, *Int. J. Pharm.*, **395**, pp. 222–231.

69. Alomrani, A. H., Shazly, G. A., Amara, A. A. and Badran, M. M. (2014). Itraconazole-hydroxypropyl-beta-cyclodextrin loaded deformable liposomes: in vitro skin penetration studies and antifungal efficacy using Candida albicans as model, *Colloids Surf. B*, **121**, pp. 74–81.

70. Kaminskas, L. M., Kelly, B. D., McLeod, V. M., Sberna, G., Owen, D. J., Boyd, B. J. and Porter, C. J. (2011). Characterisation and tumour targeting of PEGylated polylysine dendrimers bearing doxorubicin via a pH labile linker, *J. Control. Release*, **152**, pp. 241–248.

71. Sun, L., Zhou, D. S., Zhang, P., Li, Q. H. and Liu, P. (2015). Gemcitabine and gamma-cyclodextrin/docetaxel inclusion complex-loaded liposome for highly effective combinational therapy of osteosarcoma, *Int. J. Pharm.*, **478**, pp. 308–317.

72. Li, J. (2010). Self-assembled supramolecular hydrogels based on polymer–cyclodextrin inclusion complexes for drug delivery, *NPG Asia Mater.*, **2**, pp. 112–118.

73. Concheiro, A. and Alvarez-Lorenzo, C. (2013). Chemically cross-linked and grafted cyclodextrin hydrogels: from nanostructures to drug-eluting medical devices, *Adv. Drug Deliv. Rev.*, **65**, pp. 1188–1203.

74. Liu, K. L., Zhang, Z. and Li, J. (2011). Supramolecular hydrogels based on cyclodextrin-polymer polypseudorotaxanes: materials design and hydrogel properties, *Soft Matter*, **7**, pp. 11290–11297.

75. Abu Hashim, I. I., Higashi, T., Anno, T., Motoyama, K., Abd-ElGawad, A.-E. H., El-Shabouri, M. H., Borg, T. M. and Arima, H. (2010). Potential use of γ-cyclodextrin polypseudorotaxane hydrogels as an injectable sustained release system for insulin, *Int. J. Pharm.*, **392**, pp. 83–91.

76. Machín, R., Isasi, J. R. and Vélaz, I. (2012). β-Cyclodextrin hydrogels as potential drug delivery systems, *Carbohydr. Polym.*, **87**, pp. 2024–2030.

77. Glisoni, R. J., Garcia-Fernandez, M. J., Pino, M., Gutkind, G., Moglioni, A. G., Alvarez-Lorenzo, C., Concheiro, A. and Sosnik, A. (2013). beta-Cyclodextrin hydrogels for the ocular release of antibacterial thiosemicarbazones, *Carbohydr. Polym.*, **93**, pp. 449–457.

78. Morie, A., Garg, T., Goyal, A. K. and Rath, G. (2016). Nanofibers as novel drug carrier: an overview, *Artif. Cells Nanomed. Biotechnol.*, **44**, pp. 135–143.

79. Schiffman, J. D. and Schauer, C. L. (2008). A review: electrospinning of biopolymer nanofibers and their applications, *Polym. Rev.*, **48**, pp. 317–352.

80. Gang, E. H., Ki, C. S., Kim, J. W., Lee, J., Cha, B. G., Lee, K. H. and Park, Y. H. (2012). Highly porous three-dimensional poly(lactide-co-glycolide) (PLGA) microfibrous scaffold prepared by electrospinning method: a comparison study with other PLGA type scaffolds on its biological evaluation, *Fibers Polym.*, **13**, pp. 685–691.

81. Celebioglu, A. and Uyar, T. (2011). Electrospinning of polymer-free nanofibers from cyclodextrin inclusion complexes, *Langmuir*, **27**, pp. 6218–6226.

82. Jia, Y.-T., Gong, J., Gu, X.-H., Kim, H.-Y., Dong, J. and Shen, X.-Y. (2007). Fabrication and characterization of poly (vinyl alcohol)/chitosan blend nanofibers produced by electrospinning method, *Carbohydr. Polym.*, **67**, pp. 403–409.

83. Celebioglu, A. and Uyar, T. (2010). Cyclodextrin nanofibers by electrospinning, *Chem. Commun.*, **46**, pp. 6903–6905.

84. Vigh, T., Horvathova, T., Balogh, A., Soti, P. L., Dravavolgyi, G., Nagy, Z. K. and Marosi, G. (2013). Polymer-free and polyvinylpirrolidone-based electrospun solid dosage forms for drug dissolution enhancement, *Eur. J. Pharm. Sci.*, **49**, pp. 595–602.

85. Canbolat, M. F., Celebioglu, A. and Uyar, T. (2014). Drug delivery system based on cyclodextrin-naproxen inclusion complex incorporated in electrospun polycaprolactone nanofibers, *Colloids Surf. B*, **115**, pp. 15–21.

86. Cirillo, G., Parisi, O. I., Curcio, M., Puoci, F., Iemma, F., Spizzirri, U. G. and Picci, N. (2010). Molecularly imprinted polymers as drug delivery systems for the sustained release of glycyrrhizic acid, *J. Pharm. Pharmacol.*, **62**, pp. 577–582.

87. Siemoneit, U., Schmitt, C., Alvarez-Lorenzo, C., Luzardo, A., Otero-Espinar, F., Concheiro, A. and Blanco-Mendez, J. (2006). Acrylic/cyclodextrin hydrogels with enhanced drug loading and sustained release capability, *Int. J. Pharm.*, **312**, pp. 66–74.

88. Cunliffe, D., Kirby, A. and Alexander, C. (2005). Molecularly imprinted drug delivery systems, *Adv. Drug Deliv. Rev.*, **57**, pp. 1836–1853.

89. Liu, Z., Bucknall, D. G. and Allen, M. G. (2010). Absorption performance of iodixanol-imprinted polymers in aqueous and blood plasma media, *Acta Biomater.*, **6**, pp. 2003–2012.

90. Puoci, F., Cirillo, G., Curcio, M., Parisi, O. I., Iemma, F. and Picci, N. (2011). Molecularly imprinted polymers in drug delivery: state of art and future perspectives, *Expert Opin. Drug Deliv.*, **8**, pp. 1379–1393.

91. Peppas, N. A. and Huang, Y. (2002). Polymers and gels as molecular recognition agents, *Pharm. Res.*, **19**, pp. 578–587.

92. Cerchiara, T., Abruzzo, A., di Cagno, M., Bigucci, F., Bauer-Brandl, A., Parolin, C., Vitali, B., Gallucci, M. C. and Luppi, B. (2015). Chitosan based micro- and nanoparticles for colon-targeted delivery of vancomycin prepared by alternative processing methods, *Eur. J. Pharm. Biopharm.*, **92**, pp. 112–119.

93. Alvarez-Lorenzo, C. and Concheiro, A. (2004). Molecularly imprinted polymers for drug delivery, *J. Chromatogr. B*, **804**, pp. 231–245.

94. Harada, A. (1996). Preparation and structures of supramolecules between cyclodextrins and polymers, *Coord. Chem. Rev.*, **148**, pp. 115–133.

95. Dong, R., Zhou, Y., Huang, X., Zhu, X., Lu, Y. and Shen, J. (2015). Functional supramolecular polymers for biomedical applications, *Adv. Mater.*, **27**, pp. 498–526.

96. Loethen, S., Kim, J. M. and Thompson, D. H. (2007). Biomedical applications of cyclodextrin based polyrotaxanes, *Polym. Rev.*, **47**, pp. 383–418.

97. Wenz, G., Han, B. H. and Muller, A. (2006). Cyclodextrin rotaxanes and polyrotaxanes, *Chem. Rev.*, **106**, pp. 782–817.

98. Young, C., Schluep, T., Hwang, J. and Eliasof, S. (2011). CRLX101 (formerly IT-101)-a novel nanopharmaceutical of camptothecin in clinical development, *Curr. Bioact. Compd.*, **7**, pp. 8–14.

99. Jiang, L., Gao, Z.-M., Ye, L., Zhang, A.-Y. and Feng, Z.-G. (2013). A tumor-targeting nano doxorubicin delivery system built from amphiphilic polyrotaxane-based block copolymers, *Polymer*, **54**, pp. 5188–5198.

100. Jiang, L., Gao, Z.-M., Ye, L., Zhang, A.-Y. and Feng, Z.-G. (2013). A pH-sensitive nano drug delivery system of doxorubicin-conjugated amphiphilic polyrotaxane-based block copolymers, *Biomater. Sci.*, **1**, pp. 1282–1291.

Chapter 3

Hydrogels as Intelligent Drug Delivery Systems

Natassa Pippa,[a,b] Nikolaos Bouropoulos,[c] Stergios Pispas,[b] Costas Demetzos,[a] and Apostolos Papalois[d]

[a]*Section of Pharmaceutical Technology, Department of Pharmacy, School of Health Sciences, National and Kapodistrian University of Athens, Panepistimioupolis Zografou, 15771 Athens, Greece*

[b]*Theoretical and Physical Chemistry Institute, National Hellenic Research Foundation, 48 Vasileos Konstantinou Avenue, 11635 Athens, Greece*

[c]*Department of Materials Science, University of Patras, Rion, Greece, and Institute of Chemical Engineering and High Temperature Chemical Processes FORTH, Patras, Greece*

[d]*ELPEN Research -Experimental Centre, Athens, Greece*

natpippa@pharm.uoa.gr

Hydrogels are swollen nanosized networks consisting of hydrophilic or amphiphilic polymer chains. Hydrogels can protect and transfer bioactive molecules, therapeutic nucleotides, and proteins/peptides and control their release by integrating highly responsive functional groups that respond to external stimuli by configurational changes

Drug Delivery Nanosystems: From Bioinspiration and Biomimetics to Clinical Applications
Edited by Costas Demetzos, Stergios Pispas, and Natassa Pippa

ISBN 978-981-4774-92-5 (Hardcover), 978-0-429-49054-5 (eBook)
www.panstanford.com

and/or present biodegradable links in the polymer network. Like other nanosystems, nanogels can be easily administered as drug delivery formulations for parenteral and transdermal administration. Stimuli-responsive behavior offers high special triggered actuation, encapsulation, and release properties and is most of the times followed by the presence of surface functional chemical groups that are available for bioconjugation with bioactive factors for targeting special macromolecular targets on damaged tissue surface. The aim of this chapter is to discuss in depth the challenges associated with the development of hydrogels as delivery platforms and also issues that are related to their preparation process, their physicochemical properties, the drug release kinetics, and the conditions under which the system is delivered to the human body. Special attention will be given to stimuli-responsive nanogels.

3.1 Introduction

Nanotechnology is an emerging technology seeking to exploit distinct technological advances controlling the structure of nanoscale biomaterials at a nanodimensional scale approaching individual molecules and their aggregates or supramolecular structures [1–5]. The term "nanomedicine" is used to describe those technologies under the umbrella of nanotechnology with therapeutic applications in human health. Nanoscale biomaterials are totally biocompatible, nontoxic, nonimmunogenic, and biodegradable and, furthermore, have been used or have the potential to be used in personalized biomedical applications, such as drug delivery, tissue regeneration, and diagnostics [1, 2]. Nanotechnological systems are used in pharmaceutical sciences as bioactive molecule delivery systems for therapeutic and diagnostic purposes and in vivo tissue imaging for medical applications. Furthermore, new scientific studies combine nanosystem applications for simultaneously treating the disease and monitoring disease progression, helping the clinical doctor to get the most accurate diagnosis. These systems are known as theranostics (diagnostic-therapeutic products). The most important nanotechnological bioactive molecule delivery systems will be studied, from their technological development in the laboratory to their clinical use regarding their biophysics, therapeutic efficacy, and safety. The modern scientist in the broader field of pharmaceutical sciences and the health officer have a great advantage when they understand the behavior of these nanotechnological bioactive molecule delivery systems at a technological level as well as in the human organism. Pharmaceutical nanotechnology research aims to develop new drugs based on bioactive molecule delivery with nanosystems and to geometrically increase medicines that are currently in clinical studies. The pharmaceutical industry follows the same path, investing in the bioactive molecule development from the wider pharmaceutical nanotechnology point of view. According to Peppas [3]:

> Biomimetic polymeric networks can be prepared by designing interactions between the building blocks of biocompatible networks and the desired specific ligands, and by stabilizing these interactions by a three-dimensional structure. These structures are at the same time flexible enough to allow for diffusion of solvent and ligand into and out of the networks. Synthetic networks that can be designed to recognize and bind biologically significant molecules are of great importance and influence a number of emerging technologies. These artificial materials can be used as unique systems or can be incorporated into existing drug delivery technologies that can aid in the removal or delivery of biomolecules and restore the natural profiles of compounds in the body. . . . These micropatterned structures may be used for a host of applications including cell adhesion, separation processes, the so-called "factory-on-a-chip" microscale reactors, and microfluidic devices.

In other words, biomimetic materials processing is defined as the design and synthesis of new functional materials by refining the knowledge and understanding of related biological products, structures, functions, and processes (e.g., by mimicking biological systems, achieving molecular-scale control via self-assembly and directed assembly techniques) [4, 5].

The research orientation of a smart therapeutic system is one that can essentially bring the clinical practice to the patient, providing sensing and treatment without the need for human intervention [4, 6–10]. Polymer therapeutics describes a new class of drug delivery systems where polymers play a key role [9, 10]. The responsive hydrogels developed fit into both polymer and smart delivery systems and can be characterized as intelligent polymer therapeutics [11–22]. Responsive hydrogels have proven their pharmaceutical and biological effectiveness on the macro- and/or nanoscale. This will allow them to actively sense and respond to stimuli on the same scale as many biological and biochemical processes [19–22]. According to He et al. [22]:

> Stimuli-sensitive block copolymer hydrogels, which are reversible polymer networks formed by physical interactions and exhibit a sol-gel phase-transition in response to external stimuli, have great potential in biomedical and pharmaceutical applications, especially in site-specific controlled drug-delivery systems. The drug may be mixed with a polymer solution in vitro and the drug-loaded hydrogel can form in situ after the in vivo administration, such as injection; therefore, stimuli-sensitive block copolymer hydrogels have many advantages, such as simple drug formulation and administration procedures, no organic solvent, site-specificity, a sustained drug release behavior, less systemic toxicity and ability to deliver both hydrophilic and hydrophobic drugs. Among the stimuli in the biomedical applications, temperature and pH are the most popular physical and chemical stimuli, respectively.

As mentioned above, stimuli-responsive or "smart" hydrogels respond to environmental changes (pH, temperature, etc.) in ways that can be exploited for biomedical and clinical purposes. The response can be triggered by a change in temperature, pH, or light or by more specific changes, such an increase in the blood glucose level. For this reason their range of applications is broad. pH is an environmental property that changes in the compartments of cells and of the human body (i.e., stomach) as a result of many diseases (cancer, inflammation, etc.) and is highly manipulated by the human body. Hydrophilic polymer networks, known as hydrogels, which respond to changes in pH, offer a novel strategy for targeting many diseases and inflammatory conditions, too [15–22]. These "smart" hydrogels exhibit single or multiple stimuli-responsive characters that could be used in biomedical applications, including controlled drug delivery, bioengineering, or tissue engineering. Temperature- and/or pH-sensitive block copolymer hydrogels for biomedical and pharmaceutical applications have been extensively developed in the past decade [19–22]. To understand the distinct advantages of "smart" hydrogels as drug delivery platforms in nanomedicine it is necessary to look at the existing goals, properties, and applications of other nanodevices in the field: biodegradation, long circulation, targeting, intracellular/organelle delivery, stimuli responsiveness, and imaging properties.

The aim of this chapter is to discuss in depth the challenges associated with the development of hydrogels as delivery platforms, issues that are related to the preparation process, their physicochemical properties, the drug release kinetics, and the conditions under which the system is delivered to the human body. Special attention will be given to stimuli-responsive nanogels.

3.2 Hydrogels

A large number of polymeric systems under development in nanomedicine are either self-assembled systems, such as micelles, polymeric nanoparticles, and polymersomes, or bulk polymers, such as biodegradable polyesters. Cross-linked, hydrophilic polymer networks, otherwise known as hydrogels, offer certain advantages over other biomedical polymers. They are held together via covalent cross-links [23–27]. Covalent bonds provide added integrity and control. Hydrogels are also very similar to biological matter in their soft, highly hydrated nature. They can be fabricated over a wide range of sizes. They also have highly controllable material properties. Hydrogels are network structures formed by hydrophilic polymers that are mutually attached by cross-links, keeping large amounts of water in the formed matrix. From a pharmaceutical point of view, hydrogels have gained much attention in the last decades as they are considered to be attractive drug delivery platforms for a wide range of therapeutic molecules due to some unique properties. Hydrogels are considered key tools for the design of biomaterials such as wound dressings, drug reservoirs, and temporary scaffolds for cells. Despite their potential, conventional hydrogels have limited applicability under wet physiological conditions because they suffer from an uncontrollable temporal change in shape: swelling takes place immediately after the installation [23]. They can be loaded with high amounts of molecules (as the cross-links keep them entrapped in the formed matrix), and the release of the molecules can be controlled by varying the hydrogels' characteristics. Many drug molecules suffer from impediments such as low solubility, off-target toxicity, instability, or inefficient transfer across biological barriers, limiting their use in vivo. Their encapsulation into nanogels may thus offer a solution for safe and efficient delivery as encapsulation imparts to the system prolonged circulation time in biological media such as blood, excellent stability upon dilution, protection from premature degradation, enhanced permeability, and improved biodistribution and pharmacokinetics. Different chemical and physical cross-linking methods used for the design of biodegradable hydrogels are summarized and discussed next.

Chemical cross-linking is a highly versatile method to create hydrogels with good mechanical stability. However, the cross-linking agents used are often toxic compounds that have been extracted from gels before they can be applied. Moreover, cross-linking agents can give unwanted reactions with the bioactive substances present in the hydrogel matrix. Such adverse effects are avoided with the use of physically cross-linked gels. The structure of and interactions in covalently and ionically cross-linked chitosan (CS) hydrogels for biomedical applications are described in Ref. [27]. According to Berger et al. [27], covalent cross-linking leads to the formation of hydrogels with a permanent network structure, since irreversible chemical links are formed, and this type of linkage allows absorption of water and/or bioactive compounds without dissolution and permits drug release by diffusion. pH-controlled drug delivery is made possible by the addition of another polymer [27]. On the other hand, ionically cross-linked hydrogels are generally considered as biocompatible and well-tolerated and their nonpermanent network is formed by reversible links. It should be noted that ionically cross-linked CS hydrogels exhibit a higher swelling sensitivity to pH changes compared to covalently cross-linked CS hydrogels [27].

In some cases, the release profile of the encapsulated drug from hydrogels followed trends similar to the release of the drug from the soluble polymer-drug conjugates. The synthetic methodology employed does not involve the use of coupling reagents in the final conjugation between the active molecule and the polymer, excluding the presence of potential toxic residuals. For this reason, the conjugation method is relatively simple and is applicable to nearly any hydroxyl-containing drugs (i.e., paclitaxel) [28].

3.2.1 PEGylated Hydrogels

Watanabe et al. [29] developed polyethylene glycol (PEG) hydrogels cross-linked by a hydrolysable polyrotaxane, their hydrolytic erosion characterized in terms of supramolecular dissociation of the polyrotaxane. A multifunctional cross-linker composed of the hydrolysable polyrotaxane, in which many alpha-cyclodextrins (α-CDs) are threaded onto a PEG chain capped with L-phenylalanine via ester linkages, was used (the PEG network was covalently bound to hydroxyl groups of α-CDs in the polyrotaxane). The interesting finding was that the in vitro hydrolysis study revealed that the time to reach complete gel erosion was shortened on increasing the polyrotaxane content in the feed in relation to the decreased number of chemical cross-links between PEG and α-CDs in the polyrotaxane [29].

A series of PEG hydrogels cross-linked by a hydrolysable polyrotaxane was prepared, and they can be utilized as long-term-stable but actually hydrolysable hydrogels for polymeric scaffolding in tissue engineering since the time to reach complete gel erosion was found to be prolonged on decreasing the polyrotaxane content and increasing the PEG:α-CD ratio [30].

Missirlis et al. followed inverse emulsion photopolymerization of acrylated PEG-*b*-poly(propylene glycol)-*b*-PEG and PEG to prepare stable, cross-linked, amphiphilic hydrogels. The presence of hydrophobic nanodomains within was verified through the use of pyrene as a microenvironmentally sensitive probe, and the hydrophilic poly(propylene glycol)–rich domains appear to be suitable for the incorporation of bioactive compounds [31].

Hydrogels have been already used as transfection and nucleoside delivery agents in cancer chemotherapy and in vivo brain-targeting agents [32–37]. Several different nanogels consisting of interpenetrating networks composed of amphiphilic polymers and cationic polyethyleneimine were designed for encapsulation and delivery of cytotoxic nucleoside analogs, namely nucleoside 5'-triphosphates, into cancer cells [32–37]. The published data demonstrate that this carrier-based approach to delivery of cytotoxic drugs may enhance tumor specificity and significantly reduce side effects related to systemic toxicity usually observed during cancer chemotherapy [32–37].

3.2.2 Glucose-Responsive Hydrogels

A novel glucose-responsive hydrogel system based on dynamic covalent chemistry and inclusion complexation was formed by simply mixing the solutions of three different biomaterials: poly(ethylene oxide)-*b*-polyvinyl alcohol (PEO-*b*-PVA) diblock polymer, α-CD, and phenylboronic acid (PBA)-terminated PEO cross-linker [38]. Dynamic covalent bonds between PVA and PBA provided sugar-responsive cross-linking, and the inclusion complexation between PEO and α-CD promoted hydrogel formation and enhanced hydrogel stability [38]. This hydrogel with tunable glucose responsiveness is a "smart" system that finds potential applications in biomedical and pharmaceutical fields, such as treatment of diabetes [38].

An injectable and glucose-responsive hydrogel constructed from the complexation of boronic acid and glucose within a single component polymeric material was recently described in the literature [39]. The ratio of boronic acid and glucose functional groups was the critical parameter for hydrogel formation. It was found that polymers with 10%–60% boronic acid, with the balance being glucose modified, were proneto form hydrogels and these hydrogels were shear thinning and self-healing, recovering from a shear-induced flow to a gel state within seconds [39].

3.2.3 pH-Responsive Hydrogels

The first biomedical area in which pH-responsive microgels came into clinical use was the oral loading and delivery of biological macromolecules, especially peptides and proteins. The acidic pH of the stomach and the proteolytic enzymes are a formidable barrier to the oral delivery of many biomacromolecules. Peppas and coworkers investigated the use of pH-responsive, poly(methacrylic acid-grafted-ethylene glycol), or P(MAA-*g*-EG), hydrogels as oral delivery vehicles for insulin. Insulin was loaded into polymeric microspheres and administered orally to healthy and diabetic Wistar rats [40]. In the acidic environment of the stomach, the hydrogels were unswollen, in the collapsed state, due to the formation of intermolecular polymer complexes, but the insulin remained in the hydrogel, protected from proteolytic degradation. In the intestine (the pH is around 7), the complexes dissociated, which resulted in fast gel swelling and insulin burst release [40]. The above is the mechanism of insulin release from pH-responsive hydrogels [40–43]. The same team developed nanospheres of cross-linked networks of MAA grafted with PEG, and acrylic acid (AAc) grafted with PEG nanospheres for the same purpose, the oral delivery of insulin, which was entrapped at low pH (pH = 3) but was released at more neutral pH (pH = 7) [42, 43].

P(MAA-*g*-EG) is a complexation hydrogel molecularly designed for oral insulin delivery in another case [44]. This investigation demonstrated that the P(MAA-*g*-EG) hydrogel microparticles could be used as a cytocompatible carrier possessing the transport-enhancing effect of insulin on the intestinal epithelial cells [44]. The same observation was achieved when insulin was loaded into hydrogel microparticles after 2 h, with loading efficiencies greater than 70% for both P(MAA-*g*-EG) and P(MAA-*g*-EG) functionalized with wheat germ agglutinin (WGA). The pH-responsive release profile demonstrated again that the pH shift from the stomach to the small intestine can be used as a physiologic trigger to release insulin from P(MAA-*g*-EG) and P(MAA-*g*-EG)-WGA microparticles, thus limiting the release of insulin into the acidic environment of the stomach [45, 46]. The degree of intestinal permeation enhancement was found to be strongly dependent on the size of hydrogel particles [47].

An oral insulin delivery system based on copolymers of PEG dimethacrylate and MAA (formed by esterification reaction of different molecular weight PEGs with MAA in the presence of acid catalyst) was developed, and its functional activity was tested in nonobese diabetic rats, with very nice preclinical results [48]. The size of these pH-sensitive poly(ethylene glycol dimethacrylate):MAA, or PEGDMA:MAA, microparticles increased with the increasing molecular weight of the PEGDMA polymer chain. The release of insulin was found to be sensitive to different pH conditions (minimal leakage in stomach and higher release at pH = 7.4) [48].

3.2.4 Thermosensitive Hydrogels

Thermosensitive hydrogels are crucial materials used in pharmaceutical technology because they have great potential in various applications, such as drug delivery, cell encapsulation, tissue engineering, and regenerative medicine. It should be noted that injectable thermosensitive hydrogels with a lower sol-gel transition temperature around the physiological temperature have been extensively studied. By in vivo injection, the hydrogels formed nonflowing gel at body temperature. Upon encapsulation of bioactive compounds, the hydrogel systems could act as a controlled drug release depot in situ. According to Jeong et al. [50]:

> When the hydrogel is formed under physiological conditions and maintains its integrity for a desired period of time, the process may provide various advantages over conventional hydrogels. Because of the simplicity of pharmaceutical formulation by solution mixing, biocompatibility with biological systems, and convenient administration, the pharmaceutical and biomedical uses of the water-based sol-gel transition include solubilization of low-molecular-weight hydrophobic drugs, controlled release, labile biomacromolecule delivery, such as proteins and genes, cell immobilization, and tissue engineering. When the formed gel is proven to be biocompatible and biodegradable, producing non-toxic degradation products, it will provide further benefits for in vivo applications where degradation is desired. It is timely to summarize the polymeric systems that undergo sol-gel transitions, particularly due to temperature, with emphasis on the underlying transition mechanisms and potential delivery aspects.

Thermosensitive hydrogel systems, especially the injectable ones, have a great number of advantages, including simplicity of drug formulation, protective compartment for sensitive active substances, prolonged and localized drug delivery, and ease of application [49, 50]. Another advantage of thermosensitive hydrogels is the absence of organic solvents during the preparation protocol, copolymerization agents, or an externally applied trigger for gelation [51]. The physicochemical property, stability, and composition prospects of smart, thermoresponsive polymers, specifically PEG/poly(*N*-isopropylacrylamide) (PNIPAAm)-based thermoresponsive injectable hydrogels, were recently utilized for pharmaceutical purposes [52].

A series of thermosensitive copolymer hydrogel based on aminated hyaluronic acid (AHA)-*g*-PNIPAAm were synthesized by coupling carboxylic acid end–capped PNIPAAm (PNIPAAm–COOH) with AHA through amide bond linkages. These thermosensitive hydrogels have attractive properties to serve as cell or pharmaceutical delivery vehicles for a variety of tissue engineering applications [53]. PNIPAAm-*g*-methylcellulose thermoreversible hydrogel as a 3D support was also developed for cell encapsulation toward the regeneration of articular cartilage through a tissue engineering approach [54]. A new series of random poly(methyl vinyl ether-*co*-maleic anhydride) (Gantrez® AN, GZ) and Pluronic® F127 (PF127) copolymers (GZ-PF127), that formed thermosensitive hydrogels were also prepared for the controlled release of proteins, such as bovine serum albumin (BSA) and recombinant kinetoplastid membrane protein of Leishmania (rKMP-11) [55]. The gelation temperature and mechanical properties could be controlled by the molar ratio of GZ and PF127 polymers and the copolymer concentration in aqueous media [55]. Multiblock Pluronic copolymers linked by d-lactide and l-lactide oligomers with different spacer lengths were synthesized for the controlled release of human growth hormone (hGH) [56]. hGH was released in a sustained and zero-order fashion for 13 days by a coupled diffusion/erosion mechanism from this novel temperature-sensitive and in situ forming hydrogel system [56]. Triblock copolymers consisting of Pluronic copolymer end-capped with D- or L-lactic acid oligomers (PL-LA(*n*)) with various chain lengths ($n = 5, 12$, etc.) were synthesized for the controlled release of hGH, too [57]. Recently, fine intra-articular-administrated CS thermosensitive hydrogels combined with alginate microspheres were prepared as a drug delivery system for improving the therapeutic/anti-inflammatory effect of diclofenac sodium [58]. The design and characterization of injectable and thermosensitive hydrogel composites comprised of poly(lactic-*co*-glycolic acid) (PLGA)-*g*-PEG containing hydroxyapatite (HA) for potential application in bone tissue engineering were also presented [59]. CS/glycerophosphate (GP) disodium thermosensitive hydrogels were prepared for the sustained delivery of venlafaxine hydrochloride (VH), and the drug release mechanism was diffusion-controlled, fitting to the first-order model [60]. Biodegradable poly(3-hydroxybutyrate-*co*-3-hydroxyhexanoate) nanoparticles containing an insulin-phospholipid complex were loaded in CS-based thermosensitive hydrogels for long-term sustained and controlled delivery of this protein [61]. The injectable hydrogels, prepared by adding a β-GP salt solution to a CS solution while stirring, showed a rapid solution-to-gel transition at 37°C, a porous structure, and a comparative degradation and swelling rate in vitro [61]. The incorporation of ofloxacin into pH-/thermosensitive hydrogels based on acrylic acid (AAc) and *N*-isopropylacrylamide using (+)–*N,N'*-diallyltartramide as the cross-linking agent and water as the solvent are presented in Ref. [62]. A new approach by using the dissipative properties of a hydrogel matrix as an internal heat source when the material is mechanically loaded is presented in Ref. [63]. The smart delivery system consists of a highly dissipative hydrogel matrix and thermosensitive nanoparticles that shrink upon an increase in the temperature. This complex system was used for the encapsulation and controlled release of the growth factor [63].

Anticancer drugs are also encapsulated into thermosensitive hydrogels, with very nice results, for biomedical purposes. Thermosensitive poly(organophosphazenes)–bearing hydrophobic isoleucine ethyl ester groups and hydrophilic alpha-amino-omega-methoxy-PEG of molecular weight 550 along with hydrolysis-sensitive glycyl lactate ethyl esters have been synthesized for sustained delivery of doxorubicin [64]. The authors demonstrated that the hydrogel forming property of poly(organophosphazenes) was affected on incorporation of doxorubicin, resulting in an increase in the gelation temperature and a decrease in the gel strength [64]. Poly(organophosphazene) hydrogel systems showed adequate characteristics for local intratumoral delivery of doxorubicin, including dose capacity, local retention, and minimal systemic spill-over, but the safety and biocompatibility of poly(organophosphazene) should be further evaluated and its application should be extended to other anticancer agents [65]. A thermosensitive CS/β-GP hydrogel loaded with docetaxel (DTX) for intratumoral delivery was developed [66]. The in vitro release profiles, in vivo antitumor efficacy, pharmacokinetics, and biodistribution of DTX-loaded CS/β-GP hydrogel met the requirements for biomedical applications in anticancer therapy [66]. Liposomal doxorubicin was encapsulated into the hydrogel to form a novel thermosensitive formulation that prolonged the sustained release of DOX [67]. The hydrogel is composed of CS/β-GP. The encapsulation efficiency of the anticancer compound was found extremely high (98%), while the in vitro and in vivo antitumor experiments demonstrated that the liposomal-hydrogel system had a better antineoplastic effect and less toxicity than the liposomal system alone [67]. Pharmacokinetic studies showed that the prepared hydrogel exhibited a higher bioavailability in human plasma and tumor [67]. A soluble CS derivative, *N*-[(2-hydroxy-3-trimethylammonium) propyl] CS chloride, was synthesized and interacted with GP to produce a thermosensitive hydrogel as the matrix of doxorubicin-loaded liposomes for topical anticancer therapy offering reduced dosing frequency and sustained drug release [68]. Generally, the advanced development of CS hydrogels has led to new drug delivery systems that release their payloads under varying environmental stimuli [69].

An innovative biodegradable thermosensitive composite hydrogel, based on PEG-poly(ε-caprolactone)-PEG (PEG-PCL-PEG, PECE) and Pluronic F127 copolymer, was successfully prepared, and vitamin B12, honokiol, and BSA were encapsulated and released very slowly from the above delivery system [70, 71]. Thermosensitive hydrogels based on CS and its derivatives containing medicated nanoparticles were designed for transcorneal administration of 5-fluorouracil in a sustained release manner [72]. An injectable thermosensitive CS/gelatin/GP hydrogel as a sustained-release system of latanoprost for glaucoma treatment showed a good in vitro and in vivo biocompatibility [73]. Thermosensitive PLGA-PEG-PLGA triblock copolymers as in situ gelling matrices followed zero-order release kinetics for vitamin B12 over 25 days, in contrast to the Higuchi modeling for naltrexone hydrochloride over a period of 17 days [74].

Generally, smart composite hydrogels consisting of CS microspheres physically embedded within a thermoresponsive hydrogel have been synthesized and tested for their capacity of loading and controlled release of active pharmaceutical ingredients [75, 76]. Several physicochemical characteristics are crucial formulation parameters affecting the solution stability, the sol/gel transition behavior, and/or the final hydrogel structure and consequently their properties for drug delivery and tissue engineering purposes [75, 76]. According to Tahrir et al. [77]:

> [G]reat attention has been paid to in situ gel-forming chitosan/glycerophosphate (CS/Gp) formulation due to its high biocompatibility with incorporated cells and medical agents, biodegradability and sharp thermosensitive gelation. CS/Gp is in liquid state at room

temperature and after minimally invasive administration into the desired tissue, it forms a solid-like gel as a response to temperature increase. . . . This thermosensitive hydrogel has a great potential as scaffold material in tissue engineering, due to its good biocompatibility, minimal immune reaction, high antibacterial nature, good adhesion to cells and the ability to be molded in various geometries. Moreover, CS/Gp hydrogel has been utilized as a smart drug delivery system to increase patient compliance by maintaining the drug level in the therapeutic window for a long time while avoiding the need for frequent injections of the therapeutic agent.

Additionally, thermosensitive PNIPAAm hydrogels with an interpenetrating polymer network (IPN) structure were synthesized for the purpose of improving mechanical properties of the hydrogel, the response rate to temperature, and sustained release of drugs and proteins (i.e., BSA) [78]. It should be noted that the morphology of these hydrogels is quite different. Namely, the IPN hydrogels showed a fibrillar-like porous network structure that normal PNIPAAm did not have [78]. Protein/synthetic polymer hybrid IPNs of PNIPAAm with *Bombyx mori* silk fibroin have been also prepared [79].

3.3 Hydrogels for Controlled Release of Drugs and Proteins

Hydrogels and nanogels are ideal platforms for the controlled release of the encapsulated bioactive compounds (i.e., proteins, peptides, and drug molecules) [80–82]. Nanogels exhibit an excellent drug-loading capacity, high stability, biologic consistence, and response to a wide variety of environmental stimuli, as mentioned above [80–82]. Figure 3.1 presents the drug release from nanogels. Li et al. demonstrated the influence of Hofmeister ions on the size and guest encapsulation stability of polymeric nanogels. While variations in macroscopic phase transitions have been observed in response to the presence of salts, changes in the size and host-guest behavior of polymeric aggregates in the presence of salts have not been explored in any detail. Encapsulation stability of guest molecules is dependent on the nature of the salt used for the preparation of nanogels; chaotropic anions afford nanogels with a greater guest encapsulation stability [83].

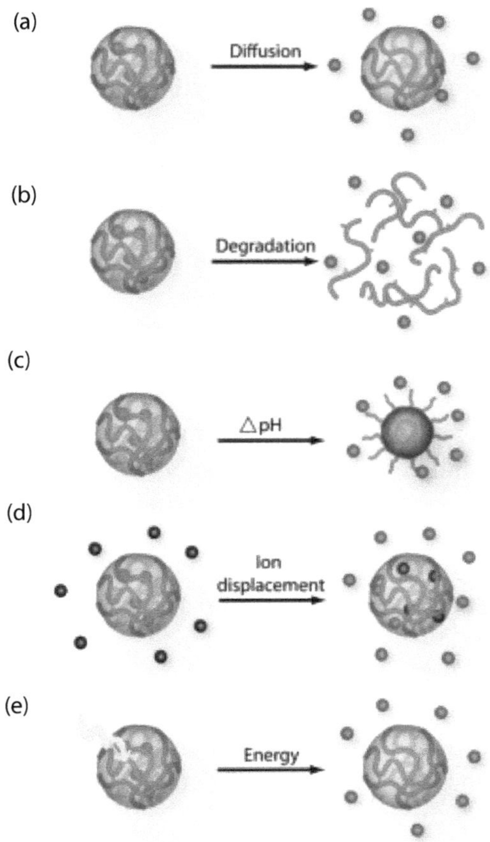

Figure 3.1 Drug release from nanogels. (a) Diffusion of the drug out of nanogels. (b) Drug release due to degradation of biodegradable polymer chains or cross-links. (c) Change in pH results in deionization of the polymer network and release of the electrostatically bound drug. (d) Multivalent low-molecular-weight cations or polyions of either charge can displace drugs having the same charge sign from electrostatic complexes with ionic nanogels. (e) Drug release can be induced by an external energy applied to nanogels that induces degradation or structural transition of the nanogel polymer chains [80].

Zalfen et al. reported on a multicomponent drug delivery biomaterial that consists of a hydrogel matrix in which drug-loaded biodegradable microcarriers are dispersed and whose potential applications could be found in the design of implantable devices with long-term activity, as required by contraceptive and hormone replacement treatments [84]. The hydrogel consisted of 2-hydroxyethyl methacrylate (HEMA) cross-linked by ethylene glycol dimethacrylate (EGDMA). The microcarriers were biodegradable PCL microspheres in which active molecules, such as levonorgestrel, were encapsulated. The developed device, due to its composite structure, has the ability to combine several release mechanisms, leading to drug release obeying zero-order kinetics for most of the time [84].

A novel copolymer hydrogel was prepared by Arica et al. [85] in the membrane form using a 2-HEMA monomer and a macromonomer p-vinyl benzyl (V)-PEO via photoinitiated polymerization. Drug release experiments were performed in a continuous release system using a model drug (vancomycin) loaded within copoly(HEMA/V-PEO) membranes. The developed transdermal antibiotic carrier exhibited high drug-loading efficiencies and controlled release properties [85].

A pH-sensitive hydrogel together with a poly(HEMA) barrier was used as a gate to control drug release [86]. In addition, poly(HEMA) coated with PEO-poly(propylene oxide) (PPO)-PEO macromolecular surfactant was utilized to enhance mucoadhesion on the device surface. The release profiles of two model drugs, acid orange 8 and BSA were studied in this assembled system, which compared with the conventional drug-entrapped carriers and enteric-coating systems [86]. The authors observed the local targeting and unidirectional release in vitro [86].

The swelling behavior and the in vitro release of the antihypertensive drug verapamil hydrochloride from calcium alginate and CS-treated calcium alginate beads were investigated by Paspasrakis and Bouropoulos [87]. Calcium-alginate beads, CS-coated alginate beads, and alginate-CS mixed beads were synthesized, and high drug loading was achieved (~80%) in both calcium-alginate and calcium alginate-CS mixed beads. The drug release mechanisms were either "anomalous transport" or "case-II transport" [87].

The release of albumin, a model protein, from alginate/hydroxypropyl-methylcellulose (HPMC) gel beads was studied by Nochos et al. [88]. The morphology, bead size, and swelling ratio were studied in different physical conditions (i.e., fully swollen, dried, and reswollen). These swelling experiments showed that the bead diameter increases with the viscosity of the alginate solution while the addition of HPMC resulted in a significant increase in the swelling ratio [88]. The addition of HPMC increased the protein-release rate, while the release mechanism fitted the Peppas model. Alginate/HPMC beads improved BSA release in a physiological saline solution, and all formulations presented a non-Fickian release mechanism described by the Peppas model [88].

The hydrogels based on homopolymers and copolymers of *N*-ethyl morpholine methacrylamide (EMA) and *N,N*-dimethylacrylamide (DMA) have been prepared in order to be applied as matrices for ibuprofen release as a method for minimizing the very low aqueous solubility of ibuprofen, the segregation of the drug into microdomains, and possible crystallization (leading to possible damage of the mucous membrane of the stomach) [89]. The hydrogels were loaded with ibuprofen, and the release over time was tested in different aqueous media. For DMA hydrogels, most of the ibuprofen was released as noncrystalline ibuprofen at pH 7.4 but it was not able to prevent crystallization at pH 2 and 5. On the other hand, the EMA hydrogels were able to prevent crystallization of the ibuprofen at all pH values investigated [89].

The investigation of Jabeen et al. highlighted the pH responsiveness of composite alginate hydrogels prepared under different conditions to be employed in drug delivery and controlled released applications [90]. The hydrogels composed of sodium alginate, PEO, and AAc with CD showed significant variations in rheological properties, drug encapsulation capability, and release kinetics. Ibuprofen was used as the model drug. The ibuprofen encapsulation capacity was low, and it was released slowly when the hydrogels were prepared at pH = 1. The hydrogels prepared at neutral pH (pH 7) showed the highest ibuprofen encapsulation capacity and also optimum drug release kinetics. The hydrogels prepared at pH = 12 were more viscous, had low tensile strength, were unstable on change in temperature, and exhibited a fast drug release rate [90]. The presence of surfactant also altered the loading efficiency and the release profile of the encapsulated ibuprofen [91].

Additionally, hydrogels composed of alginate and poloxamer were loaded with indomethacin, incorporated into the ceramic (composites of biomorphic silicon) carbides, and cross-linked [92]. The indomethacin release profile was found to be dependent on the microstructure of the ceramics selected. The most interesting finding was that the released indomethacin was able to modulate the degradation of chondrocytes' extracellular matrix and promote the formation of new collagen by osteoarthritic chondrocytes [92]. This prepared system meets all the requirements for application in bone pathologies therapy [92].

The feasibility of forming solid molecular dispersions of poorly water soluble drugs in cross-linked poly(2-hydroethyl methacrylate) (PHEMA) hydrogels has been reported in Refs. [93, 94]. This team investigated the extent of enhancement of the kinetic solubility of amorphous solid dispersions of indomethacin within cross-linked PHEMA hydrogels as compared with those based on conventional water-soluble polymer carriers [94]. The controlled release of indomethacin was achieved.

3.4 Other Applications of Hydrogels

In Ref. [95], several ciprofloxacin (CFX) imprinted and nonimprinted hydrogels were prepared and evaluated as ocular drug delivery systems in aqueous media. 2-HEMA was used as a solvent and backbone monomer, EGDMA as a cross-linker, MAA as a functional monomer, and CFX as the template molecule. In vitro antibacterial activity of hydrogels was studied and demonstrated the effect of CFX-loaded hydrogels against *Pseudomonas aeruginosa* (and *Staphylococcus aureus* isolated from patients' eyes [95]. This study indicated the antibacterial efficacy of CFX-loaded hydrogels [95].

An ocular drug delivery system for topotecan (TPT) loaded in biocompatible hydrogels of PCL-PEG-PCL block copolymers for sustained TPT release in the vitreous tumor was developed for the treatment of retinoblastoma, the most common primary ocular malignancy in children [96]. Hydrogel cytotoxicity was studied in retinoblastoma cells as a surrogate for efficacy, and TPT vitreous pharmacokinetics and systemic as well as ocular toxicity were evaluated in rabbits [96]. The pseudoplastic behavior of the hydrogels makes them suitable for intraocular administration. In vitro release profiles showed a sustained release of TPT from PCL-PEG-PCL up to a week, and drug loading did not affect the release pattern [96]. According to these findings, the novel TPT hydrogels can deliver sustained concentrations of active drug into the vitreous with excellent biocompatibility in vivo and pronounced cytotoxic activity in retinoblastoma cells and thus may become an additional strategy for intraocular retinoblastoma treatment [96].

Hybrid polyacrylamide/bacterial cellulose (PAM/BC) nanofiber cluster hydrogels with high strength, toughness, and recoverability were synthesized by in situ polymerization of acrylamide monomer in a BC nanofiber cluster suspension as biomaterials for bone and cartilage repair materials [97].

Hydrogels for dual drug release were designed and developed by Murata et al. [98]. The hydrogels covalently contained the polymeric micelles that exhibited different drug release properties. The hydrogels that were formed from polymeric micelles possessing a tightly packed (i.e., well entangled) inner core exhibited a higher storage modulus than the hydrogels that were formed from the polymeric micelles possessing a loosely packed structure. The release of two different bioactive molecules was examined with very nice results [98].

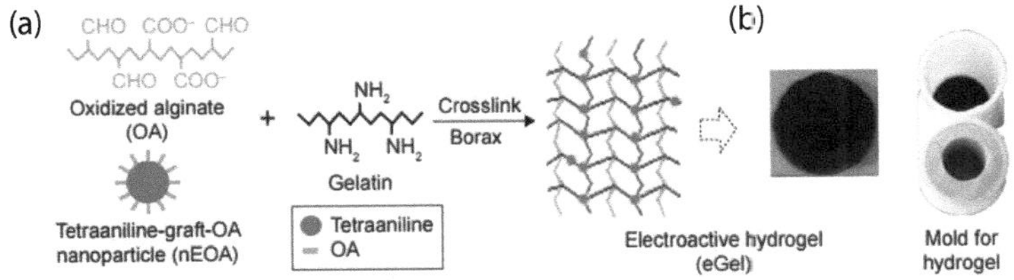

Figure 3.2 Preparation of electroactive hydrogels. Notes: (a) Scheme for preparation of electroactive hydrogels from OA/nEOA cross-linking gelatin (eGel) and (b) the real hydrogel of eGel photographed with a digital camera and the homemade mold for hydrogel preparation [99].

Furthermore, injectable electroactive hydrogels are promising in regenerative medicine and drug delivery. Figure 3.2 represents the preparation of electroactive hydrogels. The synthesis and characterization of an injectable hydrogel based on oxidized alginate (OA) cross-linking gelatin (nEOAs), reinforced by electroactive tetra-aniline-graft-OA nanoparticles, where nEOAs are expected to impart electroactivity besides reinforcement without significantly degrading the other properties of hydrogels, was reported in Ref. [99]. With considerable injectability, uniformity, degradability, electroactivity, relative robustness, and biocompatibility, these injectable electroactive hydrogels may have a huge potential as scaffolds for tissue regeneration and matrix for stimuli-responsive drug release [99].

3.4.1 Magnetic Hydrogels as Drug Delivery Systems

Magnetic hydrogels are fabricated using synthetic or natural polymers that encapsulate magnetic nanoparticles (MNPs) within the polymeric matrix. Under the influence of an external magnetic stimulus as an alternating magnetic field, MNPs produce heat and they can be used in cancer treatment (hyperthermia) or as contrast agents in magnetic resonance imaging. The most common MNPs encapsulated in polymeric networks are Fe_3O_4 (magnetite), γ-Fe_2O_3 (maghemite), FePt (iron platinum), CoFe (cobalt iron), and cobalt ferrite ($CoFe_2O_4$). Furthermore, a combination of MNPs with thermosensitive polymers such as PNIPAAm leads to the formation of thermoresponsive magnetic hydrogels with applications in drug delivery, biomedical imaging, cancer cell hyperthermia treatment, and tissue engineering [100, 101].

The addition of drugs in magnetic hydrogels can lead to a controlled release behavior under the variation of the magnetic field. The release of diclofenac sodium from kappa-carrageenan/PVA, and magnetite magnetic hydrogels showed that drug release is affected by the magnetic stimuli, hydrogel composition, and the pH of the release medium [102]. Paulino et al. studied the remote release of curcumin from natural polysaccharide–based hydrogels containing magnetite nanoparticles [103]. BSA was incorporated in hemicellulose-based magnetic hydrogels and showed excellent adsorption and controlled release profiles [104]. Finally, more intelligent magnetic hydrogels are based on pulse application of atomic force microscopy (AMF) on magnetic hydrogels, which triggers on-demand pulsatile drug release [105, 106].

3.5 Limitations for Hydrogel Administration

Extensive literature claims that hydrogels are ideal vectors for drug, vaccine, peptide, and protein delivery for two important reasons: their 3D structure allows for topological control of the solute transport and their ability to be modified by the desirable hydrophilic/hydrophobic balance allows for better control and delay or acceleration of drug transport [107–112]. Hydrogels are used for the administration of therapeutic compounds via several routes of administration (transdermal, oral, ocular, etc.), but there are some limitations for their administration. In Fig. 3.3 the complex physiology of the gastrointestinal tract is presented This complexity poses challenges for oral delivery but can be exploited to achieve controlled drug release. According to Lee et al. [113]:

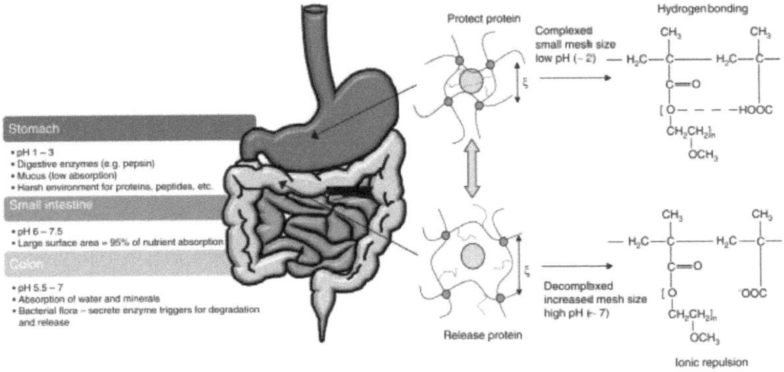

Figure 3.3 The complex physiology of the gastrointestinal tract poses challenges for oral delivery but can be exploited to achieve controlled drug release. Complexation hydrogels can deliver a therapeutic through the harsh environment of the stomach, protecting it from denaturation by acidic pH or digestive enzymes. The drug is released in the upper small intestine, which has a lower population of enzymes, neutral pH, and a large surface area accounting for 95% of nutrient absorption, due to decomplexation and an increase in mesh size triggered by ionic repulsion and swelling of the polymer at high pH. The colon is another commonly targeted site due to neutral pH and lower enzymatic activity [103].

> Hydrogels are particularly important as carriers for oral delivery because they can be rendered anionic, cationic or amphiphilic by appropriate copolymerization processes with ionic components. Although this incorporation of ionic moieties leads to environmentally sensitive structures, and therefore often intelligent systems, there are numerous unanswered questions concerning the hydrogels' use as oral delivery vehicles. Below, we summarize a number of important

problems that need to be addressed and solved in the next few years of drug delivery research.

- Although design of hydrogel carriers is based on a three-component thermodynamic behavior (hydrogel/drug/water), design equations must incorporate the importance of other components in the studied systems, such as electrolytes.
- Intelligent systems are often designed without consideration of possible interaction of the solute (drug/protein) with other secondary components such as electrolytes, etc.
- Phenomena of segregation or agglomeration of hydrogel particles are not taken into consideration, when studying drug delivery.
- Significant changes in local osmotic effects due to associated changes in salt concentration and ionic strength variations are rarely taken into consideration during design.
- Other well-known gel-related phenomena are not taken into consideration, such as Donnan equilibrium, electroneutrality of charges, and the like.
- Our knowledge of the mechanisms of drug/protein/peptide transport across an underlying mucosal or cellular structure after initial drug release is still not well understood for a large number of large molecular weight solutes. For these reasons, future research on the development and understanding of solute transport through hydrogels under 'real' conditions must be further understood. Still, the previous analysis has shown that the so-called environmentally sensitive or intelligent hydrogels are very useful in a large number of applications and will continue to be important, especially for protein delivery.

3.6 Conclusions and Future Perspectives

Most studies on hydrogels show that there are a significant number of parameters that can be tuned in order to control the thermodynamics, morphology, stability, and properties of these drug delivery systems. Several examples already highlight interesting properties of hydrogels, which increase the demand for the design and development of multifunctional vector systems to improve targeted drug delivery, tumor targeting, and imaging or to enhance cellular interactions and internalization. Figure 3.4 illustrates the current approaches in hydrogel research and its application in developing clinical products in comparison with the suggested future efforts on hydrogel research. Hydrogels are drawing increased attention as a novel platform that combines the best properties of polymeric materials, with promising applications as controlled release and stimuli-responsive drug delivery systems that overcome the existing limitations of other vectors. For instance, the stability, drug loading and release, and permeability of mixed systems are important aspects for drug-delivery applications that have shown to be individually adjustable for hydrogel systems in terms of several parameters, such as the molar composition, the molar mass, and the preparation protocol. Hydrogel platforms can be considered as new therapeutic platforms in pharmaceutical technology that may be able to deliver active pharmaceutical ingredients to specific tissues. Additionally, they can improve the pharmacokinetics/pharmacodynamics of drugs and affect their total bioavailability, due to their physicochemical and mechanical properties, which depend on the chemical nature of the components utilized. Next generations of drug delivery systems will incorporate "smart" biosensing and stimuli-responsive functionalities that will enable unaided in vivo feedback control. Furthermore, a state-of-the-art technology for the fabrication of smart hydrogels is 3D printing. Encapsulation of drugs or cells in 3D-printed smart hydrogels is an emerging technology with potential applications in tissue engineering [114, 115].

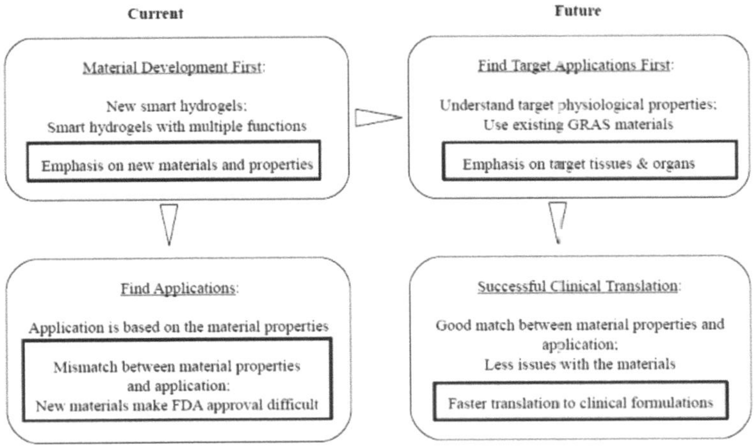

Figure 3.4 The current approaches in hydrogel research and its application in developing clinical products in comparison with the suggested future efforts on hydrogel research [106].

References

1. Koutsopoulos, S. (2012). Molecular fabrications of smart nanobiomaterials and applications in personalized medicine, *Adv. Drug Deliv. Rev.*, **64**, pp. 1459–1476.
2. Venugapal, J., Prabhakaran, M. P., Low, S., Choon, A. T., Zhang, Y. Z., Deepika, G. and Ramakrishna, S. (2008). Nanotechnology for nanomedicine and delivery of drugs, *Curr. Pharm. Des.*, **14**, pp. 2184–2200.
3. Peppas, N. A. (2004). Intelligent therapeutics: biomimetic systems and nanotechnology in drug delivery, *Adv. Drug Deliv. Rev.*, **56**, pp. 1529–1531.
4. Takai, O. (2006). Biomimetic nanotechnology, *Ann. N.Y. Acad. Sci.*, **1093**, pp. 84–97.
5. Hilt, J. Z. (2004). Nanotechnology and biomimetic methods in therapeutics: molecular scale control with some help from nature, *Adv. Drug Deliv. Rev.*, **56**, pp. 1533–1536.
6. Caruthers, S. D., Wickline, S. A. and Lanza, G. M. (2007). Nanotechnological applications in medicine, *Curr. Opin. Biotechnol.*, **18**, pp. 26–30.
7. Grzybowski, B. A. and Huck, W. T. (2016). The nanotechnology of life-inspired systems, *Nat. Nanotechnol.*, **11**, pp. 585–592.
8. Nayak, S. and Lyon, L. A. (2005). Soft nanotechnology with soft nanoparticles. *Angew. Chem. Int. Ed. Engl.*, **44**, pp. 7686–7708.
9. Demetzos, C. and Pippa, N. (2014). Advanced drug delivery nanosystems (aDDnSs): a mini-review, *Drug Deliv.*, **21**, pp. 250–257.
10. Pippa, N., Pispas, S. and Demetzos, C. (2016). Polymer self-assembled nanostructures as innovative drug nanocarrier platforms, *Curr. Pharm. Des.*, **22**, pp. 2788–2795.
11. Kopecek, J. (2007). Hydrogel biomaterials: a smart future?, *Biomaterials*, **28**, pp. 5185–5182.
12. Kopeček, J. and Yang, J. (2012). Smart self-assembled hybrid hydrogel biomaterials, *Angew. Chem. Int. Ed. Engl.*, **51**, pp. 7396–7417.
13. Drury, J. L. and Mooney, D. J. (2003). Hydrogels for tissue engineering: scaffold design variables and applications, *Biomaterials*, **24**, pp. 4337–4351.
14. Jiang, Y., Chen, J., Deng, C., Suuronen, E. J. and Zhong, Z. (2014). Click hydrogels, microgels and nanogels: emerging platforms for drug delivery and tissue engineering, *Biomaterials*, **35**, pp. 4969–4985.

15. Peppas, N. A., Bures, P., Leobandung, W. and Ichikawa, H. (2000). Hydrogels in pharmaceutical formulations, *Eur. J. Pharm. Biopharm.*, **50**, pp. 27–46.

16. Patel, G. C. and Dalwadi, C. A. (2013). Recent patents on stimuli responsive hydrogel drug delivery system, *Recent Pat. Deliv. Formul.*, **7**, pp. 206–215.

17. Gupta, P., Vermani, K. and Garg, S. (2002). Hydrogels: from controlled release to pH-responsive drug delivery, *Drug Discov Today*, **7**, pp. 569–579.

18. Dalwadi, C. and Patel, G. (2015). Application of nanohydrogels in drug delivery systems: recent patents review, *Recent Pat. Nanotechnol.*, **9**, pp. 17–25.

19. Sood, N., Bhardwaj, A., Mehta, S. and Mehta, A. (2016). Stimuli-responsive hydrogels in drug delivery and tissue engineering, *Drug Deliv.*, **23**, pp. 758–780.

20. Soppimath, K. S., Aminabhavi, T. M., Dave, A. M., Kumbar, S. G. and Rudzinski, W. E. (2002). Stimulus-responsive "smart" hydrogels as novel drug delivery systems, *Drug Dev. Ind. Pharm.*, **28**, pp. 957–974.

21. Prabajaran, M. and Mano, J. F. (2006). Stimuli-responsive hydrogels based on polysaccharides incorporated with thermo-responsive polymers as novel biomaterials, *Macromol. Biosci.*, **6**, pp. 991–1008.

22. He, C., Kim, S. W. and Lee, D. S. (2008). In situ gelling stimuli-sensitive block copolymer hydrogels for drug delivery, *J. Control. Release*, **127**, pp. 189–207.

23. Kamata, H., Li, X., Chung, U. I. and Sakai, T. (2015). Design of hydrogels for biomedical applications, *Adv. Healthcare Mater.*, **4**, pp. 2360–2374.

24. Patenaude, M., Smeets, N. M. and Hoare, T. (2014). Designing injectable, covalently cross-linked hydrogels for biomedical applications, *Macromol. Rapid. Commun.*, **35**, pp. 598–617.

25. Van Tomme, S. R., Storm, G. and Hennink, W. E. (2008). In situ gelling hydrogels for pharmaceutical and biomedical applications, *Int. J. Pharm.*, **355**, pp. 1–18.

26. Hennink, W. E. and van Nostrum, C. F. (2002). Novel crosslinking methods to design hydrogels, *Adv. Drug Deliv. Rev.*, **54**, pp. 13–36.

27. Berger, J., Reist, M., Mayer, J. M., Felt, O., Peppas, N. A. and Gurny, R. (2004). Structure and interactions in covalently and ionicallycrosslinked chitosan hydrogels for biomedical applications, *Eur. J. Pharm. Biopharm.*, **57**, pp. 19–34.

28. Schoenmakers, R. G., van de Wetering, P., Elbert, D. L. and Hubbell, J. A. (2004). The effect of the linker on the hydrolysis rate of drug-linked ester bonds, *J. Control. Release.*, **95**, pp. 291–300.

29. Watanabe, J., Ooya, T., Park, K. D., Kim, Y. H. and Yui, N. (2000). Preparation and characterization of poly(ethylene glycol) hydrogels cross-linked by hydrolysable polyrotaxane, *J. Biomater. Sci. Polym. Ed.*, **11**, pp. 1333–1345.

30. Ichi, T., Watanabe J., Ooya, T. and Yui, N. (2001). Controllable erosion time and profile in poly(ethylene glycol) hydrogels by supramolecular structure of hydrolysable poltrotaxane, *Biomacromolecules*, **2**, pp. 204–210.

31. Missirlis, D., Tirelli, N. and Hubbell, J. A. (2005). Amphiphilic hydrogel nanoparticles. Preparation, characterization, and preliminary assessment as new colloidal drug carriers, *Langmuir*, **21**, pp. 2605–2613.

32. Liu, F. and Huang, L. (2002). Development of non-viral vectors for systemic gene delivery, *J. Control. Release*, **78**, pp. 259–266.

33. Vinogradov, S. V. and Kabanov, A. V. (2004). Synthesis of nanogels carriers for delivery of active phosphorylated nucleoside analogues, *Polym. Prepr.*, **228**, p. 298.

34. Vinogradov, S. V., Kohli, E. and Zeman, A. D. (2005). Cross-linked polymeric nanogels formulations of 5'-triphosphates of nucleoside analogues: role of the cellular membrane in drug release, *Mol. Pharmaceutics*, **2**, pp. 449–461.

35. Vinogradov, S. V., Zeman, A. D., Batrakova, E. K. and Kabanov, A. V. (2005). Polyplexnanogels formulations for drug delivery of cytotoxic nucleoside analogs, *J. Control. Release*, **107**, pp. 143–157.

36. Vinogradov, S. V., Kohli, E. and Zeman, A. D. (2006). Comparison of nanogels drug carriers and their formulations with nucleoside 5'-triphosphates, *Pharm. Res.*, **23**, pp. 920–930.

37. Vinogradov, S. V., Batrakova, E. K. and Kabanov, A. V. (2004). Nanogels for oligonucleotide delivery to the brain, *Bioconjugate Chem.*, **15**, pp. 50–60.

38. Yang, T., Ji, R., Deng, X. X., Du, F. S. and Li, Z. C. (2014). Glucose-responsive hydrogels based on dynamic covalent chemistry and inclusion complexation, *Soft Matter*, **10**, pp. 2671–2678.

39. Dong, Y., Wang, W., Veiseh, O., Appel, E. A., Xue, K., Webber, M. J., Tanh, B. C., Yang, X. W., Weir, W., Langer, R. and Anderson, D. G. (2016). Injectable and glucose-responsive hydrogels based on boronic acid-glucose complexation, *Langmuir*, **32**, pp. 8743–8747.

40. Lowman, A. M., Morishita, M., Kajita, M., Magai, T. and Peppas, N. A. (1999). Oral delivery of insulin using pH-responsive complexation gels, *J. Pharm. Sci.*, **88**, pp. 933–937.

41. Babu, V. R., Patel, P., Mundargi, R. C., Rangaswamy, V. and Aminabhavi, T. M. (2008). Developments in polymeric devices for oral insulin delivery, *Expert Opin. Drug Deliv.*, **5**, pp. 403–415.

42. Foss, A. C., Goto, T., Morishita, M. and Peppas, N. A. (2004). Development of acrylic-based copolymers for oral insulin delivery, *Eur. J. Pharm. Biopharm.*, **57**, pp. 163–169.

43. Foss, A. C. and Peppas, N. A. (2004). Investigation of cytotoxity and insulin transport of acrylic-based copolymer protein delivery systems in contact with Caco-2 cultures, *Eur. J. Pharm. Biopharm.*, **57**, pp. 447–455.

44. Ichikawa, H. and Peppas, N. A. (2003). Novel complexation hydrogels for oral peptide delivery: in vitro evaluation of their cytocompatibility and insulin-transport enhancing effects using Caco-2 cell manolayers, *J. Biomed. Mater. Res. Part A*, **67**, pp. 609–617.

45. Wood, K. M., Stone, G. M. and Peppas, N. A. (2008). Wheat germ agglutinin functionalized complexation hydrogels for oral insulin delivery, *Biomacromolecules*, **9**, pp. 1293–1298.

46. Wood, K. M., Stone, G. M. and Peppas, N. A. (2010). The effect of complexation hydrogels on insulin transport in intestinal epithelial cell models. *Acta Biomater.*, **6**, pp. 48–58.

47. Morishita, M., Goto, T., Peppas, N. A., Joseph, J. I., Toriman, M. C., Nakmura, K., Yamagata, K. and Lowman, A. M. (2004). Mucosal insulin delivery systems based on complexation polymer hydrogels: effect of particle size on insulin enteral absorption, *J. Control. Release*, **97**, pp. 115–124.

48. Kumar, A., Lahiri, S. S. and Singh, H. (2006). Development of PEGDMA:MAA based hydrogel microparticles for oral insulin delivery, *Int. J. Pharm.*, **323**, pp. 117–124.

49. Cong, C., Qi, T., Wei, X., Qu, Y., Wu, Q., Luo, F. and Qian, Z. (2013). Thermosensitive polymeric hydrogels as drug delivery systems, *Curr. Med. Chem.*, **20**, pp. 79–94.

50. Jeong, B., Kim, S. W. and Bae, Y. H. (2002). Thermosensitive sol-gel reversible hydrogels, *Adv. Drug Deliv. Rev.*, **54**, pp. 37–51.

51. Ruel-Gariépy, E. and Leroux, J. C. (2004). In situ-forming hydrogels: review of temperature-sensitive systems, *Eur. J. Pharm. Biopharm.*, **58**, pp. 409–426.

52. Alexander, A., Ajazuddin, K., Khan, J., Saraf, S. and Saraf, S. (2014). Polyethylene glycol(PEG)-Poly(N-isopropylacrylamide) (PNIPAAm) based thermosensitive injectable hydrogels for biomedical applications, *Eur. J. Pharm. Biopharm.*, **88**, pp. 575–585.

53. Tan, H., Ramirez, C. M., Miljkovic, N., Li, H., Rubin, J. P. and Marra, K. G. (2009). Thermosensitive injectable hyaluronic acid hydrogel for adipose tissue engineering, *Biomaterials*, **30**, pp. 6844–6853.

54. Sá-Lima, H., Tuzlakoglu, K., Mano, J. F. and Reis, R. L. (2011). Thermoresponsivepoly(N-isopropylacrylaminde)-g-methylcellulose hydrogel as a three-dimensional extracellular matrix for cartilage-engineered applications, *J. Biomed. Mater. Res. Part A*, **98**, pp. 596–603.

55. Moreno, E., Schwartz, J., Larrañeta, E., Nquewa, P. A., Sanmartín, C., Agüeros, M., Irache, J. M. and Espuelas, S. (2014). Thermosensitive hydrogels of poly(methyl vinyl ether-co- maleic anhydride) -Pluronic (®) F127 copolymers for controlled protein release, *Int. J. Pharm.*, **459**, pp. 1–9.

56. Chung, H. J, Lee, Y. and Park, T. G. (2008). Thermo-sensitive and biodegradable hydrogels based on stereocomplexedPluronic multi-block copolymers for controlled protein delivery, *J. Control. Release*, **127**, pp. 22–30.

57. Park, S. Y., Chung, H. J., Lee, Y. and Park, T. G. (2008). Injectable and sustained delivery of human growth hormone using chemically modified Pluronic copolymet hydrogels, *Biotechnol. J.*, **3**, pp. 669–675.

58. Qi, X., Qin, X., Yang, R., Qin, J., Li, W., Luan, K., Wu, Z. and Song, L. (2016). Intra-articular administration of chitosan thermosensitive in situ hydrogels combined with diclofenac sodium-loaded alginate microspheres, *J. Pharm. Sci.*, **105**, pp. 122–130.

59. Lin, G., Comsimbescu, L., Karrin, N. J. and Tarasevicj, B. J. (2012). Injectabe and thermosensitibe PLGA-g-PEG hydrogels, containing hydroxyapatite: preparation, characterization and in vitro release behavior, *Biomed. Mater.*, **7**, p. 024107.

60. Peng, Y., Li, J., Li, J., Fei, Y., Dong, J. and Pan, W. (2013). Optimization of thermosensitive chitosan hydrogels for the sustained delivery of venlafaxine hydrochloride, *Int. J. Pharm.*, **441**, pp. 482–490.

61. Peng, Q., Sun, X., Gong, T., Wu, C. Y., Zhang, T., Tan, J. and Zhang, Z. R. (2013). Injectable and biodegradable thermosensitive hydrogels loaded with PHBHHx nanoparticles for the sustained and controlled release of insulin, *Acta Biomater.*, **9**, pp. 5063–5069.

62. Cuggino, J. C., Contreras, C. B., Jimerez-Kairuz, A., Maletto, B. A. and Alvarez-Igarzabal, C. I. (2014). Novel poly(NIPA-co-AAc) functional hydrogels with potential application in drug controlled release, *Mol. Pharmaceutics*, **11**, pp. 2239–2249.

63. Moghadam, M. N., Kolesov, V., Vogel, A., Klok, H. A. and Pioletti, D. P. (2014). Controlled release from a mechanically-stimulated thermosensitive self-heating composite hydrogel, *Biomaterials*, **35**, pp. 450–455.

64. Kang, G. D., Cheon, S. H. and Song, S. C. (2006). Controlled release of doxorubicin from thermosensitivepoly(organophosphazene) hydrogels, *Int. J. Pharm.*, **319**, pp. 29–36.

65. Al-abd, A. M., Hong, K. Y., Song, S. C. and Kuh, H. J. (2010). Pharmacokinetics of doxorubicin after intratumoral injection using a thermosensitive hydrogel in tumor-bearing mice, *J. Control. Release*, **142**, pp. 101–107.

66. Li, C., Ren, S., Dai, Y., Tian, F., Wang, X., Zhou, S., Deng, S., Liu, Q., Zhao, J. and Chen, X. (2014). Efficacy, pharmacokinetics, and biodistribution of thermosensitive chitosan/β-glycerophosphate hydrogel loaded with docetaxel, *AAPS Pharm. Sci. Tech.*, **15**, pp. 417–422.

67. Ren, S., Dai, Y., Li, C., Qiu, Z., Wang, X., Tian, F., Zhou, S., Liu, Q., Xing, H., Lu, Y., Chen, X. and Li, N. (2016). Pharmacokonetics and pharmacodynamics evaluation of a thermosensitive chitosan based hydrogel containing liposomal doxorubicin, *Eur. J. Pharm. Sci.*, **92**, pp. 137–145.

68. Wang, W., Zhang, P., Shan, W., Gao, J. and Liang, W. (2013). A novel chitosan-based thermosensitive hydrogel containing doxorubicin liposomes for topical cancer therapy, *J. Biomater. Sci. Polym. Ed.*, **24**, pp. 1649–1659.

69. Bhattarai, N., Gunn, J. and Zhang, M. (2010). Chitosan-based hydrogels for controlled, localized drug delivery, *Adv. Drug Deliv. Rev.*, **62**, pp. 83–99.

70. Gong, C. Y., Shi, S., Dong, P. W., Zheng, X. L., Fu, S. Z , Guo, G., Yang, J. L., Wei, Y. Q. and Qian, Z. Y. (2009). In vitro drug release behavior from a novel thermosensitive composite hydrogel based on Pluronic F127 and poly(ethylene glycol)-poly(epsilon-caprolactone)-poly(ethylene glycol) copolymer, *BMC Biotechnol.*, **9**, p. 8.

71. Gong, C. Y., Dong, P. W., Shi, S., Fu, S. Z., Yang, J. L., Guo, G., Zhao, X., Wei, Y. Q. and Qian, Z. Y. (2009). Thermosensitive PEG-PCL-PEG hydrogel controlled drug delivery system: sol-gel-sol transition and in vitro drug release study, *J. Pharm. Sci.*, **98**, pp. 3707–3717.

72. Fabiano, A., Bizzarri, R. and Zambito, Y. (2017). Thermosensitive hydrogel based on chitosan andits derivatives containing medicated nanoparticles for transcoorneal administration of 5-fluorouracil, *Int. J. Nanomed.*, **12**, pp. 633–643.

73. Cheng, Y. H., Hung, K. H., Tsai, T. H., Lee, C. J., Ku, R. Y., Chiu, A. W., Chiou, S. H. and Liu, C. J. (2014). Sustained delivery of layanoprost by thermosensitive chitosan-gelatin-based hydrogel for controlling ocular hypertension, *Acta Biomater.*, **10**, pp. 4360–4366.

74. Khodaverdi, E., Tekie, F. S., Mohajeri, S. A., Ganji, F., Zohuri, G. and Hadizadeh, F. (2012). Preparation and investigation of sustained drug delivery systems using and injectable, thermosensitive, in situ forming hydrogel composed of PGLA-PEG-PLGA, *AAPS Pharm. Sci. Tech.*, **13**, pp. 590–600.

75. Constantin, M., Bucatariu, S. M., Doroftei, F. and Fundueanu, G. (2017). Smart composite materials based on chitosan microspheres embedded in thermosensitive hydrogel for controlled delivery of drugs, *Carbohydr. Polym.*, **157**, pp. 493–502.

76. Supper, S., Anton, N., Seidel, N., Riemenschnitter, M., Curdy, C. and Vandamme, T. (2013). Thermosensitive chitosan/glycerosphosphate-based hydrogel and its derivatives in pharmaceutical and biomedical applications, *Expert Opin. Drug Deliv.*, **11**, pp. 249–267.

77. Tahrir, F. G., Ganji, F. and Ahooyi, T. M. (2015). Injectable thermosensitive chitosan/ glycerophosphate-based hydrogels for tissue engineering and drug delivery applications: a review, *Recent Pat. Drug Deliv. Formul.*, **9**, pp. 107–120.

78. Zhang, Z. X., Wu, D. Q. and Chu, C. C. (2004). Synthesis, characterization and controlled drug release of thermosensitive IPN-PNIPAAm hydrogels, *Biomaterials*, **25**, pp. 3793–3805.

79. Gil, E. S. and Hudson, S. M. (2007). Effect of silk fibroin interpenetrating networks on swelling/deswelling kinetics and rheological propertied of poly(N-isopropylacrylamine) hydrogels, *Biomacromolecules*, **8**, pp. 258–264.

80. Kabanov, A. V. and Vinogradov, S. V. (2009). Nanogels as pharmaceutical carriers: finite networks of infinite capabilities, *Angew. Chem. Int. Ed. Engl.*, **48**, pp. 5418–5429.

81. Chacko, R. T., Ventura, J., Zhuang, J. and Thayumanavan, S. (2012). Polymer nanogels: a versatile nanoscopic drug delivery platform, *Adv. Drug Deliv. Rev.*, **64**, pp. 836–851.

82. Zhang, H., Zhai, Y., Wang, J. and Zhai, G. (2016). New progress and prospects: the application of nanogels in drug delivery, *Mater. Sci. Eng. C*, **60**, pp. 560–568.

83. Li, L., Ryu, J. H. and Thayumanavan, S. (2013). Effect of Hofmeister ions on the size and the encapsulation stability of polymer nanogels, *Langmuir*, **29**, pp. 50–55.

84. Zalfen, A. M., Nizet, D., Jérôme, C., Jérôme, R., Frankenne, F., Foidart, J. M, Maguet, V., Lecomte, F., Hubert, P. and Evrard, B. (2008). Controlled release of drugs from multi-component biomaterials, *Acta Biomater.*, **4**, pp. 1788–1796.

85. Arica, M. Y., Bayramoglu, G., Arica, B., Yalcin, E., Ito, K. and Yagci, Y. (2005). Novel hydrogel membrane based on copoly(hydroxyelthyl methacrylate/p-vinylbenzyl-poly(ethylene oxide)) for biomedical applications: propertied and drug release characteristics, *Macromol. Biosci.*, **5**, pp. 983–992.

86. He, H., Cao, X. and Lee, L. J. (2004). Design of a novel hydrogel-based intelligent system for controlled drug release, *J. Control. Release*, **95**, pp. 391–402.

87. Paspasrakis, G. and Bouropoulos, N. (2006). Swelling studies and in vitro release of verapamil from calcium alginate and calcium alginate-chitosan beads, *Int. J. Pharm.*, **323**, pp. 34–42.

88. Nochos, A., Douroumis, D. and Bouropoulos, N. (2008). In vitro release of bovine serum albumin from alginate/HPMC hydrogel beads, *Carbohydr. Polym.*, **74**, pp. 451–457.

89. Velasco, D., Danoux, Ch. B., Redondo, J. A., Elvira, C., San Román, J., Wray, P. S. and Kazarian, S. G. (2011). pH-sensitive polymer hydrogels derived from morpholine to prevent the crystallization of ibuprofen, *J. Control. Release*, **149**, pp. 140–145.

90. Jabeen, S., Maswal, M., Chat, O. A., Rather, G. M. and Dar, A. A. (2016). Rheological behavior and ibuprofen delivery applications of pH responsive composite alginate hydrogels, *Colloids Surf. B*, **139**, pp. 211–218.

91. Jabeen, S., Chat, O. A., Maswal, M., Ashraf, U., Rather, G. M. and Dar, A. A. (2015). Hydrogels of sodium alginate in cationic surfactants: surfactant dependent modulation of encapsulation/release toward ibuprofen, *Carbohydr. Polym.*, **133**, pp. 144–153.

92. Díaz-Rodríguez, P. and Landin, M. (2015). Controlled release of indomethacin from alginate-poloxamer-silicon carbide composites decrease in-vitro inflammation, *Int. J. Pharm.*, **480**, pp. 92–100.

93. Zahedi, P. and Leem, P. I. (2007). Solid molecular dispersions of poorly water-soluble drugs in poly(2-hydroxyethyl methacrylate) hydrogels, *Eur. J. Pharm. Biopharm.*, **65**, pp. 320–328.

94. Sun, D. D., Ju, T. C. and Lee, P. I. (2012). Enhanced kinetic solubility profiles of indomethacin amorphous solid dispersions in poly(2-hydroxyethyl methacrylate hydrogels, *Eur. J. Pharm. Biopharm.*, **81**, pp. 149–158.

95. Kiomars, S., Heidari S., Malaekeh-Nikouei, B., Shayani Rad, M., Khameneh, B. and Mohajeri, S. A. (2017). Ciprofloxacin-improted hydrogels for drug sustained release in aqueous media, *Pharm. Dev. Technol.*, **22**, pp. 122–129.

96. Taich, P., Moretton, M. A., Del Sole, M. J., Winter, U., Bernabeu, E., Croxatto, J. O., Oppezzo, J., Williams, G., Chantada, G. L., Chiappetta, D. A. and Schaiquevich, P. (2016). Sustained-release hydrogels of topotecan for retinoblastoma, *Colloids Surf. B*, **146**, pp. 624–631.

97. Yuan, N., Xu, L., Zhang, L., Ye, H., Zhao, J., Liu, Z. and Rong, J. (2016). Superior hybrid hydrogels of poltacrylamide enhanced by bacterial cellulose nanofiber clusters, *Mater. Sci. Eng. C*, **67**, pp. 221–230.

98. Murata, M., Uchida, Y., Takami, T., Ito, T., Anzai, R., Sonotaki, S. and Murakami, Y. (2017). Dual drug release from hydrogels covalently containing polymeric micelles that possess different drug release properties, *Colloids Surf. B*, **153**, pp. 19–26.

99. Wang, Q., Wang, Q. and Teng, W. (2016). Injectrable, degradable, electroactivenanocomposite hydrogels containing conductive polymer nanoparticles for biomedical applications, *Int. J. Nanomed.*, **11**, pp. 11–144.

100. Jalili, N. A., Muscarello, M. and Gaharwar, A. K. (2016). Nanoengineered thermoresponsive magnetic hydrogels for biomedical applications, *Bioeng. Transl. Med.*, **1**, pp. 297–305.

101. Giani, G., Fedi, S. and Barbucci, R. (2012). Hybrid magnetic hydrogel: a potential system for controlled drug delivery by means of alternating magnetic fields, *Polymers*, **4**, pp. 1157–1169.

102. Mahdavinia, G. R. and Etemadi, H. (2014). In situ synthesis of magnetic CaraPVA IPN nanocomposite hydrogels and controlled drug release, *Mater. Sci. Eng. C*, **45**, pp. 250–260.

103. Paulino, A. T., Pereira, A. G., Fajardo, A. R., Erickson, K., Kipper, M. J., Muniz, E. C., Belfiore, L. A. and Tambourgi, E. B. (2012). Natural polymer-based magnetic hydrogels: potential vectors for remote-controlled drug release, *Carbohydr. Polym.*, **90**, pp. 1216–1225.

104. Zhao, W., Odelius, K., Edlund, U., Zhao, C. and Albertsson, A. C. (2015). In situ synthesis of magnetic field-responsive hemicellulose hydrogels for drug delivery, *Biomacromolecules*, **16**, pp. 2522–2528.

105. Satarkar, N. S. and Hilt, J. Z. (2008). Magnetic hydrogel nanocomposites for remote controlled pulsatile drug release, *J. Control. Release*, **130**, pp. 246–251.

106. Campbell, S., Maitland, D. and Hoare, T. (2015). Enhanced pulsatile drug release from injectable magnetic hydrogels with embedded thermosensitive microgels, *ACS Macro Lett.*, **4**, pp. 312–316.

107. Saboktakin, M. R. and Tabatabaei, R. M. (2015). Supramolecular hydrogels as drug delivery systems, *Int. J. Biol. Macromol.*, **75**, pp. 426–436.

108. Lee, S. G., Kim, S. R., Cho, H. I., Kang, M. H., Yeam, D. W., Lee, S. H. and Choi, Y. W. (2014). Hydrogel-based ultra-moisturizing cream formulation for skin hydration and enhanced dermal drug delivery, *Biol. Pharm. Bull.*, **37**, pp. 1674–1682.

109. Ashley, G. W., Henise, J., Reid, R. and Santi, D. V. (2013). Hydrogel drug delivery system with predictable and tunable drug release and degradation rates, *Proc. Natl. Acad. Sci. U.S.A.*, **110**, pp. 2318–2323.

110. Sharpe, L. A., Daily, A. M., Horava, S. D. and Peppas, N. A. (2014). Therapeutic applications of hydrogels in oral drug delivery, *Expert Opin. Drug Deliv.*, **11**, pp. 901–915.

111. Shi, Y., Wang, Z., Zahng, X., Xu, T., Ji, S., Ding, D., Yang, Z. and Wang, L. (2015). Multi-responsive supramolecular hydrogels for drug delivery, *Chem. Commun. (Camb)*, **51**, pp. 15265–15267.

112. Salatin, S., Barar, J., Barzegar-Jalali, M., Adibkia, K., Milani, M. A. and Jelvehgari, M. (2016). Hydrogel nanoparticles and nanocomposites for nasal drug/vaccine delivery, *Arch. Pharm. Res.*, **39**, pp. 1181–1192.

113. Lee, S. C., Kwon, I. K. and Park, K. (2013). Hydrogels for delivery of bioactive agents: a historical perspective, *Adv. Drug Deliv. Rev.*, **65**, pp. 17–20.

114. Wang, S., Lee, J. M. and Yeong, W. Y. (2015). Smart hydrogels for 3D bioprinting, *Int. J. Bioprint.*, **1**, pp. 3–14.

115. Ozbolat, I. T. (2017). *3D Bioprinting: Fundamentals, Principles and Applications*, Academic Press, London, pp. 1–11.

Chapter 4

Ocular Drug Delivery Nanosystems: Recent Developments and Future Challenges

Elena A. Mourelatou, Yiannis Sarigiannis, and Christos C. Petrou
Department of Life and Health Sciences, School of Sciences and Engineering, Pharmacy Program, University of Nicosia, 46 Makedonitissas Avenue, CY-2417, Nicosia, Cyprus
petrou.c@unic.ac.cy

Nanotechnology today offers a modern arsenal of well-defined nanostructured drug carriers that can be employed for targeted drug delivery to the eye, which constitutes one of the major challenges of current scientific research. Drug delivery in the anterior segment of the eye is hindered due to bioavailability issues, attributed to the various ocular barriers that result in early elimination, low permeability, and low corneal residence time. Regarding drug delivery to the posterior segment, poor patient compliance, short drug retention time, and side effects associated with invasive routes of administration limit the treatment effectiveness of sight-

Drug Delivery Nanosystems: From Bioinspiration and Biomimetics to Clinical Applications
Edited by Costas Demetzos, Stergios Pispas, and Natassa Pippa

ISBN 978-981-4774-92-5 (Hardcover), 978-0-429-49054-5 (eBook)
www.panstanford.com

threatening diseases, such as age-related macular degeneration (AMD), diabetic retinopathy (DR), glaucoma, and retinitis pigmentosa. In this chapter, the various nanotechnology formulation approaches to ocular drug delivery presented in the last few years are reviewed and their benefits, as well as limitations, are outlined.

4.1 Introduction

Ocular drug delivery, especially to the posterior segment of the eye, is one of the most challenging fields of drug delivery today. This is attributed to the ocular anatomy and the existence of several protective mechanisms and barriers that result in drug elimination and low bioavailability. Three different categories of ocular barriers exist: the static, dynamic, and metabolic barriers (enzymatic degradation). The cornea, the blood-aqueous barrier, and the blood-retinal barrier (BRB) belong to the static barriers; and the conjunctival and choroidal blood flow, the lymph flow, the tear turnover, and the nasolacrimal drainage belong to the dynamic barriers [1–3].

Regarding the treatment of anterior segment diseases (keratitis, conjunctivitis, dry eye syndrome [DES], etc.), topical administration is the most commonly used route (Fig. 4.1), where formulations such as solutions, suspensions, ointments, and hydrogels are applied [4]. Although this route is characterized by high patient compliance (no pain), low production cost, and easy formulation and production processes, it suffers from low bioavailability, with less than 5% of the administered dose being able to overcome the ocular barriers and reach the target site. This creates the need for repeated administration in order to achieve a therapeutic effect, which leads to poor patient compliance and side effects caused by systemic absorption of the administered drug [5, 6]. On the other hand, the treatment of posterior segment diseases (glaucoma, age-related macular degeneration [AMD], uveitis, diabetic retinopathy [DR], endophthalmitis, diabetic macular edema, etc.) requires more invasive approaches, such as intravitreal, subconjunctival, subtenon, and posterior juxtascleral routes (Fig. 4.1), with the most prevalent being intravitreal injection [5]. The latter, especially when repeated at regular intervals for maintaining the desired drug's concentration (e.g., for glaucoma treatment), is associated with significant patient discomfort and nonconformance, as well as sight-threatening complications, including a risk of infections, endophthalmitis, retinal tear or detachment, lens damage, and cataract [2, 7]. Reaching the posterior segment through systemic administration (oral and intravenous) is impractical, since the volume of the eye is extremely small compared to the whole body and the presence of blood retinal barriers limits its accessibility [3].

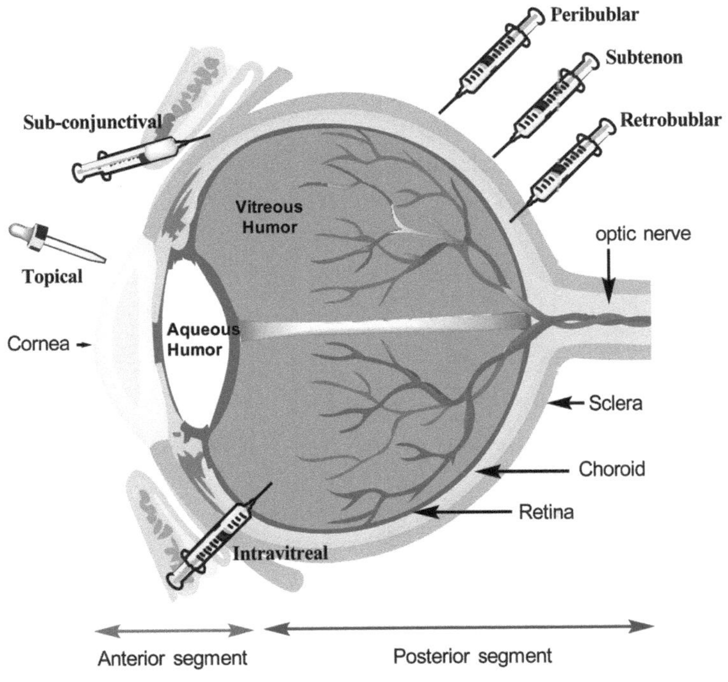

Figure 4.1 Ocular anatomy and different routes of ocular administration.

As a result, research in ocular drug delivery has focused on the development of novel noninvasive drug carriers that will be able to overcome the ocular barrier and result in increased drug bioavailability. Especially, targeting the posterior segment of the eye through noninvasive topical administration is in the forefront of ocular drug delivery research. An ideal ocular carrier should have the ability to target the disease site, control and/or sustain drug release, prolong the ocular residence time, and provide an administration frequency that will ensure patient conformance [8].

Therefore, carriers based on nanotechnology (liposomes, dendrimers, liquid crystals, polymeric nanoparticles [NPs], etc.) (Fig. 4.2) can contribute significantly to ocular drug delivery due to their ability to protect bioactive molecules from the ocular environment (enzymes in lacrimal fluids, proteins in tears, etc.), improve drug stability, reduce retinal toxicity caused by the administered drug, and provide controlled and sustained drug release. Moreover, they can enhance the drug's bioavailability by prolonging precorneal retention time and increasing transcorneal permeability, reduce the administration frequency and consequently improve patient adherence to therapy, and target the diseased tissues or cells via attachment of targeting molecules to their surface [9]. The scope of this chapter is to outline the recent advances of pharmaceutical nanotechnology in ocular drug delivery by reviewing all categories of nanosystems that have been formulated and studied for the enhancement of ocular drug bioavailability.

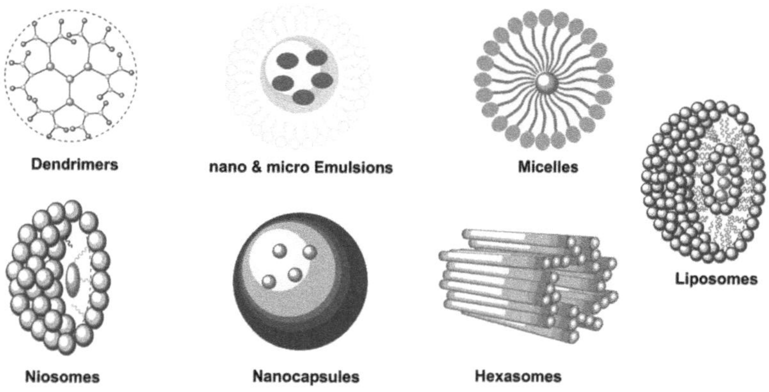

Figure 4.2 Nanocarriers used in ocular drug delivery.

4.2 Ocular Drug Delivery Nanosystems

4.2.1 Dendrimers

Dendrimers belong to a class of nanoarchitectures with wide biopharmaceutical applicability [10]. They were synthesized successfully for the first time in 1978 by Vögtle and coworkers [11], but Tomalia and coworkers [12] later on baptized them "dendrimers" from two Greek words, "dendros," meaning "tree" or "branch," and "meros," meaning "part." These monodisperse 3D polymeric structures, typically water soluble, display unique physicochemical properties due to their nanosize (3–20 nm) and their ability to have multiple functional surface groups, often seen in naturally occurring systems, that is, globular proteins. They are composed of a main core, interior layers of several moieties (generations), and a multifunctional terminal surface area incorporating groups such as $-NH_2$, $-COOH$, and $-OH$, most of them responsible for the electrostatic or covalent bonds with the drugs [13]. This structural pluralism lends peculiar properties enabling high drug payload by encapsulation in the interior cavities or electrostatic interactions or even formation of covalent bonds with the functional groups of the outer surface of the dendrimers.

Cationic molecules absorb drugs better than the uncharged and the anionic ones, while they display increased permeability due to their interaction with lipid bilayers. However, cationic dendrimers are more toxic, which renders the modification of the outer surface more than compulsory for reducing toxicity [14]. Two main methods are generally used for the preparation of dendrimers: a divergent method and a convergent one (Fig. 4.3). In the divergent method, the dendrimer grows outward using a main core molecule. On the opposite hand, in the convergent method, the dendrimer is built stepwise, starting from the terminal groups and progressing inward. When the branched polymeric arms (dendrons) have grown enough, they are attached to the main core molecule [15].

To date, over 100 structurally different dendrimer families have been synthesized. Various dendrimer structures have been used for the treatment of glaucoma, ocular hypertension, cataract incisions, mydriasis, conjunctivitis, intraocular infections, retinoblastoma, and retinal neuroinflammation [16]. Polyamidoamine (PAMAM) dendrimers, offering high aqueous solubility and lack of immunogenicity, are the most investigated family of dendrimers. In addition, modified PAMAM dendrimers with polyethylene glycol (PEG) moieties or other functional groups exhibit low cytotoxicity and increased biocompatibility [17]. Dendrimers have been useful in ocular drug delivery as they exhibit moderate antimicrobial activity, increase corneal residence time, enhance corneal transport, and promote adhesion and proliferation of human corneal epithelial cells. As a result, the uptake of drugs increases and the wound healing is expedited [18].

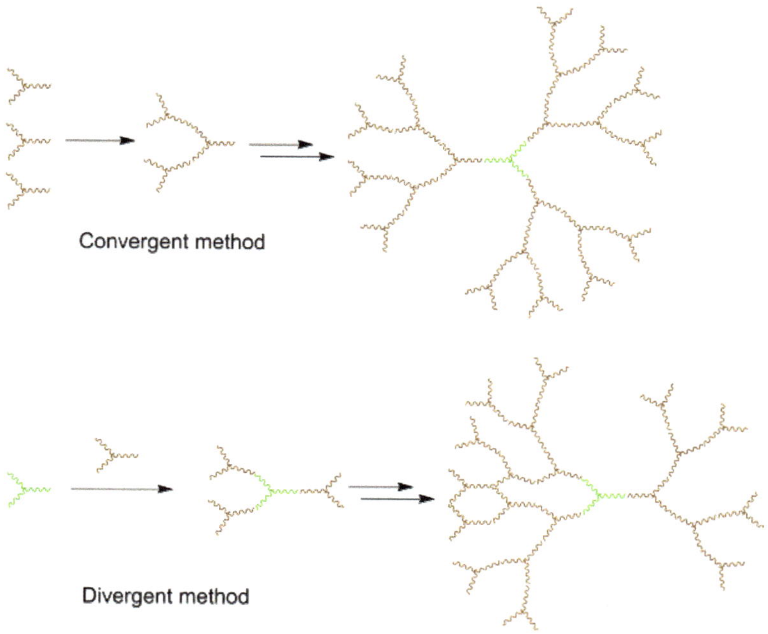

Figure 4.3 Convergent and divergent growth methods.

Regarding anterior ocular drug delivery, in vivo studies, performed in New Zealand albino rabbits with several dendrimer solutions of the PAMAM family applied topically, showed weak irritation with minor lesions in anterior ocular tissues (concentrations up to 2% w/v) [19]. Most of the clinical studies reveal a side effect of cloudiness in the vitreous of all the animals treated with a high dendrimer dose (100 ug) per eye. The cloudiness conforms with necropsy and is found to be systematic and dose dependent. Poupot and coworkers [20] defined the no-observed-adverse-effect level (NOAEL) as 20 ug of dendrimer per eye. Recently, Kannan and coworkers [21] explored a subconjunctival injectable gel based on the G4-PAMAM dendrimer and hyaluronic acid (HA) incorporated with dendrimer-dexamethasone (DEX) conjugates as a potential strategy for sustained delivery and enhanced bioavailability of corticosteroids. In addition, in a recent publication, Richichi and coworkers [22] reported the synthesis of the PAMAM-based matrix metalloproteinase (MMP) inhibitor 5, a high-affinity inhibitor of MMP-9, which is the most relevant MMP responsible for ocular damages in DES. This treatment merges the impressive properties of PAMAM–type dendrimers in terms of water solubility with the highly active MMP inhibitor, leading to remarkable topical activity, with no symptoms of corneal desiccation being observed.

In posterior ocular drug delivery, dendrimeric systems may enhance the effective delivery of therapeutic agents to intraocular tissues, such as the retina or the choroid, using noninvasive delivery methods [23]. Wei and coworkers reported recently a facile and friendly approach with the development of a noninvasive gene therapy for the posterior segment by using a simple dendrimeric system, G3 PAMAM, combined with penetratin, a cell-penetrating peptide (CPP), for topical gene delivery [24]. The compact complex has 150 nm diameter and a zeta potential about 30 mV. The complex was evaluated in vitro and in vivo when instilled in the conjunctival sac of rats. The intact complexes resided in the retina for more than 8 h, resulting in the efficient expression of red fluorescent protein plasmid in the posterior segment. Previously, Sun et al. [25] had reported the synthesis and evaluation of a hybrid nonviral dendrimeric system, G4/ECO/pDNA; plasmid DNA (pDNA) was condensed firstly by octa(3-aminopropyl) silsesquioxane (POSS-G4, where POSS stands for polyhedral oligomeric silsesquioxane), and then (1-aminoethyl)iminobis[*N*-(oleicylcysteinyl-1-amino-ethyl) propionamide] (ECO) lipid was incorporated into the delivery system through electrostatic interactions between the cationic head group of ECO and the negatively charged surface of the G4-pDNA complexes. Depending on the different ratio of the moieties, the sizes were distributed from 50 to 200 nm whereas the ζ-potentials were in the 25–30 mV range. The synthesized dendrimers exhibited high stability, low cytotoxicity, and efficient intracellular gene transfection and expression in ARPE-19 (human retinal pigmented epithelium [RPE] cells) in 10% serum media. These modules also mediated significant gene transfection in both mouse retina and RPE layers ex vivo. The same group recently published the use of the same type of dendrimeric systems for the treatment of Leber's congenital amaurosis type 2, a genetic disease causing retinal degeneration with severe vision loss at an early age [26]. Furthermore, Kannan and coworkers [27] used hydroxyl PAMAM-type dendrimers to deliver high payload (~21%) of triamcinolone acetonide (TA), a potent steroid with anti-inflammatory and antiangiogenic activity, for the treatment of retinal diseases. The dendrimers were 4–5 nm in size and depended on the conjugated TA, while the ζ-potentials were in the range of 5–6 mV due to the presence of three to four primary amine groups on the dendrimer surface. The synthesized dendrimeric systems exhibited a satisfactory release of TA (~2% per day for a period for ~21 days), enhanced cellular uptake, and significantly more efficacious anti-inflammatory (activated microglial cells) and anti–vascular endothelial growth factor (VEGF) activity (retinal pigment epithelial cells) compared to free TA. However, this study lacks any in vivo experiments. In another recent study, Yavuz et al. [28] used various PAMAM-type dendrimers to deliver DEX for the treatment of DR. Several DEX-PAMAM complexes were prepared, with a particle size range of 125–250 nm, and evaluated for their cytotoxicity and cell permeability in ARPE-19 cells, as well as for their ex vivo transportation across cornea and sclera-choroid-retina pigment epithelium. The ocular distribution of the complexes was evaluated in Sprague–Dawley rats following topical and subconjunctival administration. Results have shown that DEX-PAMAM G3.5 and G4.5 (dendrimers with –COOH) enhance in vitro permeability and ex vivo transport of DEX, as well as in vivo ocular distribution, in comparison with DEX suspension.

In general, no clinical data of ocular safety of dendrimers in humans have been published to date, and in animals there is a lack of complete reports of in vivo toxicological investigations. Only partial results have been reported during efficacy assays. With ongoing clinical trials studying the use of gene therapy in various retinal diseases, this is an exciting area of drug development, and further advances could change the way clinicians treat these and other sight-threatening conditions.

4.2.2 Liposomes

Liposomes are vesicles composed of lipid bilayers of amphiphilic molecules, mainly phospholipids (natural or synthetic), entrapping aqueous phases. A vast variety of different liposomal carriers can be produced by adjusting a number of structural parameters (the number and composition of their lipid bilayers, their size, etc.) or by modifying their surface (e.g., conjugation of polymers or targeting molecules). The advantages that they offer as drug delivery systems render them promising carriers in ocular drug delivery. Specifically, liposomes are biocompatible (due to the phospholipids used); biodegradable; able to encapsulate polar, nonpolar, and amphiphilic active ingredients due to the simultaneous existence of lipophilic (lipid bilayer) and hydrophilic (aqueous core) regions in their structure; and able to reduce drug toxicity and degradation. Moreover, with their use drug release can be controlled through appropriate selection of the lipid bilayer components; cells/tissues can be targeted through surface modification and conjugation of targeting molecules; and ocular retention time can be increased by adjusting their size, surface charge (e.g., positively charged liposomes have the ability to form electrostatic interactions with the negatively charged ocular mucosa, leading to prolonged precorneal retention), and surface properties (e.g., polymer coating). Finally, they have exhibited enhanced corneal permeability and uptake, leading to improved bioavailability [4, 29, 30].

However, their clinical application is limited due to problems related to their stability (hydrolysis or oxidation of their structural components, aggregation phenomena, drug leakage, etc.) and limited encapsulation capacity (especially for lipophilic drugs), which decreases the amount of time following administration in which the therapeutic concentration of the active ingredient can be maintained. Moreover, sterilization of liposomal formulations while maintaining their integrity can be difficult and administration through intravitreal injection can lead to rapid clearance from the posterior segment of the eye due to the leaky BRB present in patients with specific disorders, like DR [8]. Stability issues can be dealt with appropriate lipid selection (e.g., charged liposomes avoid aggregation due to electrostatic repulsion and there is reduced drug leakage from rigid lipid bilayers) and/or surface modification (e.g., PEGylation) [31]. Nowadays, there are only a few approved ocular products based on liposomal technology, such as Visudyne® and OPTO lipo spray. Visudyne is a liposomal formulation of verteporfin used in photodynamic therapy, administered via intravenous infusion for the treatment of choroidal neovascularization due to AMD, pathologic myopia, or presumed ocular histoplasmosis [1].

OPTO lipo spray, consisting of vitamins A and E encapsulated in liposomes, is sprayed on closed eyelids for relief from DES [32].

Nowadays, significant research activity is carried out on improving ocular drug delivery with the use of liposomes, as illustrated by the formulations shown in Table 4.1. The main focus is the improvement of drug bioavailability by increasing the ocular residence time and transcorneal permeation. For this purpose, liposomes are formulated with a positive surface charge or coated with mucoadhesive polymers. The latter has been performed with the use of chitosan, which is a natural, positively charged mucoadhesive polymer that also acts as a penetration enhancer by affecting the tight junctions of epithelial cells. The amount of chitosan that was used for coating liposomes needed to be optimized for producing vesicles with the desirable physicochemical characteristics [33]. In a study by Lin et al., HA was used for liposome coating performed by developing electrostatic interactions of the negatively charged polymer with the positively charged liposomes [34]. The same polymer was used for coating phytosomes, that is, supramolecular complexes formed between phospholipids and drug molecules, where electrostatic interactions or hydrogen bonds are formed between the drug molecules and the phospholipids' head groups. These novel carriers were studied for the ocular delivery of L-carnosine, as an alternative to the use of *N*-acetyl-L-carnosine (prodrug), for overcoming drawbacks associated with age-related variations of ocular esterase activity. The encapsulation efficiency was affected by the phospholipid:drug ratio and the presence of HA [35]. In a study by Dong et al., silk fibroins (SFs) extracted from the cocoons of *Bombyx mori* were used as novel mucoadhesive materials. Coating affected the liposomes' size, ζ-potential, encapsulation efficiency, release rate, and in vitro corneal permeation, with the last two depending on the SF concentration and molecular weight (SFs with different molecular weights had different dissolving times) [36]. Positively charged liposomes encapsulating both hydrophilic and lipophilic active ingredients were prepared for the enhancement of retinal drug delivery after intravitreal injection. The carriers should have the ability to diffuse through the vitreous humor and reach the retina. Then the encapsulated active ingredient should be released and penetrate across the retina to reach the outer retinal layer, where the disordered cells are located. Liposome PEGylation improved their diffusion ability at a specific surface charge. The penetration of lipophilic agents across the retina was greatly influenced by the chain length of the main phospholipid used for liposome preparation (the shorter the chain length, the deeper the penetration) and the agent's lipophilicity. Hydrophilic molecules could only penetrate deeper into the retina if they were first conjugated to phospholipids, with the phospholipid that demonstrated the best penetration being diphytanoylphosphatidylethanolamine (DPhPE) [37].

A formulation strategy for targeting the posterior eye segment through topical administration is to modify the composition of the liposomes' lipid bilayer in an attempt to increase their elasticity and ultimately enhance their transcorneal permeability. For this purpose, edge activators (e.g., surfactants) have been incorporated in liposomal vesicles, leading to the production of novel deformable liposomal carriers. In this context, a new class of carriers, called proglyosomes (i.e., vesicles composed of propylene glycol [PG] as edge activator, phospholipids, and water), were developed for the intraocular delivery of tacrolimus. PG was selected due to its biocompatibility and plasticizing effect and the drug's solubilizing properties. The addition of specific concentrations of PG to both the organic and aqueous phase during vesicle preparation resulted in small, stable, nontoxic, deformable vesicles with prolonged drug release (12 h) and corneal retention (8 h) and increased corneal permeation [38]. In another study, a mixture of surfactants and liquid lipids was incorporated in soybean phosphatidylcholine vesicles for fluidizing their bilayer and ultimately increasing their elasticity. The vesicles' characteristics depended on the type and concentration of surfactants and liquid lipids used but remained unchanged by gamma ray sterilization. When the surfactant Transcutol® was used alone, the formulation exhibited the most prolonged activity (lasted for 24 h) and the highest drug release, due to the turbulence produced in the bilayer lipid packing by the shorter surfactant chain [39]. Chen et al. prepared chitosan-coated deformable liposomes from Egg phosphatidylcholine (EggPC) and Solutol® HS-15. The polymer concentration was optimized in terms of vesicle physicochemical characteristics, stability, and drug loading. Chitosan's mucoadhesiveness resulted in prolonged retention time, and its effect on the corneal epithelial cell junctions combined with the liposomes' increased bilayer elasticity increased the formulation's transcorneal permeation [40].

Table 4.1 Liposomal ocular drug delivery systems

Composition	Drug / Indication	Preparation method	Administration route	Advantages offered	Ref.
SoyPC/Chol and chitosan	Timolol maleate/ Lowering of IOP in glaucoma	Lipid film hydration method, sonication for sizing, ammonium sulfate and pH gradient for drug encapsulation, incubation in chitosan solution for coating	Topical	High EE, controlled drug release, increased in vitro transcorneal penetration and corneal retention, more pronounced and prolonged therapeutic activity in vivo (vs. drug solution or uncoated liposomes), enhanced BA, no ocular irritation	[33]
PC/Chol/SA (15:3:2 wt/wt ratio) and hyaluronic acid	Doxorubicin/ Proliferative retinopathy	Solvent evaporation method, sonication and extrusion for sizing, incubation for drug loading and polymer coating	Ocular instillation	Sustained DR, prolonged in vivo precorneal retention and in vitro transcorneal permeation, enhanced in vivo aqueous humor absorption, HCE cell nucleus targeting	[34]
L-carnosine complexed with SoyPC (1:2 molar ratio)	L-carnosine/ Prevention of cataractogenesis associated with diabetes	Dispersion of drug-phospholipid complexes in appropriate aqueous buffer with dissolved hyaluronic acid, under specific conditions of temperature and agitation	Topical	Sustained ex vivo transcorneal permeation, significant inhibition of lens browning as well as formation of advanced glycation end products	[35]

Composition	Drug / Indication	Preparation method	Administra-tion route	Advantages offered	Ref.
PC/Chol/SA (30:10:1:1 molar ratio) and silk fibroins	Ibuprofen/Ocular inflammation	Ethanol injection method, incubation for polymer coating	-	Increased and prolonged in vitro corneal permeation to HCE cells, significant HCE uptake, no cytotoxicity	[36]
HSPC/DSPE-PEG/ DOTAP or DMPC/ DSPE-PEG/ DOTAP (76,2:3,8:20 molar ratio)	NBD-DPhPE, CF NHS ester/-	Lipid film hydration method followed by extrusion for size adjustment	Intravitreal injection	In vivo diffusion through vitreous humor, accumulation in the retina's inner limiting membrane, release and transportation of loaded agents to deeper retina layers, prolonged retention time in outer retinal layers	[37]
HSPC and propylene glycol	Tacrolimus/ Immune-mediated inflammatory intraocular disorders	Film hydration method, sonication for sizing	Topical	High EE (>96% of 0,1% w/v), prolonged DR (12 h) and in vivo corneal retention (8 h), higher ex vivo transcorneal permeation and in vivo BA compared to drug solution and conventional liposomes, no ocular irritation	[38]

(Continued)

Table 4.1 *(Continued)*

Composition	Drug / Indication	Preparation method	Administration route	Advantages offered	Ref.
SoyPC, surfactants (Transcutol®, Labrasol®, Tween® 80, etc.), and liquid lipids (Labrafac® lipophile WL1349)	Acetazolamide/ Glaucoma (lowering of IOP)	Thin film hydration method	Topical	High EE (>90%), sustained DR, increased in vivo therapeutic effectiveness and prolonged lowering of IOP (vs. conventional liposomes), no ocular irritation	[39]
EggPC and Solutol® HS-15 (7,5:1 molar ratio) and chitosan (0,1% w/v)	Flurbiprofen/ Ocular inflammation	Modified ethanol injection method, sonication for sizing, coating via incubation	Topical	High ex vivo corneal permeation and in vivo ocular retention time, no ocular irritation	[40]
DOPE/DPPC/ CHEMS (4:2:4 molar ratio)	Fusidic acid/ Bacterial infections	Reverse-phase evaporation, sizing via extrusion	-	Increased in vitro antimicrobial activity	[41]

Composition	Drug / Indication	Preparation method	Administration route	Advantages offered	Ref.
DPPC/DSPC/lyso PC/DSPE-PEG/1,3-diolein/CHEMS	Calcein/-	Reverse-phase evaporation method, sizing via sonication	-	Internalization by HRPE cells (ARPE-19) and vascular endothelial cells in vitro, no cytotoxicity, light- and pH-sensitive DR in the cytosol	[42]
Nanocomposites of betaxolol HCl in montmorillonite and PC/chol/octadecylamine liposomes	Betaxolol hydrochloride/Lowering of IOP	Montmorillonite acidification, ethanol injection using ammonium sulfate gradient	Ocular instillation	Controlled DR, reduced drug toxicity, longer in vivo maintenance of drug levels in the aqueous humor, prolonged in vivo ocular retention time and therapeutic activity	[44]
Deacetylated gellan gum and soyPC/chol liposomes	Timolol maleate/Lowering of IOP	Reverse evaporation method followed by sonication and pH-gradient formation	Topical	Decreased DR rate, increased in vivo retention time and in vitro apparent permeability coefficient, enhancement of the IOP reduction in vivo	[45]

(Continued)

Table 4.1 (*Continued*)

Composition	Drug / Indication	Preparation method	Administration route	Advantages offered	Ref.
DOTAP/DOPE (1:1 molar ratio) and targeting peptide (ME27 or Y) (liposome/peptide/siRNA 1:4:1 weight ratio)	siRNA for the silencing of the MRTF-B gene/ Prevention of conjunctival fibrosis responsible for glaucoma surgery failure	Incubation of liposomes with siRNA	-	MRTF-B gene silencing and blockage of collagen matrix contraction in vitro	[47]
HSPC/Chol/ DSPE-PEG-Trf/ ATTO-DOPE liposomes (2:1:0,02:0,005 molar ratio)	Luciferase pDNA/-	Thin film hydration method followed by microfluidizer processing	Ocular instillation	Improved in vivo accumulation in target cells (human Tenon's fibroblast cells)	[48]

Composition	Drug / Indication	Preparation method	Administration route	Advantages offered	Ref.
DOTAP/DOPE/Chol liposomes (1:1:1 molar ratio), protamine, and TAT peptide (1:20 DNA/liposomes ratio)	GFP pDNA or chicken Rpe65 complementary DNA, base pair mouse rhodopsin promoter/Expression of Rpe65 gene	Thin film hydration method	Subretinal injection	Enhanced gene delivery to specific cells, prolonged transgene expression in Rpe65 knockout mice	[49]

SoyPC, soybean phosphatidylcholine; PC, phosphatidylcholine; chol, cholesterol; IOP, intraocular pressure; GFP, green fluorescent protein; Rpe65, retinal pigment epithelium protein 65; EE, encapsulation efficiency; DR, drug release; BA, bioavailability; HCE, human corneal epithelial cell; DOTAP, 1,2-dioleoylphosphatidylethanolamine; SA, stearylamine; DMPC, 1,2-dimyristoyl-sn-glycero-3-phosphocholine; HSPC, hydrogenated soy L-a phosphatidylcholine; DSPE-PEG, 1,2-distearoyl-sn-glycero-3-phosphoethanolamine-*N*-[methoxy(polyethylene glycol)-2000]; Trf, transferrin; ATTO-DOPE, 1,2-dioleoyl-sn-glycero-3-phosphoethanolamine-Atto 647N; NBD-DPhPE, 2-diphytanoyl-sn-glycero-3-phosphoethanolamine-*N*-(7-nitro-2-1,3-benzoxadiazol-4-yl); CF NHS ester, carboxyfluorescein *N*-hydroxysuccinimide ester; DPPC, dipalmitoylphosphatidylcholine; CHEMS, cholesteryl hemisuccinate; HRPE, human retinal pigment epithelial; DSPC, 1,2-distearoyl-sn-glycero-3-phosphocholine; lysoPC, 1-stearoyl-2-hydroxy-sn-3-glycero-3-phosphocholine; MRTF-B, myocardin-related transcription factor B.

Liposomes can also be modified to carry out site-specific content release by responding to external and/or internal stimuli. For this purpose, fusogenic liposomes loaded with fusidic acid have been prepared for increasing the permeability of the active ingredient through the microbes' cell membranes and subsequently improve its antimicrobial activity. The liposomes' composition allowed them to be in a liquid crystalline (LC) state when found in an acidic environment or in the presence of cations, interact with cell membranes, and release their contents in the cytoplasm [41]. Another approach is to prepare pH-sensitive liposomes encapsulating gold (Au) NPs. Drug release in the cytosol of target cells can be achieved through the application of light (visible or near infrared) to Au NP–loaded liposomes located in an acidic environment (endosomes, lysosomes, etc.), which results in heat production and increase of liposomal lipid bilayer fluidity. Moreover, the low pH of the acidic environment results in phase separation phenomena in the lipid bilayer that are associated with drug release. These phenomena are induced by components added in the liposomal bilayer (e.g., diolein and cholesteryl hemisuccinate) [42].

Hybrid systems based on liposomes have also been studied. Au NPs were used as contrast agents for the capping of flucytosine-loaded liposomes [43]. After topical administration, the formulation's intraocular penetration was studied and its therapeutic efficacy in treating the experimental intravitreal *Candida albicans* infection (endophthalmitis) of the rabbit cornea was evaluated and found to be effective. The liposomes' positive surface charge (attributed to stearylamine) played a key role in both intraocular penetration and antifungal efficacy. Huang et al. encapsulated nanocomposites of betaxolol hydrochloride in montmorillonite into liposomes [44], while Yu et al. incorporated liposomes loaded with timolol maleate ™ into ion-sensitive in situ forming gels prepared from deacetylated gellan gum [45]. In both cases, the ocular retention time was prolonged, the drug's release rate was controlled, and its bioavailability or therapeutic efficacy was enhanced.

Regarding ocular gene therapy, liposomes have also been utilized as carriers of small interfering RNA (siRNA) or pDNA. In this case, positively charged phospholipids (e.g., 1,2-dioleoyl-3-trimethylammonium-propane [DOTAP]) are incorporated in the liposomal lipid bilayer for lipoplex formation (i.e., DNA-liposome complexes) through the development of electrostatic forces between the positively charged lipid head group and the negatively charged phosphate groups of the RNA backbone [46]. For improved therapeutic efficiency, cell targeting can be achieved via the use of cell-specific peptides [47], the chemical conjugation of transferrin to phospholipids, or and the control of the lipoplex size [48]. In another study, liposomes complexed with protamine and pDNA, bearing a CPP (TAT peptide) and a nuclear localization signaling peptide, were used for enhancing gene expression. Protamine was found to protect the pDNA that was loaded in the liposomal carriers from enzymatic degradation, while nuclear localization and CPPs enhanced the gene delivery to specific cells and prolonged the transgene expression [49].

4.2.3 Niosomes

Niosomes are vesicles composed of nonionic surfactants that self-assemble in bilayers when found in an aqueous environment [2]. They are studied as ocular drug delivery systems due to their ability to prolong precorneal retention time, enhance drug bioavailability, control drug release, encapsulate active ingredients of different polarities and protect them from various environmental conditions, reduce drug toxicity, and increase drug absorption (e.g., corneal permeation) by being able to pass through cell membranes and be endocytosed [4, 50]. Compared to liposomes, they have lower cost and higher stability [51]. Examples of nanogel ocular drug delivery systems are demonstrated in Table 4.2.

The niosomes' physicochemical characteristics, encapsulation efficiency, and drug release were found to be affected by their composition (type and concentration of surfactants used, surfactant:cholesterol ratio, etc.) [52, 53]. The surfactants' acyl chain length and saturation degree were identified as key factors. Moreover, the niosomes' transcorneal permeation depended on the vesicles size and membrane fluidity, with the latter being affected by the type, quantity, and transition temperature of the surfactants used [50, 54]. Moreover, cholesterol content modulates the niosomes' bilayer fluidity, where an increased cholesterol concentration increases drug encapsulation efficiency and reduces the release rate [50]. Mucoadhesive polymers, such as HA, have been used for niosome coating in order to increase mucosal adherence and prolong ocular retention time [55]. Additionally, incorporation of drug-loaded niosome in polymeric gels can control drug release and prolong the ocular retention time, thus improving the drug's therapeutic efficacy [56]. In this context, in situ forming gels, that is, gels that have the ability to convert from solution to gel (sol-gel transition) when found in a biological environment due to the effect of stimuli such as pH, temperature, and presence of ions, have also been used for niosome incorporation [53]. Usually, the thermoresponsive polymers Poloxamer 407 and Poloxamer 188 are combined with a mucoadhesive polymer, such as a cellulose derivative, to enhance drug bioavailability. The polymer type and concentration are optimized to obtain sol-gel transition at corneal temperature. In some cases, proniosomal gels, which transform to niosomes when they get hydrated, were used due to their easier production process (surfactant dissolution in a minimal organic solvent amount) and ability to adhere to the cornea and/or conjunctiva [50, 57].

For gene delivery, niosome transfection efficiency depends on their size, morphology, surface charge, and composition, which affect the cellular uptake pathway and intracellular fate [51]. Nioplexes (complexes of niosomes and DNA) are formed through the development of electrostatic forces between the negatively charged DNA and the positively charged niosomes, which is attributed to a cationic lipid incorporated in the niosomal bilayer. The physicochemical characteristics and the subsequent transfection efficiency of the nioplexes depend on the cationic lipid:DNA mass ratio and the addition of helper lipids and/or other ingredients. Specifically, nioplexes' transfection efficiency was found to be increased by the incorporation of lycopene [58], helper lipids such as cholesterol and squalene [51], and protamine [59] and was affected by the polar head group of the cationic lipid used [60]. In the case of protamine, the protamine:DNA mass ratio affected the vesicles' characteristics (size, ζ-potential, etc.), DNA condensation, protection from enzymatic degradation, and release. Finally, the administration route determined the retinal cells that exhibited protein expression, with a more uniform protein expression distribution through the retina's inner layers obtained via intravitreal injections versus a more localized protein expression produced via subretinal injections (photoreceptors and retinal pigment epithelial cells at the site of injection) [59].

Table 4.2 Niosome applications in ocular drug delivery

Composition	Active ingredient/ Indication	Preparation method	Administration route	Advantages offered	Ref.
Various Tween®, Span®, Brijs®, Pluronic®, lecithin, and chol	Ketoconazole/ Ocular keratitis	Modified coacervation-phase method	Topical	Biphasic DR, high ex vivo transcorneal permeation and in vivo BA in the aqueous humor (higher than the drug's suspension) that depends on composition, no in vivo ocular irritation	[50]
Tween 80, 1-(2-dimethylaminoethyl)-3-[2,3-di(tetradecyloxy) propyl] urea, and chol or lecithin	pCMS-EGFP (plasmid DNA)	Oil-in-water emulsion method	-	Squalene increased in vitro transfection efficiency in ARPE-19 cells	[51]
Span 20, 40, and 60; Tween 80; and chol	Lomefloxacin hydrochloride/ Bacterial conjunctivitis	Thin film hydration	Topical	Biphasic DR (initial burst release followed by a sustained release), superior in vivo therapeutic efficacy (vs. commercially available solution), no ocular irritation	[52]

(*Continued*)

Table 4.2 (*Continued*)

Composition	Active ingredient/ Indication	Preparation method	Administration route	Advantages offered	Ref.
Span 60/Chol, P407, and HPMC	Natamycin/Fungal keratitis	Thin film hydration method followed by sonication	Ocular instillation	Decreased rate of DR, high precorneal retention ability and ex vivo transcorneal permeation, sustained DR, no irritation	[53]
Span 20, 60, and 80; chol; Pluronic F127; Pluronic F68; and HPMC	Lomefloxacin hydrochloride/ Bacterial conjunctivitis	Film hydration followed by sonication	Ocular instillation	Increased precorneal retention time and transcorneal permeation, enhanced BA and in vivo antibacterial activity (vs. drug solution), no in vivo ocular irritation	[54]
Poloxamer 188/SoyPC/ Chol (9:9:1 weight ratio) and HA	Tacrolimus/ Prevention of graft rejection after corneal allograft	Niosome preparation, via proniosome reconstitution; HA coating, via incubation	Topical	Prolonged in vivo ocular retention, increased transcorneal permeability and drug concentration in aqueous humor (vs. uncoated niosomes)	[55]

Composition	Active ingredient/ Indication	Preparation method	Administration route	Advantages offered	Ref.
Span 60/Chol and 1% w/w Carbopol® 934 gel	Flurbiprofen/ Ocular inflammation	Film hydration method	Topical	Decreased rate of DR, increased BA in aqueous humor, enhanced therapeutic efficiency (vs. the drug's solution)	[56]
DOTMA, polysorbate 60, and lycopene	pCMS-EGFP (plasmid DNA)	Reverse phase evaporation method	Subretinal injection	Lycopene-increased in vitro TE in ARPE-19 cells, compared to Lipofectamine^{tm}: lower TE but higher cell viability, transfection of photoreceptors in the outer segments of the retina	[58]
2,3-Di(tetradecyloxy) propan-1-amine, squalene, Tween 80, and protamine	pCMS-EGFP (plasmid DNA)	Solvent emulsification technique, nioplexes: incubation of niosomes with protamine–pDNA complex	Intravitreal and subretinal injection	Protamine-improved DNA condensation, in vitro transfection efficiency and cell viability, and in vivo protein expression	[59]

(*Continued*)

Table 4.2 (*Continued*)

Composition	Active ingredient/ Indication	Preparation method	Administration route	Advantages offered	Ref.
Tween 80, squalene, and synthetized cationic amino lipids	pCMS-EGFP (plasmid DNA)	Oil-in-water emulsification and thin film hydration techniques	Intravitreal and subretinal injection	In vitro and in vivo transfection efficiency in retinal cells depending on the cationic lipids polar head group	[60]
Cremophor® RH 40, Cremophor EL, chol, Span 60, and sodium taurocholate	Terconazole/ Ocular fungal infections	Ethanol injection method followed by sonication	Topical	Superior ex vivo cornea permeability (vs. conventional bilosomes or niosomes), good in vivo ocular tolerability	[61]
Span 60 and Tween 20 or Tween 80	Itraconazole/ Ocular fungal infections	Modified ethanol injection method	Topical	Increased apparent permeation coefficient in vitro, enhanced in vivo antifungal activity	[62]

DR, drug release; soyPC, soybean phosphatidylcholine; chol: cholesterol; HA, hyaluronic acid; P407, Poloxamer 407; HPMC, hydroxypropyl methylcellulose; Pluronic F127, Poloxamer 407; Pluronic F68, Poloxamer 188; Tweens, polyoxyethylene sorbitan esters; Span, sorbitan fatty acid esters; Brijs, polyoxyethylene alkyl ethers; Pluronic, polyoxyethylene-polyoxypropylene block copolymers; DOTMA, *N*-[1-(2,3-dioleoyloxy)propyl]-*N*,*N*,*N*-trimethylammonium chloride; TE, transfection efficiency; pCMS-EGFP, promoter-cloning multiple site–enhanced green flouorescent protein.

In other formulation approaches, the niosome composition was slightly modified to increase the vesicles' elasticity and thus transcorneal permeability. In a study performed by Abdelbary et al. ultradeformable vesicles with increased ex vivo cornea permeability were prepared by the combination of edge activators and bile salts [61]. ElMeshad and Mohsen prepared spanlastics, that is, elastic vesicles consisting of Tween and Span® 60 [62]. Drug encapsulation efficiency and release, as well as vesicles' characteristics, depended on their composition.

4.2.4 Nanoparticles

NPs typically consist of 1–100 nm particles composed of various polymers, lipids, or other materials. Several NP-based drug delivery systems have been proposed, and these systems can improve the delivery of poorly water-soluble drugs while significantly reducing toxicity compared to the free drug. Increasing attention has been paid particularly to this aspect due to the clear therapeutic implications. NPs can become a great choice for the ocular delivery of drugs since topical delivery into the eye is preferred over systemic administration.

For NP preparation, a vast variety of different materials can be used, which include but are not limited to polyacrylates, polyalkylcyanoacrylates, polycaprolactones, polylactide, poly(lactic-*co*-glycolic acid) (PLGA), dextran, albumin, gelatin, alginate, collagen, HA, and chitosan. Moreover, NPs with large surface areas, multifunctional surface groups, and different physicochemical properties (size, ζ-potential, polydispersity index, etc.) can be prepared. As a result, they offer great flexibility in terms of drug delivery [63, 64]. Furthermore, the above-mentioned features of NPs are responsible for their in vivo fate by affecting processes such as cellular uptake and intracellular trafficking [65]. Topical administration of NPs can be employed for targeting various ocular sites and/or increasing the precorneal residence time obtained via their entrapment in the ocular mucus layer. The latter is achieved through the development of interactions between the functional groups of the NPs and the groups of mucin found in the extraocular tissue (mucoadhesiveness), leading to increased drug bioavailability [66]. During the last years, several NP systems have been developed for the ocular delivery of drugs, of polymeric, metal, or lipidic nature, which will be further described in this section.

4.2.4.1 Solid lipid nanoparticles and nanostructured lipid carriers

Solid lipid nanoparticles (SLNs) are considered to be the first generation of lipid nanoparticles (LNs), while nanostructured lipid carriers (NLCs) the second generation. SLNs are formed in an aqueous environment, with their structure consisting of a solid lipid matrix, created by lipids that are in a solid state at both room and body temperature, covered by a surfactant layer. They are also described as solidified oil-in-water (o/w) emulsions, where the oil globule has been replaced by solidified lipids [29]. NLCs have a different core composition compared to SLNs. They are composed of both solid and liquid lipids, while the core remains solid at room temperature. As a result, a higher number of crystal imperfections can be found in their structure, which increases drug loading and reduces drug expulsion during storage [67]. Three types of NLCs (imperfect, amorphous, and multiple) can be prepared by varying the production method and lipid composition, with different encapsulation efficiencies and long-term stability [68].

SLNs and NLCs have been studied as drug and gene ocular drug delivery systems (Table 4.3) due to the following attributes: (a) biocompatibility, which arises by the use of lipids approved by the European Medicines Agency and the Food and Drug Administration and generally regarded as safe (triglycerides, diglycerides, monoglycerides, capric/caprylic triglycerides, aliphatic alcohols, polyalcohol esters, fatty acids of C10–C12 chains, etc.), (b) stability (maintaining physicochemical characteristics and controlling drug leakage), (c) ability to be loaded with active ingredients of different hydro- or lipophilicity and protect them from environmental conditions (e.g., enzymes), (d) ability to increase the corneal absorption and ocular retention time, leading to enhanced bioavailability, (e) ability to control and sustain drug release, and (f) easy production and sterilization with steam sterilization, without their stability being compromised [1, 9, 29, 68, 69].

However, SLNs have drawbacks that limit their application, such as reduced drug loading capacity and drug expulsion during storage. To overcome these issues, surface modifications can be performed on SLNs or NLCs can be used alternatively due to their ability to encapsulate higher drug amounts and control more efficiently their release [70].

Table 4.3 SLN and NLC ocular drug delivery systems

Carrier	Composition	Active ingredient/ Indication	Preparation method	Administration route	Advantages offered	Ref.
SLN	Soy phospholipids, Compritol® 888 ATO, and Myrj® 52, with SA (positively charged) and without SA (negatively charged)	Tetrandrine/Posterior lens opacification, glaucoma, retinopathy, and ocular inflammation	Emulsion evaporation-solidification at low temperature	Topical	High EE (>91%), prolonged DR, BA enhancement, no cytotoxicity, more efficient cellular uptake by negatively charged SLNs	[73]
SLN	Stearic acid or palmitic acid and different concentrations of PVA	Itraconazole/Fungal corneal infections	Melt-emulsion sonication and low-temperature solidification	Topical	SLNs prepared from steric acid showing higher EE, higher corneal permeability (in vitro), and antimicrobial efficacy (in vitro)	[74]

(*Continued*)

Table 4.3 (*Continued*)

Carrier	Composition	Active ingredient/ Indication	Preparation method	Administration route	Advantages offered	Ref.
SLN	GMS and PVA or Tween® 80 or Pluronic® F68	Celecoxib/Ocular inflammations	Melt-emulsion sonication and low-temperature solidification	Topical	Increased drug EE, prolonged ocular retention and effective reduction of inflammation parameters in vivo, high in vitro transcorneal permeability, good in vivo ocular tolerability	[75]
SLN	Glycerol (37,5 wt%), hydrogenated coco-glycerides (4,5 wt%), soyPC (0,5 wt%), ascorbic acid (0,25 wt%), P188 (1,0 wt%) and CTAB or DDAB (0,5 wt%)	Epigallocatechin gallate/Age-related macular edema, diabetic retinopathy, and inflammatory disorders due to anti-inflammatory and antioxidant activity	Multiple emulsion	Ocular instillation	Increased ocular retention time, protection of drug, no ocular irritation	[76]
					Prolonged DR, enhanced cornea permeability tested ex vivo, no ocular irritation	[77]

Carrier	Composition	Active ingredient/ Indication	Preparation method	Administration route	Advantages offered	Ref.
SLN	Precirol® ATO 5, DOTAP, and Tween 80, complexed with P and HA (HA-P-DNA-SLN at a 0.5:2:1:2 weight ratio)	Plasmid containing the human RS1 gene with mOPS promoter /X-linked juvenile retinoschisis (retinal degenerative disorder associated with gene mutation)	Solvent emulsification-evaporation	Intravitreal injection	Increased cell transfection in retinal photoreceptors and improvement of retinal structure in Rs1h-deficient mice	[78]
SLN	Stearic acid (4%–8% w/w), Tween 80 (2%–4% w/w), and sodium deoxycholate (1%–3% w/w)	Levofloxacin/ Conjunctivitis	Solvent evaporation	Topical	Increased EE, biphasic DR (initial burst release followed by sustained release), same in vitro antimicrobial activity as commercially available eye drops, no irritation	[79]

(Continued)

Table 4.3 (*Continued*)

Carrier	Composition	Active ingredient/ Indication	Preparation method	Administration route	Advantages offered	Ref.
SLN	Compritol 888 ATO (2,5%), soya lecithin (0,4%), PEG 600 (4,2%), and Tween 80 (5,8%)	Ketoconazole/Fungal posterior ocular infections (e.g., keratitis and endophthalmitis)	Hot high-pressure homogenization	Topical	High drug EE, enhanced permeability through cornea (ex vivo), significant antifungal activity, increased drug BA in the aqueous and vitreous humor, good ocular tolerability	[80]
NLC	Precirol ATO5, Lutrol® F68, squalene, and 1-oleoyl-glycerol (lipophilic surfactant)	Triamcinolone acetonide/Treatment of posterior segment diseases, like macular edema, neovascularization, and other ocular inflammatory disorders, due to its antiangiogenic activity	High-pressure homogenization method	Topical	Controlled DR (first-order kinetics), enhanced ex vivo transcleral permeation (zero-order kinetics) and scleral accumulation, prolonged ex vivo ocular retention, no toxicity or irritation	[81]

Carrier	Composition	Active ingredient/ Indication	Preparation method	Administration route	Advantages offered	Ref.
NLC	Lipid phase: Precirol ATO5, Gelucire® 44/14, Gelucire 43/01, Gelucire 50/13, Lipocire® DM, Witepsol E85, Imwitor 900K, Imwitor 491, Dynasan 114, Dynasan 118, Softisan 142, cetyl palmitate, stearic acid, Miglyol® 812, Softisan 645, and Perhidrosqualene, Aqueous phase: Tween 80, CTAB, Pluronic F127, and chitosan	Ibuprofen/Ocular inflammatory diseases	Melt-emulsification and ultrasonication cold method for chitosan and Pluronic F127 addition	Topical	Prolonged precorneal retention time, sustained DR, biocompatibility with Y-79 human retinoblastoma cells	[82]

(*Continued*)

Table 4.3 (*Continued*)

Carrier	Composition	Active ingredient/ Indication	Preparation method	Administration route	Advantages offered	Ref.
NLC	Synthetized HACC, β-GP Compritol 888 ATO, Miglyol 812N, GMS, Kolliphor® HS15, and Cremophor® EL	Dexamethasone/Ocular inflammation	NLC, via melt-emulsification; thermogel, via polymer mixing	Topical	High EE, sol-gel transition at 35°C, sustained DR	[83]
NLC	GMS, polysorbate 80, lauroyl macrogolglycerides, caprylocaproyl macrogolglycerides, and caprylic/capric triglycerides	Magniferin/Treatment of cataract, diabetic retinopathy, age-related macular degeneration, and other oxidative stress-related ocular diseases	Ultrasonication method	Topical	Sustained DR, increased corneal permeation, prolonged corneal retention, good ocular tolerability, enhanced ocular BA	[84]

EE, entrapment efficiency; DR, drug release; BA, bioavailability; Compritol 888 ATO, glyceryl behenate; Myrj 52, PEG (40) stearate; P, protamine; mOPS, murine opsin; HA, hyaluronic acid; SA, stearylamine; soyPC, soybean phosphatidylcholine; GMS, glyceryl monostearate; P188, Poloxamer 188; CTAB, cetyltrimethylammonium bromide; DDAB, dimethyldioctadecylammonium bromide; PVA, polyvinyl alcohol; PEG, polyethylene glycol; Precirol ATO5, glyceryl distearate; Lutrol F68, Poloxamer 188; DOTAP, 1,2-dioleoyil-3-trimethylammonium-propane chloride salt; HACC, hydroxypropyltrimethyl ammonium chloride chitosan; β-GP, β-glycerophosphate.

The in vivo behavior and drug encapsulation efficiency of the above-mentioned LNs depend on their size, surface characteristics (surface charge, surface modifications, etc.), and lipid composition [71]. The size of LNs was found to be related with cornea uptake, where the smaller the size the higher is the observed uptake [9]. LNs with a positive surface charge exhibit increased ocular retention time due to the development of electrostatic forces with the negatively charged mucosa [29], an effect that can also be produced by coating LNs with positively charged polymers [72]. Moreover, surface charge was found to affect the cellular uptake of tendrandrine-loaded SLNs into human lens epithelial cells (SRA 01/04), with anionic vesicles providing better results [73]. The lipid composition affected the amount of itraconazole loaded in SLNs, as well as the in vitro permeability of the final formulation through the cornea [74]. Apart from lipids, the surfactants and/or added polymers used in NP formulation also affect drug loading, drug release, and NP size, as demonstrated by the study by Sharma et al., who prepared celecoxib SLNs with varying compositions (polyvinyl alcohol [PVA], Tween 80, or Poloxamer 188) [75].

To increase drug bioavailability from topically administered SLNs or NLCs, thermosensitive polymers have been employed, such as Poloxamer 188 and 407 [81]. These polymers have the ability to undergo a transition from the solution phase to the gel phase (sol-gel transition) at specific temperatures. If this transition happens at ocular temperature, prolonged residence time can be obtained. In a study performed by Almeida et al. ibuprofen-loaded NLCs were combined with Poloxamer 407 (i.e., Pluronic® F127) and the mucoadhesive polymer chitosan. The final formulation exhibited sustained drug release and prolonged precorneal retention time, which was the result of the combined polymer activity [82]. In another study, positively charged SLNs, which contained Poloxamer 188, were loaded with epigallocatechin gallate. It was observed that their ocular retention time was prolonged and the type of cationic ingredient used (cetyltrimethylammonium bromide [CTAB] or dimethyldioctadecylammonium bromide [DDAB]) affected the transcorneal permeability and the permeation kinetics [77]. Furthermore, Tan et al. incorporated NLCs into a thermoresponsive and biodegradable hydrogel prepared by the synthesized hydroxypropyltrimethyl ammonium chloride chitosan (HACC), which is a water-soluble chitosan derivative, and β-glycerophosphate (β-GP). Gelation was found to be affected by HACC's degree of substitution, and the overall hybrid system was found to sustain DEX release [83]. Due to HACC's quaternized nature, stronger electrostatic interactions can be developed with the anionic corneal surface, and thus prolonged precorneal retention can be obtained [85, 86].

In terms of gene delivery, complexation of DNA with protamine increased the transfection efficacy of DNA-loaded carriers. This was attributed to the nuclear localization induced by protamine, the release of the DNA-protamine complex from SLNs due to the lysosomal activity, and the stabilization of DNA against enzymatic degradation [87]. Moreover, the combination of the mucoadhesive polymer HA with protamine in SLNs complexed with DNA resulted in increased cell transfection and specific gene expression [78].

4.2.4.2 Polymeric nanoparticles

Polymeric NPs have been utilized in an increasing number of fields during the last years. Their preparation can be conducted via either the dispersion of preformed polymers or the polymerization of monomers. For the production of such drug delivery formulations, several techniques are applied, like solvent evaporation, supercritical fluid technology, salting-out, dialysis, microemulsion (ME), miniemulsion, surfactant-free emulsion, and interfacial polymerization. In ocular drug delivery, polymeric NPs have attracted the interest of scientists in the last few years. Various polymeric systems have been developed and tested against glaucoma, intraocular pressure (IOP), conjunctivitis, inflammation, retinopathies, DR, AMD, etc., some examples of which are presented in Table 4.4.

Singh and coworkers [88], in a recent publication, have reported the development of a pH-triggered in situ forming gel with incorporated NPs for the ophthalmic delivery of acetazolamide. In situ gels can be considered advantageous as they offer an accurate and reproducible quantity of drug and enhanced precorneal residence time [89, 90], while NPs can increase conjunctival permeation. The mucoadhesive polymer Carbopol® 934P (polyacrylic acid derivative) was used for gel formation since it displays a sol-gel transition at specific pH values (neutral to basic pH) [91–93]. The polymer concentration was optimized in order to provide sol-gel transition upon ocular instillation (0,5% w/v). Moreover, the polymer used for NP formation affected their characteristics (size, polydispersity index, etc.), encapsulation efficiency, and in vitro permeability, with the best formulation being the one prepared by PLGA. This formulation demonstrated sustained action of acetazolamide with a significant decrease in the IOP.

A dispersion of polymeric NPs from Eudragit® RL100 and PVA was found to increase ketotifen fumarate's corneal permeation coefficient. The drug-to-polymer ratio affected the NPs' characteristics (size, polydispersity index, ζ-potential, etc.), drug loading, release rate, and ocular penetration. Moreover, the produced NPs had a positive surface charge, attributed to Eudragit RL100, which helps increase the ocular retention time [94]. In another study, Eudragit RL100 polymeric NPs of ketoroloac tromethamine were incorporated into an in situ forming gel consisting of the thermosensitive polymer Pluronic F127 and the mucoadhesive polymer hydroxypropyl methylcellulose (HPMC). The formulation parameters (i.e., type of aqueous phase, drug-to-polymer ratio, organic-to-aqueous-phase ratio, and organic phase type) affected drug loading and release rate, as well as the particle characteristics (e.g., size) [95]. Moreover, Shi et al. prepared cationic NPs from a self-assembling block copolymer, synthesized by the chemical conjugation of chitosan with methoxy PEG-poly(ε-caprolactone). Chitosan properties (i.e., cationic charge, mucoadhesiveness, and penetration enhancement) contributed to the improvement of drug bioavailability [96]. Chitosan and its various derivatives have been investigated extensively as ocular delivery systems [97], since they can overcome the problems of low ocular bioavailability and retention time.

In a study performed by Maged et al., cyclodextrins that are also used in commercially available eye products (i.e., methyl-β-cyclodextrin and hydroxypropyl-β-cyclodextrin) were employed as econazole nitrate carriers, to overcome problems associated with the nanosuspension (NS) preparation method (e.g., stickiness and drug loss) and obtain NPs with the desired characteristics and improved drug release properties. The optimum cyclodextrin and stabilizing polymer or surfactant was chosen in terms of production yield, particle size, drug release, and stability [98]. Gelatin NPs have also been prepared for ocular delivery of the lipophilic drug moxifloxacin. The amount of glutaraldehyde that was used in this study as a cross-linking agent affected the particle size and drug loading [99].

Table 4.4 Polymeric nanoparticles in ocular drug delivery

Composition	Active ingredient/ Indication	Preparation method	Advantages offered	Ref.
Eudragit® RS100 or Eudragit RL100 or PLGA, Tween® 80, PVA, and Carbopol® 934P	Acetazolamide/ Lowering of IOP, open angle glaucoma	Nanoprecipitation method	Sustained action (8 h), increased preocular residence time and ex vivo transcorneal permeation, enhanced in vivo lowering of IOP (vs. eye drops), no in vivo ocular irritation	[88]
Eudragit RL100, polyvinyl alcohol, and ethanol	Ketotifen fumarate	o/w Solvent diffusion method	High EE, positive surface charge, biphasic DR profile (initial burst release followed by a sustained release), increased corneal permeation coefficient	[94]
Eudragit RL100 in citrate-phosphate buffer, Pluronic® F127 (14% w/v), HPMC (1,5% w/v), and ethanol	Ketoroloac tromethamine/ Postoperative inflammation	Nanoprecipitation (solvent displacement) method	Sustained DR, prolonged precorneal retention time, improved ex vivo and iv vivo transcorneal permeation (vs. commercial eye drops), improved iv vivo BA in the aqueous humor, no ocular irritation	[95]
MPEG-PCL-CS (self-assembling block copolymer)	Diclofenac/Ocular inflammation		Sustained DR (8 h), prolonged precorneal retention time and increased transcorneal penetration both in vitro and in vivo, improved BA in the aqueous humor (vs. commercial formulation), no ocular irritation or cytotoxicity	[96]

Composition	Active ingredient/ Indication	Preparation method	Advantages offered	Ref.
Methyl-β-cyclodextrin or hydroxypropyl-β-cyclodextrin as drug carriers PEO, PVP K 30, P407, Tween 80 or Cremophor® EL as the stabilizer, and chitosan	Econazole nitrate/Topical ocular infections	Nano-spray-drying technique	Optimum results produced by Tween 80 and hydroxypropyl-β-cyclodextrin, higher drug bioavailability iv vivo compared to the drug's suspension, no ocular irritation	[98]
Gelatin type A and glutaraldehyde	Moxifloxacin/ Acute bacterial conjunctivitis	Two-step desolvation technique	Biphasic DR, no in vivo ocular irritation, enhanced in vivo antimicrobial activity (vs commercial product)	[99]

PEO, polyethylene oxide; PVP, polyvinyl pyrrolidone; PVA, polyvinyl alcohol; PLGA, poly(lactic-*co*-glycolic acid); IOP, intraocular pressure; HPMC, hydroxypropyl methylcellulose; DR, drug release; BA, bioavailability; EE, entrapment efficiency; CS, chitosan; MPEG-PCL, methoxy polyethylene glycol-poly(ε-caprolactone); o/w, oil-in-water.

Of paramount interest is also the research on the delivery of siRNA with polymeric NPs. Gene therapy, through the application of these tools, can become an efficient option against severe conditions (of genetic or pathological origin). However, several considerations regarding stability, formulation, and efficacy need to be taken into account until these systems can be considered for authorization as medicinal products in order to extended siRNA application to clinical practice, even though polymeric NPs can overcome a lot of these obstacles. In addition, a major obstacle in siRNA-based therapy of corneal neovascularization (CNV) is the severe cytotoxicity caused by repeated drug treatment [102]. Current nonviral polymers investigated as efficient carriers for siRNA include synthetic polyamines such as polyethylenimine (PEI), polysaccharides such as chitosan, inulin (INU), and polyaminoacids such as α,β-poly(*N*-2-hydroxyethyl)-d,l-aspartamide and poly-L-lysine [103]. Han et al., in their recent study, examined the ocular delivery of therapeutic siRNA in corneal CNV therapy. A reducible NP system based on branched polyethylenimine (rBPEI) was studied as a new siRNA carrier. High-molecular-weight rBPEI was produced by the self-cross-linking of thiolated BPEI in mild conditions. As a result, stable siRNA/rBPEI NPs were created. When the NPs are located in the reductive cytosol, the rBPEI polymeric matrix can be degraded into nontoxic low-molecular-weight BPEI and release the encapsulated siRNA. Significant gene knockdown of angiogenesis was observed in vivo after subconjuctival injection in rats [102].

4.2.4.3 Polymeric nanocapsules

Polymeric nanocapsules are small sized (<1 μm) vesicular drug delivery systems that have been studied for both topical and systemic drug delivery. Their structure is characterized by a central core (oil droplet) enclosed in a polymeric film [104, 105]. Aggregation phenomena can be avoided through the use of steric agents and/or surfactants, since a unimodal size distribution with a low polydispersity index is a necessary characteristic for safe and effective drug delivery [106].

Reimondez-Troitino and coworkers [107] have recently reported on the preparation of polymeric nanocapsules loaded with cyclosporine A or vitamin A, with or without mitomycin C, and evaluated their effectiveness in healing corneal injuries.

The nanocapsule's polymeric shell was produced by the CPPs polyarginine or protamine, via the solvent displacement technique, and facilitates the interaction of the nanocapsules with the cornea [108]. The nanocapsules, both loaded and unloaded, were found to accelerate corneal wound healing after instillation when tested in vivo, with the most efficient in terms of healing rate being those prepared by protamine and loaded with mitomycin C.

4.2.4.4 Polymeric micelles

Several proposed methods for the ocular delivery of drugs show limitations in regard to the administration site and the frequency of the injections. Polymeric micelles (10–200 nm, having a hydrophobic core and a hydrophilic corona) have increasingly shown their potential as nanocarriers to overcome such limitations and provide therapeutic drug concentrations in the ocular tissues of the anterior and posterior segments following topical administration [109, 110]. Most of the polymeric micelles used in drug delivery consist of amphiphilic diblock (hydrophilic-hydrophobic) polymers, triblock (hydrophilic-hydrophobic-hydrophilic) polymers, and graft (hydrophilic-hydrophobic) and ionic (hydrophilic-ionic) copolymers.

Polymeric micelles are self-assembling colloidal systems obtained by amphiphilic copolymers with distinct hydrophobic and hydrophilic segments. The polymer self-assembles to form micelles in aqueous media, wherein water-insoluble segments form the core and hydrophilic segments form the corona. This hydrophobic core allows effortless encapsulation of several poorly water-soluble drugs, like corticosteroids. Polymeric micelles seem to be very promising in ocular drug delivery since they can improve drug permeability across ocular epithelia [111, 112].

Di Prima and coworkers [113], in their review, described the production of novel polymeric micelles by synthesizing a new amphiphilic polymer based on the biocompatible material INU. For increasing the formulation's interactions with mucin and consequently the ocular retention time, new functional groups were introduced in INU by ethylenediamine (EDA). Functionalization was performed by activating the hydroxyl groups of INU via microwave and then reacting it with an excess quantity of EDA [114]. Subsequently, conjugation of activated retinoic acid (RA) to the INU-EDA complex was performed in order to introduce hydrophobic domains and create the amphiphilic polymer INU-EDA-RA. The polymeric micelles were loaded with corticosteroids (DEX, triamcinolone, and TA) and were reported to present increased in vitro mucoadhesion, transcorneal permeation, and drug fluxes across human endometrial adenocarcinoma (HEC) cells [113].

4.2.4.5 Inorganic gold and silver nanoparticles

Au and silver (Ag) NPs, that is, metal NPs, are characterized by a large surface area to volume ratio, which is responsible for their superior properties [115]. Their small size, providing them with the ability to overcome the ocular barriers, has rendered them attractive for use in ophthalmology. However, the size of metal NPs needs to be adjusted in order to obtain high transcorneal permeation and targeted drug delivery. Especially, Ag NPs have been proposed as an alternative for the treatment of retinal diseases due to their low cost [116] and ability to affect VEGF cellular functions [117]. Colloidal Au and Ag NPs, commercially available and stabilized with citrate, are often utilized in various delivery systems.

Natesan and coworkers [118] incorporated Au NPs and hypocrellin B (HB) in PLGA NPs (HBS-NPs) for the treatment of AMD via photodynamic therapy. The results obtained demonstrated that intravenous administration of HBS-NPs resulted in posterior segment accumulation, enhanced reactive oxygen species (ROS) generation, and singlet oxygen production, as well as an antiangiogenic effect, rendering them promising for the treatment of ocular vascular diseases.

Anbukkarasi and coworkers [119] biosynthesized Ag NPs by using an ethanolic extract of *Tabernaemontana divaricata* leaves. These Ag NPs were found to have a concentration-dependent antioxidant activity, when tested in vitro for radical-scavenging activity, and reducing power. Furthermore, they partly prevented cataract formation induced by selenite when tested in vivo, which is associated with damage by free radicals. This was demonstrated by the retention of the antioxidant enzymes mean activities, the retention of the levels of reduced glutathione, and by the prevention of malondialdehyde elevation.

Recently, Au NPs have been introduced in cancer radiotherapy as a new approach. Tumor damage caused by radiation can be enhanced with the use of Au NPs due to their high atomic number, which changes photon interactions [120]. Therefore, an increased photoelectric effect can be produced, leading to an increased radiation dose in the ocular tumor. At the same time, lower doses were observed to normal tissues. Nevertheless, toxicity issues limit their clinical application in eye brachytherapy [121].

Utilization of small-sized (20 and 80 nm) Au and Ag NPs for the treatment of retinal diseases or even the retinal accumulation of such NPs from the use of cosmetic products and/or exposure to the environment need to be evaluated in terms of safety, due to potential in vitro neuronal retinal toxicity, as demonstrated in the study of Söderstjerna and coworkers [122].

4.2.5 Nanosuspensions

NSs are colloidal dispersion systems consisting of particles with nanodimensions [30]. They are being studied as ocular drug delivery systems due to their ability to enhance drug solubility and therapeutic efficacy, reduce the amount of administered drug and its systemic toxicity, and prolong ocular retention time and drug release, hence improving lipophilic drug bioavailability [123]. NSs can be prepared either with top-down techniques that use mechanical forces (e.g., milling and high-pressure homogenization) or with bottom-up techniques (e.g., particle precipitation from an organic solvent solution and spray-drying) [98]. Some examples of NSs studied for ocular drug delivery via topical administration and the observed outcomes that they have shown are presented in Table 4.5.

For the improvement of drug bioavailability, positively charged nanocrystals were produced for the ocular delivery of DEX acetate and polymyxin B sulfate by Romero et al. [101]. The nanocrystals' charge, which contributes to the nanocrystals stability and prolonged ocular retention time, was generated from polymyxin B sulfate (a positively charged drug) and the use of preservatives, for example, cetylpyridinium chloride (CPC) and benzalkonium chloride (BAC). The small size of the nanocrystals contributes to an increase in the drug saturation solubility and ocular retention time [101].

Table 4.5 Nanosuspensions studied as ocular drug delivery systems

Composition	Active ingredient/Indication	Preparation method	Advantages offered	Ref.
Carboxymethyl chitosan and Poloxamer 407 and 188	Sparfloxacin/Bacterial conjunctivitis	Solvent diffusion method followed by probe sonication	Prolonged in vitro drug release (9 h), no ocular irritation and toxicity, enhanced in vitro and in vivo antimicrobial activity	[100]
Positively charged nontoxic stable drug nanocrystals with CPC or BAC	Dexamethasone acetate and polymyxin B sulfate/Ocular inflammation and bacterial infections, respectively	Small-scale method for wet bead milling	Prolonged ocular retention time, increased drug saturation solubility	[101]

CPC, cetylpyridinium chloride; BAC, benzalkonium chloride.

A combination of mucoadhesive polymers with NSs was applied by Ambhore et al. [101] for the ocular delivery of the water-insoluble antimicrobial drug sparfloxacin, where the water-soluble chitosan derivative carboxymethyl chitosan was used together with Poloxamer 407 and 188. The type and concentration of mucoadhesive polymers and stabilizing surfactants used for the preparation of the NS were found to be affecting the NPs' characteristics, drug loading, and release rate [100].

4.2.6 Nanogels

Nanogels are 3D nanoscale networks of hydrogel particles that are cross-linked either physically (noncovalent interactions, i.e., hydrogen bonds, electrostatic interactions, and/or hydrophobic interactions) or chemically (covalent interactions) [124]. They have the ability to uptake large amounts of water or other physiological fluids, due to the existence of hydrophilic groups (e.g., hydroxyl, amide, and sulfonic groups) on the polymeric chains, while maintaining their internal network structure [125]. There are two different approaches that can be employed for nanogel synthesis. The first one is the synthesis of polymeric molecules that self-assemble (physical cross-linking) or that have groups that can be chemically cross-linked (disulfide, amide, or imine cross-linking). The second one involves polymerization procedures followed by purifications steps [126]. Nanogels prepared through chemical cross-linking of the polymeric chains are considered to be more stable than the ones prepared through physical cross-linking, but the conditions used for their preparation (organic solvent usage, high temperatures, etc.) can damage sensitive bioactive molecules. Apart from this disadvantage, another problem related to the use of nanogels is the initial burst release of the entrapped active ingredient [127]. Drug release can be controlled by diffusion, swelling, or chemical reactions, depending on the nanogel physicochemical properties and drug-loading mechanism [126, 128]. Moreover, nanogels can exhibit a stimuli-responsive behavior, where the drug is released from the nanogel matrix as a response to changes in the temperature, pH, or the presence of enzymes. This behavior can be easily monitored by the selection of polymer and cross-linker components, leading to drug release at the target site [129]. In terms of ocular drug delivery, nanogels are gaining attention due to their biocompatibility, design flexibility, ability to incorporate or attach on their surface large amounts of bioactive molecules, and exhibit controlled or triggered drug release characteristics and mucoadhesive properties, with the latter leading to increased ocular retention time and thus increased bioavailability and patient compliance [130]. Various studies have been performed for topical ocular drug delivery of active pharmaceutical ingredients with the use of nanogels, such as antibiotics [131], antifungal agents [132], and other poorly water-soluble drugs [133]. Moreover, the use of nanogels has been observed to increase drug permeability through the cornea [132].

Novel formulation approaches, as the ones presented in Table 4.6, are oriented toward the formulation of mucoadhesive and/or in situ forming nanogels. Mucoadhesive nanogels can interact with the ocular mucosa through electrostatic, covalent, or hydrophobic interactions and prolong the ocular retention time [134, 135]. In the study of Brannigan and Khutoryanskiy [2017], a nanogel with mucoadhesive properties was prepared through the synthesis of poly((2-dimethylamino)ethyl methacrylate) quaternized with acryloyl chloride and the use of *N,N'*-methylene-bis-acrylamide for polymer cross-linking. Mucoadhesiveness depended on the degree of acryloyl chloride quaternization. Nasr and Khoee [134] developed a nanogel that apart from being mucoadhesive was also biodegradable (fitting of drug-loaded dendrimerized poly(butylene adipate) NPs to *N*-succinyl chitosan). In this study, drug loading depended on the molecular weight of the hydrophobic polymer segment and drug release depended on the degradation rate of poly(butylene adipate). In situ forming nanogels exhibit a transition from solution to gel upon ocular instillation as a response to temperature and/or pH changes. These systems have advantages such as accurate dosing and prolonged precorneal retention due to gel formation. For this purpose, thermosensitive and mucoadhesive polymers, such as Poloxamer 407 and 188, and *N*-isopropylacrylamide, have been used alone [136] or in combination with polymers sensitive to pH, for example, poly(methacrylic acid) [137]. In the study by Liu et al. [137], drug release was controlled by the gradual dissolution of Poloxamer hydrogel and the subsequent decomposition of drug-loaded NPs.

Table 4.6 Nanogel ocular drug delivery systems

Composition	Active ingredient/ Indication	Preparation method	Administration route	Advantages offered	Ref.
MC-*g*-PNtBAm	Dexamethasone/ Ocular inflammation	Polymer grafting procedure with the use of cerium ammonium nitrate	Topical administration	High drug EE (>95%), controlled biphasic DR, in vitro biocompatibility with HEC	[127]
Drug-loaded dendrimerized poly(butylene adipate) nanoparticles and S-Cs	Loteprednol etabonate/Ocular inflammation	Nanoparticle preparation, single oil-in-water emulsion/solvent technique; S-Cs grafting, carbodiimide reaction; nanogel stabilization, chitosan self-crosslinking	Topical administration	Biphasic DR (initial burst release followed by sustained release), good in vitro mucoadhesiveness	[134]
Synthesized PDMAEMA, MBA as cross-linker, and acryloyl chloride	Pilocarpine hydrochloride/ Reduction in IOP	Surfactant-free-radical polymerization in aqueous conditions, quaternized with acryloyl chloride	Topical administration	High EE (>20% of the nanogel's total weight), sustained DR (6 h), good ex vivo mucoadhesiveness to conjunctive tissues	[135]

(*Continued*)

Table 4.6 (*Continued*)

poly(NIPAAm-MAA-VP)	Ciprofloxacin/ Bacterial keratitis	Free-radical polymerization for polymer synthesis, drug loading via incubation	Ocular instillation	High EE (>95%), $T_{sol\text{-}gel}$ > 36°C and at pH 3 and 7, biphasic DR, superior in vitro antibacterial effect (vs. drug solution), in vivo enhanced efficacy in severe forms of bacterial keratitis	[136]
Amphipathic polymer QACMC and Poloxamer 407 and 188	Curcumin/ Inhibition of proliferation of HLE cells and protection of RC, RGC, and HEC	Drug-.loaded nanoemulsion formation by the film-ultrasonication method and Poloxamer addition	Ocular instillation	$T_{sol\text{-}gel}$ at 34 ± 1°C, controlled DR with a zero-order kinetics, increased in vitro corneal permeation and in vivo BA in the aqueous humor, no in vivo irritation	[137]

PDMAEMA, poly((2-dimethylamino)ethyl methacrylate); MBA, *N,N'*-methylene-bis-acrylamide; S-Cs, *N*-succinyl chitosan; IOP, intraocular pressure; EE, encapsulation efficiency; DR, drug release; BA, bioavailability; QACMC, octadecyl-quaternized carboxymethyl chitosan; HLE, human lens epithelial; RC, retinal cells; RGC, retinal ganglion cells; HEC, human corneal epithelial cells; $T_{sol\text{-}gel}$, solution-to-gel transition temperature; poly(NIPAAm-MAA-VP), poly(*N*-isopropylacrylamide-methacrylic acid-vinylpyrrolidone); MC-*g*-PNtBAm, methylcellulose modified through grafting of poly(*N-tert*-butylacrylamide) (PNtBAm) molecules.

Another approach is the formulation of self-assembled nanogels. These nanogels are formed by polymers with a hydrophilic and a hydrophobic moiety, usually produced by polymer grafting, due to hydrophobic interactions [127]. In a study by Jamard et al. [127], the grafting procedure of poly(*N-tert*-butylacrylamide) (hydrophobic moiety) to methylcellulose molecules (hydrophilic moiety) was optimized in terms of grafting degree and nanogel properties, with the degree of hydrophobization affecting the drug release rate. DEX was entrapped in the hydrophobic domains of nanogels during the self-assembly.

4.2.7 Lipid-based liquid crystals (cubosomes, hexasomes)

Lipid-based lyotropic LC NPs are drug delivery systems prepared by the addition of amphiphilic lipids (natural or synthetic) in an aqueous medium, leading to the formation of LC phases, which are then dispersed into structured NPs [140]. Several different LC phases can be produced (lamellar, hexagonal, cubic, nematic, gel, etc.), depending on the combination of different types and concentrations of amphiphilic molecules and solvent, as well as on the existing conditions, such as temperature, pressure, addition of other ingredients, pH, and ionic strength [141]. These parameters can be varied in order to accomplish the formation of thermodynamically stable LC structures under physiological conditions, even without providing energy for NP dispersion, and the triggered release of the encapsulated active ingredient [140]. The LC NPs that are most commonly studied as drug delivery systems are cubosomes and hexasomes. Cubosomes are obtained from 3D inversed bicontinuous cubic (V_2) phases. They consist of a network of aggregates that form curved bicontinuous lipid bilayers with a curvature directed toward the aliphatic chains, separating two distinct, nonintersecting hydrophilic regions [142, 143]. Hexasomes are obtained from inverse hexagonal (H_2) phases, which consist of a hexagonal lattice created by the packing of cylindrical micelles of amphiphilic molecules [142]. Their key difference, compared to other vesicular systems with lamellar phases, such as liposomes and niosomes, is their highly ordered internal molecular organization, which is characterized by a network of internal aqueous channels separated from the external aqueous environment.

Table 4.7 Ocular drug delivery systems based on liquid crystalline nanoparticles

LC NP type	Composition	Active ingredient/ Indication	Preparation method	Administration route	Advantages offered	Ref.
Hexasomes	GMO, P407, Gelucire 44/14, and QACMC	Tetrandrine/ Chronic keratitis, cataracts, retinopathy, and glaucoma	High-shear emulsification followed by ultrasonication	Topical	High EE (>90%), biphasic DR profile (initial burst release followed by sustained release), increased in vitro transcorneal permeation and longer preocular retention (vs. drug solution) resulting in increased BA in the aqueous humor	[73]
Cubosomes	GMO/P407 (9:1 weight ratio)	Timolol maleate/ Lowering of intraocular pressure	High-pressure homogenization	Topical	High EE, enhanced in vitro corneal penetration, and improved in vivo therapeutic efficacy due to longer ocular retention (vs. drug solution)	[138]
Cubosomes	Monoolein, P407	Tropicamide/ Diagnostic purposes before and after eye surgery	Ultrasonication	Topical	High EE (>95%), good physicochemical stability and biocompatibility, high in vitro corneal permeation, faster onset and a higher intensity, prolonged in vivo mydriatic effect (vs. drug solution)	[139]

P407, Poloxamer 407; QACMC, octadecyl-quaternized carboxymethyl chitosan; GMO, glyceryl monooleate; EE, encapsulation efficiency; DR, drug release; BA, bioavailability.

As ocular drug delivery systems, LC NPs, and especially cubosomes, have several advantages, such as biocompatibility (arising from the utilization of nontoxic amphiphilic lipids that have the ability to form LC phases); bioadhesiveness; ability to be loaded with active ingredients of different characteristics (e.g., lipophilic, hydrophilic, and/or amphiphilic) with a high loading capacity due to their increased internal surface area; and ability to control and sustain the release of the active ingredient, increase drug stability, and reduce drug toxicity. Moreover, they have increased physicochemical stability compared to other colloidal carriers, such as liposomes [138, 141]. Drug loading in LC NPs can result in enhanced drug bioavailability and improved therapeutic efficacy, attributed to the higher transcorneal permeation and/or prolonged ocular retention observed, as demonstrated by the examples presented in Table 4.7 [73, 138, 139]. Their similarity to biological membranes and their ability to fuse with cell lipid bilayers are the parameters that account for their permeability. Another important characteristic is their size, which is correlated with the produced ocular irritation, in vitro stability, and penetration efficiency. Finally, when a biphasic drug release profile is obtained with the use of LC NPs, characterized by an initial burst release that is followed by a period of sustained release, a faster onset of drug activity can be observed, followed by a prolonged therapeutic effect.

The cubosome's internal structure (e.g., dimensions of the hydrophilic regions located inside the cubic phase) can be controlled by the appropriate selection of amphiphilic lipids used, environmental conditions, and preparation method. Consequently, the drug encapsulation efficiency and release can be adjusted [144]. The most commonly used preparation methods are high-pressure homogenization and high-pressure sonication (top-down techniques), which employ high energy for amphiphile dispersion. However, other low-energy alternatives (bottom-up techniques, like the hydrotope method and the "salt-induced" technique) have been developed and utilized, especially for the encapsulation of sensitive macromolecules, such as proteins. Glyceryl monooleate (GMO) and phytantriol are the most commonly used amphiphilic lipids for cubic LC NPs, with the latter providing higher stability, and oleyl glycerate and phytanyl glycerate for hexagonal LC NPs [140, 141]. For preventing LC NPs' aggregation, a stabilizer is commonly added to the formulation, with the most commonly used stabilizers being Pluronic copolymers (e.g., Poloxamer 407) and polyoxyethylene stearates (Myrj series) [140].

4.2.8 Microemulsions

Microemulsions (MEs) are dispersions of an oil and an aqueous phase with a mixture of surfactants and cosurfactants as stabilizers. They are spontaneously formed, thermodynamically stable, transparent, and with a very small droplet diameter of the dispersed phase (<100 nm). As ocular drug delivery systems, they offer several advantages, such as high drug loading, easy preparation (due to their thermodynamic stability) and sterilization (due to their small droplet size and viscosity), and ability for sustained drug release. Their high content in surfactants and cosurfactants results in low surface tension, which allows good corneal spreadability, high ocular absorption, and drug transcorneal permeation [4]. Ocular MEs are usually prepared with the phase titration method by a mixture of medium chain oils and lipids with nonionic surfactants [145].

Few o/w MEs have been studied as ocular drug delivery systems (Table 4.8), for improving drug bioavailability and enhancing the therapeutic activity of the drug, through sustaining drug release, prolonging ocular retention time and increasing transcorneal permeation [146–148]. Another approach is the preparation of a drug-loaded water-in-oil (w/o) ME that undergoes phase transition upon dilution with water following ocular instillation and transforms into a bicontinuous ME or viscous liquid crystals. This behavior leads to increased preocular retention time. The globule size, viscosity, and drug release from this formulation were affected by the water content [149].

4.2.9 Nanoemulsions

Nanoemulsions (NEs) are dispersions of two immiscible liquid phases (a lipidic one and an aqueous one) with a very small mean droplet diameter (<500 nm). They can either have two phases (o/w or w/o) or multiple phases (w/o/w), depending on the volumes of the liquid phases and the type and amount of surfactants used. Apart from surfactants, cosurfactants (e.g., PG and glycerin) are often used because they can reinforce the interfacial layer created by surfactant molecules and assist in the formation and stabilization of NEs. The structure and thermodynamic stability of NEs are different to the ones observed for MEs. For their preparation, high-energy methods (e.g., high pressure homogenization) or low-energy methods (e.g., spontaneous emulsification and phase inversion) can be used alone or in combination.

In ocular drug delivery, they offer advantages such as high encapsulation efficiency, enhanced stability, controlled drug release (by variation in composition), protection and delivery of lipophilic drugs, and enhancement of drug bioavailability through increase in transcorneal permeation time and preocular retention time [150]. Moreover, their low surface tension allows them to spread evenly on the surface of the cornea and mix with the tear film, thus enhancing drug contact with the corneal epithelium [151]. Although they have advantages, their use as drug delivery systems is often limited due to problems associated with high production costs, use of increased concentrations of surfactants when low-energy production methods are employed (which can cause irritation), inability to encapsulate lipophilic active ingredients with high melting points, and limited number of ingredients that are accepted for use [150].

For improving drug bioavailability and enhancing the therapeutic efficacy of the drug, various formulation approaches have been examined (Table 4.8). One of them includes the incorporation of NE into in situ forming gels [151, 152]. In a study by Morsi et al. [151], the combination of gellan gum and xanthan gum resulted in the in situ formation of a mucoadhesive NE gel, with the gelation process being induced by ions. In another study, Patel et al. [152] used a combination of the thermoresponsive polymers Poloxamer 407 and 188 in order to achieve sol-gel transition at corneal temperature, along with a cationic agent (cetalkonium chloride) to further increase the ocular retention time. The globule size, which affects drug release and ocular absorption and irritation, of the spontaneously emulsified NE incorporated in the formulation was found to be depended on the oil phase concentration and the amount of surfactants.

Table 4.8 Microemulsions and nanoemulsions studied as ocular drug delivery systems

Carrier	Composition	Active ingredient/ Indication	Administration route	Advantages offered	Ref.
o/w ME	Oleic acid, Tween® 80, ethanol, sodium hydroxide, and COL	Ofloxacin/Bacterial keratitis	Ocular instillation	Increased preocular residence time (not affected by COL), decreased rate of DR, decreased ex vivo transcorneal permeation rate, higher in vivo antimicrobial efficacy vs. commercial drug solution	[146]
o/w ME	Isopropyl myristate, Tween 80, and propylene glycol	Voriconazole/Fungal infections	Ocular instillation	Biphasic DR profile (initial burst release followed by sustained release), enhanced ex vivo transcorneal permeation	[147]
o/w ME	Isopropyl myristate, Tween 80, Transcutol® P, and benzalkonium chloride	Gatifloxacin/ Conjunctivitis, keratitis, keratoconjunctivitis, and endophthalmitis	Ocular instillation	Controlled DR (first-order kinetics), prolonged in vivo ocular retention time and increased ex vivo transcorneal permeation, no in vivo ocular irritation, BA improvement in aqueous humor in vivo	[148]
w/o ME	Isopropyl myristate, Tween 80, and Span® 20 in an acetate buffer	Moxifloxacin/ Bacterial keratitis	Ocular instillation	Enhanced in vivo antimicrobial efficacy (vs. drug solution), sustained DR, prolonged ocular residence time, improved BA, no ocular irritation	[149]

Carrier	Composition	Active ingredient/ Indication	Administration route	Advantages offered	Ref.
o/w NE	Peanut oil, Tween 80, Cremophor® EL and Transcutol P, gellan gum with xanthan gum, and HPMC or Carbopol® 940	Acetazolamide/ Glaucoma	Topical	Reduced rate of DR, prolonged IOP lowering in vivo (vs. commercial formulation); gellan gum–xanthan gum combination: optimum mucoadhesiveness and stability	[151]
o/w NE	Capryol 90, Tween 80, Transcutol P, cetalkonium chloride, and Poloxamer 407 and 188	Loteprednol etabonate/Ocular inflammation	Topical	Sol-gel transition at corneal temperature, zero-order DR, reduced rate of DR, improved in vivo pharmacokinetics in aqueous humor and enhanced BA (vs. commercial formulations), no ocular irritation	[152]
NE	Oleic acid, Tween 20, Transcutol P, and chitosan (1% w/w)	Cyclosporine A/ Keratoconjunctivitis sicca, dry eye disorders, or for the prevention of corneal allograft rejection	Topical	Increased in vivo ocular retention, enhanced pharmacokinetics and biodistribution, no ocular irritation	[153]

(*Continued*)

Table 4.8 (*Continued*)

Carrier	Composition	Active ingredient/ Indication	Administration route	Advantages offered	Ref.
NE	Eutanol G, Lipoid S 100, Poloxamer 407 or Tween 80, and cetylpyridinium chloride	Dexamethasone acetate and polymyxin B sulfate/ Ocular infections	Topical	Prolonged precorneal retention, no cytotoxicity	[154]
NE	Transcutol HP, corn oil, Span 20, Pluronic® F68, and hydroxyethyl β-cyclodextrins	Lutein/Macular degeneration and prevention of ocular inflammation diseases	Topical	High EE (>95%), low in vitro retinal cytotoxicity, increased in vitro sclera accumulation	[155]

ME, microemulsion; NE, nanoemulsion; DR, drug release; COL, chitosan oligosaccharide lactate; Cremophor EL, polyoxyl 35 castor oil; Transcutol P, diethylene glycol monoethyl ether; HPMC, hydroxypropyl methylcellulose; IOP, intraocular pressure; Pluronic F68, Poloxamer 188.

Another approach involves the preparation of mucoadhesive NEs. These formulations can be prepared by using mucoadhesive polymers such as chitosan [153]. In a study by Akhter et al. [153], the lipid used was selected for maximum active ingredient solubilization and enhanced corneal permeation, while the mass ratio of the surfactant/cosurfactant mixture, as well as the oil phase concentration, affected the system's phase behavior and physicochemical characteristics (e.g., droplet size, ζ-potential, viscosity, and refractive index). Alternatively, mucoadhesive NEs can be prepared with the incorporation of cationic ingredients, such as the cationic drug polymyxin B sulfate and the positively charged preservative CPC [154]. Finally, a more advanced formulation strategy concerned the preparation of a hybrid system that combined cyclodextrins and NE [155]. This combination resulted in the increase of drug encapsulation efficiency and in vitro sclera accumulation of lutein.

4.2.10 Quantum Dots

Quantum dots (QDs) can be incorporated in various NPs without altering their characteristics, due to their small size and adaptable surface chemistry. Their structure consists of a semiconductor core coated by a shell providing ameliorated optical properties. Higher aqueous solubility can be obtained through capping. Targeting of diseased tissues by QDs can be performed by functionalization, that is, conjugation of targeting ligands to their surface. There are several different core/shell combinations that can be used to produce QDs, such as CdSe/ZnS, CdTe/CdSe, InP/ZnS, and CdSe/CdS/ZnS [156]. Moreover, QDs can be used for gene therapy and the delivery of siRNA for blocking the expression of genes responsible for a specific disease. However, their use in drug delivery and diagnostics is still under consideration due to issues related with long-term safety [157].

Henning and coworkers [158] studied the in vivo blockade of angiotensin II receptor type 1 (AT1R) in the eye, via the intravenous administration of novel multivalent NPs. The NPs tested were fluorescent PEGylated QDs that had attached to their surface, via covalent bonds, the active metabolite of losartan, EXP3174. The QDs prepared were characterized by intense fluorescence and a monodisperse size distribution [159]. The results of the study showed that QDs accumulated in the posterior eye segment and specifically in blood vessels of the retina and choroid. Moreover, they increased AT1R blockade, demonstrating their potential application in treating diseases such as DR and AMD [158].

4.2.11 Contact Lenses

For a decade, contact lenses (CLs) were almost exclusively used to provide clear vision by correcting focusing errors. Advances in materials and technologies have resulted in revolutionary proposals for CL applications, promising new ways for ocular drug delivery, as well as to detect, monitor, and treat diseases such as DR, DES, glaucoma, ocular allergy, and cornea infection. Nowadays, extensive research is underway for optimum modifications resulting in prolong residence time and bioavailability of drugs within therapeutic levels on the ocular surface [160]. CLs have been discussed as potential reservoirs to deliver drugs to the eye, since the mid-1960s. However, the insufficient oxygen transmission to the cornea through them leads to the development of cornea edema, making the use of CLs impossible. Later, after the invention of poly(hydroxyethyl methacrylate) (pHEMA) as hydrogel and the creation of soft CLs, it was discovered that they were responsible for the adherence of bacteria, leading to eye infections. Hence, the next step was to invent hydrophobic materials, such as cellulose acetate butyrate and siloxane-containing hydrogels, to overcome the above-mentioned obstacles and advance CLs as ocular drug control release systems (DCRSs) [161]. Drug incorporation into CLs faces many challenges before such CLs reach the market, especially due to the CLs' classification as medical devices by the regulatory boards and agencies [162]. CLs as DCRSs have to overcome the main limitation, which is the rapid drug release and the inability to sustain drug particles into the polymer matrix. As a result, CL fabrication focuses on the improvement of the bioavailability and enhancement of patient compliance; reduction of overdosing and unwanted side effects, especially in chronic diseases such as glaucoma and DES; and promotion of the safe and comfortable wearing of CLs. Ideally, CL-based drug delivery systems should involve high drug loading and controllable drug release without compromising the CLs' biomaterial properties. There is great ongoing research on techniques to increase drug retention on the ocular surface and obtain a sustained release within therapeutic levels. Pintor and coworkers reviewed the ongoing research in the field of manufacturing CLs for the treatment of DES [163]. Due to DES's multidisciplinary etiology, anti-inflammatory compounds (cyclosporine A, DEX, or diclofenac), lubricants (HA), and secretagogues (diadenosine tetraphosphate, Ap_4A) have been proposed as main pharmacological approaches. Nevertheless, in several cases these approaches only temporarily relieve symptoms, and consequently, dry eye patients continue to meet unresolved problems. Novel bioinspired materials (cyclodextrins, liposomes, surfactants, specific monomers, etc.) and techniques (i.e., molecular imprinting) are combined toward systems development that will not only prolong the contact time of the vehicle at the ocular surface but also, at the same time, slow down the drug's clearance [164]. However, most of these reports lack analytical in vivo studies. In addition, Huang et al. [165] reported the design and fabrication of a hybrid hydrogel-based CL consisting of quaternized chitosan (HTCC), graphene oxide (GO), and Ag NPs and exhibited antibacterial and antifungal functions. Furthermore, the antifungal drug voriconazole was loaded onto GO for drug retention and promotion of its sustained release. Voriconazole-loaded CLs exhibit excellent efficacy in vitro and in vivo on a fungus-infected mouse model, indicating that this CL system might be a promising therapeutic approach for the effective treatment of fungal keratitis. Design of drug-loaded multilayered CLs is a novel approach for the manufacturing lenses that ensure controlled drug release. Pimenta et al. introduced a mathematical model based on a numerical solution of Fick's second law of diffusion, useful for predicting the behavior of the drug-loaded multilayered lenses. The model shows that the proper combination of materials as well as the manipulation of the system's characteristics (thickness of the layers, diffusivity of the drugs, etc.) allow for the design of optimum multilayered therapeutic CLs for controlled drug delivery [166]. In addition, the same group developed and investigated a microfluidic cell simulating the hydrodynamic conditions of the eye, namely the low volume of tear fluid and its continuous renovation during the release of diclofenac from a conventional HEMA-based hydrogel for CLs [167]. Another artificial in vitro model mimicking tear fluid composition was also developed and investigated moxifloxacin release from some common daily disposal and silicone hydrogel CLs. Their results underline the importance of considering various ocular parameters when determining drug release from CLs [168]. However, the drug's properties (i.e., size, structure, polarity, and solubility) are not considered in any of these studies. On the opposite hand, Mahomed and coworkers [169] investigated, in vitro and in vivo, the potential use of in-eye triggered mechanisms to supplement the details of drug release from CLs under passive release conditions, by employing ophthalmic dyes and surrogates. CLs are ideally suited for controlled drug delivery for eye diseases like glaucoma that are commonly treated using eye drops, which is an inefficient method due to the rapid clearance of the drug. However, drug loading affects the optical and physical properties of CLs. Maulvi and coworkers [170] reported a study demonstrating the potential of implantation technology to treat glaucoma using CLs. In particular, they developed a sandwich system by dispersing TM-encapsulated ethyl cellulose NPs in acrylate hydrogel and implanted the same in hydrogel CLs. In vitro release kinetic data showed sustained drug release within the therapeutic window for 168 h, while in vivo pharmacokinetic studies in rabbit tear fluid showed a significant increase in the mean residence time and the area under curve with TM-implant CLs, in comparison to eye drop therapy. In addition, Ciolino et al. [171], by using female cynomolgus monkeys with glaucoma, found that sustained delivery of latanoprost by CLs is at least as effective as daily latanoprost eye drops. However, they did not determine the optimal continuous-release dose that would be effective as well as tolerated. In addition, Brandt and coworkers demonstrated the results of a long-term safety study of a bimatoprost ocular ring (BIM ring) that delivers bimatoprost over a six-month period [172]. A BIM ring is a novel system designed to release IOP-lowering medication to the surface of the eye in a sustained manner. The overall safety profile was extremely good and consistent with data from prior Phase I.

Lee et al. [173] reported the development of a vitamin E–loaded pHEMA-hydrogel CLs, which increased significantly the loading of two hydrophilic glaucoma drugs (timolol and brimonidine). The main etiology for the high loading of the drugs seems to be the vitamin E loading. Coloading of the lipophilic vitamin A resulted, as previously, in high loading of the drugs, supporting their hypothesis.

However, the release duration time was not significantly altered in all cases. In another study, Otero-Espinar and coworkers [174] showed that the use of NSs of TA significantly increases drug-loading capacity and release of soft pHEMA CLs in comparison to the drug-saturated solution.

To conclude, despite their limitations CLs undoubtedly still show great potential as an ocular drug delivery system. New polymers increase the number of CLs specific for several target groups of consumers. Ideally, CLs will be the ocular drug delivery system for the masses, for treating diseases such as glaucoma, allergy, and other photosensitive conditions. However, different regulatory bodies and agencies are very vigilant regarding these new approaches.

4.2.12 Proteins and Peptides

Corneal epithelial cells express several transporters and receptors on their surface, which aid in the transfer of various natural organic compounds (vitamins, lipids, amino acids, etc.) across the cell membrane. Nowadays, peptide transport systems in the eye have gained attention as they are potentially involved in targeted ocular drug delivery. Hence, peptides and proteins, besides their significant therapeutic role for the treatment of ocular diseases, are called to play another important role as nanocarriers for ocular drug delivery. They are highly biocompatible and biodegradable carriers and could be easily modified to link surface ligands [175]. In the next paragraphs, peptides and proteins are going to be evaluated for their role as carriers in ocular drug delivery.

CPPs are able to cross easily membrane barriers; this ability makes them the perfect candidates for delivering drugs through ocular barriers. Hence, therapeutic peptides and CPPs could perfectly complement each other, forming an optimal formula for ocular topical administration. This noninvasive delivery and cost-effective method offers great advantages for early treatment and long-term therapy to avoid chronic irreversible vision loss. CPPs are mainly short peptides incorporating polar amino acids, mostly with positive charge, that is, Lys or Arg [176]. A peptide for ocular delivery (POD), that is also a CPP, with the sequence GGG(ARKKAAKA)$_4$, was used to deliver small and large molecules across the plasma membrane. A POD compacts pDNA, achieving transgene expression in >50% of human embryonic retinoblasts. In addition, a POD rapidly enters the neutral retina and localizes to the retinal pigment epithelium (RPE), photoreceptors, and ganglion cells [177]. The same peptide penetrates the retina, cornea, and skin for delivering recombinant proteins [178]. Another CPP, TAT conjugated to aFGF-His (TAT-aFGF-His) peptide, was used to deliver acidic fibroblast growth factor (FGF) to the retina, offering protection against ischemia-reperfusion injury following topical administration to the ocular surface in rats [179]. In addition, Mousa and coworkers [180] used a nanochitosan peptide incorporating Ser, Thr, and Tyr as the signal peptide to cross and deliver active ingredients to the retina, thus providing a targeted approach for the treatment of AMD. This peptide has the potential to promote RPE binding, leading to the engulfment process essential for phagocytosis. Penetratin is another CPP, RQIKIWFQNRRMKWKKK-FAM, used to cross the defensive barriers of the eye. Liu and coworkers [181] studied the ocular permeability of this peptide. Human conjunctival epithelial cells (NHC) were exposed to several CPPs to determine the cytotoxicity and cellular uptake. Among all, penetratin exhibited an outstanding cellular uptake compared to the control peptide (polyserine–8), while the toxicity was surprisingly low. Significantly, penetratin displayed a rapid and wide distribution in both anterior and posterior segments of the eye. Furthermore, the same group [24] used penetratin for ocular gene delivery to the posterior segment of the eye and retina targeting, following a noninvasive administration route. Unfortunately, penetratin alone failed to condense the plasmid. Thus, a G3 PAMAM dendrimer, nontoxic to the ocular cells, was incorporated in a complex with penetratin, condensing the plasmid more compactly. Following instillation in the conjunctival sac of rats, the intact complexes penetrated rapidly from the ocular surface into the fundus and resided in the retina for more than 8 h, which resulted in the efficient expression of RFP in the posterior segment. Recently, Pescina et al. [182] described the synthesis of new CPPs and their diffusion and distribution inside the cornea. By using labeling techniques with 5-carboxyfluorescein and a validated ex vivo model they evaluated their diffusion behavior and distribution inside the cornea. Furthermore, confocal microscopy experiments proved the localization of the peptides in the intercellular space and/or the plasma membrane. Most of the synthesized analogs were safe and well tolerated on the human conjunctival cell line. Another recent publication came to light [183] that demonstrated a novel platform eye drop technology for ocular drug delivery of anti-VEGF drugs to the posterior segment of the eye. In particular de Cogan et al. used CPPs to deliver known anti-VEGF drugs, such as ranibizumab and bevacizumab, to the posterior segment of the eye. CPPs have also been used for siRNA delivery in the intraocular segment of the eye [184].

Another class of peptides used for ocular drug delivery is self-assembled peptides [185]. In particular, Liang et al. reported the fabrication of a peptide-based supramolecular hydrogel (Nap-GFFY) and the delivery of diclofenac sodium (DIC) as a model drug [186]. Encapsulation was achieved by simple mixing and thorough characterization by transmission electron microscopy, and rheology was performed. Release experiments as well as toxicity in vitro studies were performed, indicating that the developed nanogel was nontoxic against several cell lines (HCEC, HLEC, and L929 cells) after incubation for 24 h, a rather short period of time. Corneal penetration and ophthalmic bioavailability studies were also performed in comparison with the commercial DIC eye drops, suggesting that this formulation could be a promising system in the treatment of anterior segment disorders.

Peptide amphiphile nanofibers are also special potential tools for ocular delivery applications due to their ability to remain on the site of interest for extended periods of time, facilitating the long-term presentation of bioactive sequences [187]. These peptide nanofibers exhibited promising antiangiogenic effects for the treatment of corneal angiogenesis and were investigated in vitro and in vivo. In addition, silk hydrogels and silk fibroin were used for the delivery of (anti-VEGF) therapeutics, for example, bevacizumab, for sustained ocular drug delivery [188]. The results demonstrated a sustained release of more than 90 days in vitro as well as in vivo experiments using an intravitreal injection model in Dutch-belted rabbits.

The number of therapeutic peptides and proteins investigated for drug delivery and the treatment of ocular diseases is constantly growing, thanks to the considerable contribution of chemistry and biotechnology.

4.3 Future Challenges and Perspectives

The complex nature of the eye challenges scientists to continue their research for an ideal ocular drug delivery system. Posterior and anterior segments of the eye are anatomically different from each other in terms of the diseases affecting them, as well as medication and duration of treatment. It is crucial to understand in depth the transport, disposition, and sustained-release mechanisms in addition to the toxicological effects in every eye segment warranted for the various nanomedicine systems. Despite the numerous studies in terms of clinical translation, sustained drug delivery to the posterior segment of the eye remains an elusive target. Properties of the carriers, such as biodegradability, release mechanisms from the carriers, and duration of release, in addition to the mode of administration and patient comfort and compliance, are distinguishing features of each carrier system. Improvement in loading capacity and efficiency, without compromising on safety and toxicity of the formulations, is imperative and also of critical importance. Biodegradable implants seem more promising for prolonged release of hydrophilic entities, antibodies, peptides, and siRNA, but the necessity of an invasive placement limits their application. Macromolecule drug delivery to the eye is also challenging due to size, stability, surface charge, nonspecificity, and toxicity. Furthermore, minimally invasive approaches to sustained posterior delivery systems are expected to gain more interest in the near future.

References

1. Bisht, R., Mandal, A., Jaiswal, J. K. and Rupenthal, I. D. (2017). Nanocarrier mediated retinal drug delivery: overcoming ocular barriers to treat posterior eye diseases, *Wiley Interdiscip. Rev. Nanomed. Nanobiotechnol.*, doi: 10.1002/wnan.1473.
2. Bravo-Osuna, I., Andrés-Guerrero, V., Pastoriza Abal, P., Molina-Martínez, I. T. and Herrero-Vanrell, R. (2016). Pharmaceutical microscale and nanoscale approaches for efficient treatment of ocular diseases, *Drug Deliv. Transl. Res.*, **6**, pp. 686–707.
3. Patel, A., Cholkar, K., Agrahari, V. and Mitra, A. K. (2013). Ocular drug delivery systems: an overview, *World J. Pharmacol.*, **2**, pp. 47–64.

4. Ameeduzzafar, Ali, J., Fazil, M., Qumbar, M., Khan, N. and Ali, A. (2016). Colloidal drug delivery system: amplify the ocular delivery, *Drug Deliv.*, **23**, pp. 700–716.

5. Gaudana, R., Ananthula, H. K., Parenky, A. and Mitra, A. K. (2010). Ocular drug delivery, *AAPS J.*, **12**, pp. 348–360.

6. Almeida, H., Amaral, M. H., Lobao, P., Frigerio, C. and Sousa Lobo, J. M. (2015). Nanoparticles in ocular drug delivery systems for topical administration: promises and challenges, *Curr. Pharm. Des.*, **21**, pp. 5212–5224.

7. Sampat, K. M. and Garg, S. J. (2010). Complications of intravitreal injections, *Curr. Opin. Ophthalmol.*, **21**, pp. 178–183.

8. Witting, M., Obst, K., Friess, W. and Hedtrich, S. (2015). Recent advances in topical delivery of proteins and peptides mediated by soft matter nanocarriers, *Biotechnol. Adv.*, **33**, pp. 1355–1369.

9. Sánchez-López, E., Espina, M., Doktorovova, S., Souto, E. B. and García, M. L. (2017). Lipid nanoparticles (SLN, NLC): overcoming the anatomical and physiological barriers of the eye – Part I – Barriers and determining factors in ocular delivery, *Eur. J. Pharm. Biopharm.*, **110**, pp. 70–75.

10. Rodríguez Villanueva, J., Navarro, M. G. and Rodríguez Villanueva, L. (2016). Dendrimers as a promising tool in ocular therapeutics: latest advances and perspectives, *Int. J. Pharm.*, **511**, pp. 359–366.

11. Buhleier, E., Wehner, W. and Vögtle, F. (1978). "Cascade" and "nonskid-chain-like" syntheses of molecular cavity topologies, *Synthesis*, **1978**, pp. 155–158.

12. Tomalia, D. A., Baker, H., Dewald, J., Hall, M., Kallos, G., Martin, S., Roeck, J., Ryder, J. and Smith, P. (1985). A new class of polymers: starburst-dendritic macromolecules, *Polym. J.* **17**, pp. 117–132.

13. Kambhampati, S. P. and Kannan, R. M. (2013). Dendrimer nanoparticles for ocular drug delivery, *J. Ocul. Pharmacol. Ther.*, **29**, pp. 151–165.

14. Yavuz, B., Pehlivan, S. B. and Ünlü, N. (2013). Dendrimeric systems and their applications in ocular drug delivery, *Sci. World J.*, **2013**, Article ID 732340 (13 pp.).

15. Sorsak, E., Valh, J. V., Urek, S. K. and Lobnik, A. (2015). Application of PAMAM dendrimers in optical sensing, *Analyst*, **140**, pp. 976–989.

16. Bravo-Osuna, I., Vicario-de-la-Torre, M., Andrés-Guerrero, V., Sánchez-Nieves, J., Guzmán-Navarro, M., de la Mata, F. J., Gómez, R., de las Heras,

B., Argüeso, P., Ponchel, G., Herrero-Vanrell, R. and Molina-Martínez, I. T. (2016). Novel water-soluble mucoadhesive carbosilane dendrimers for ocular administration, *Mol. Pharmaceutics*, **13**, pp. 2966–2976.

17. Kompella, U. B., Amrite, A. C., Ravi, R. P. and Durazo, S. A. (2013). Nanomedicines for back of the eye drug delivery, gene delivery, and imaging, *Prog. Retin. Eye Res.*, **36**, pp. 172–198.
18. Mastorakos, P., Kambhampati, S. P., Mishra, M. K., Wu, T., Song, E., Hanes, J. and Kannan, R. M. (2015). Hydroxyl PAMAM dendrimer-based gene vectors for transgene delivery to human retinal pigment epithelial cells(), *Nanoscale*, **7**, pp. 3845–3856.
19. Vandamme, T. F. and Brobeck, L. (2005). Poly(amidoamine) dendrimers as ophthalmic vehicles for ocular delivery of pilocarpine nitrate and tropicamide, *J. Control. Release*, **102**, pp. 23–38.
20. Fruchon, S., Caminade, A.-M., Abadie, C., Davignon, J.-L., Combette, J.-M., Turrin, C.-O. and Poupot, R. (2013). An azabisphosphonate-capped poly(phosphorhydrazone) dendrimer for the treatment of endotoxin-induced uveitis, *Molecules*, **18**(8), pp. 9305–9316.
21. Soiberman, U., Kambhampati, S. P., Wu, T., Mishra, M. K., Oh, Y., Sharma, R., Wang, J., Al Towerki, A. E., Yiu, S., Stark, W. J. and Kannan, R. M. (2017). Subconjunctival injectable dendrimer-dexamethasone gel for the treatment of corneal inflammation, *Biomaterials*, **125**, pp. 38–53.
22. Cerofolini, L., Baldoneschi, V., Dragoni, E., Storai, A., Mamusa, M., Berti, D., Fragai, M., Richichi, B. and Nativi, C. (2017). Synthesis and binding monitoring of a new nanomolar PAMAM-based matrix metalloproteinases inhibitor (MMPIs), *Bioorg. Med. Chem.*, **25**, pp. 523–527.
23. Weng, Y., Liu, J., Jin, S., Guo, W., Liang, X. and Hu, Z. (2017). Nanotechnology-based strategies for treatment of ocular disease, *Acta Pharm. Sin. B*, **7**, pp. 281–291.
24. Liu, C., Jiang, K., Tai, L., Liu, Y., Wei, G., Lu, W. and Pan, W. (2016). Facile noninvasive retinal gene delivery enabled by penetratin, *ACS Appl. Mater. Interfaces*, **8**, pp. 19256–19267.
25. Sun, D., Maeno, H., Gujrati, M., Schur, R., Maeda, A., Maeda, T., Palczewski, K. and Lu, Z.-R. (2015). Self-assembly of a multifunctional lipid with core-shell dendrimer DNA nanoparticles enhanced efficient gene delivery at low charge ratios into RPE cells, *Macromol. Biosci.*, **15**, pp. 1663–1672.
26. Sun, D., Sahu, B., Gao, S., Schur, R. M., Vaidya, A. M., Maeda, A., Palczewski, K. and Lu, Z.-R. (2017). Targeted multifunctional lipid ECO plasmid

DNA nanoparticles as efficient non-viral gene therapy for Leber's congenital amaurosis, *Mol. Ther. Nucleic Acids*, **7**, pp. 42–52.

27. Kambhampati, S. P., Mishra, M. K., Mastorakos, P., Oh, Y., Lutty, G. A. and Kannan, R. M. (2015). Intracellular delivery of dendrimer triamcinolone acetonide conjugates into microglial and human retinal pigment epithelial cells, *Eur. J. Pharm. Biopharm.*, **95**, pp. 239–249.

28. Yavuz, B., Pehlivan, S. B., Vural, İ. and Ünlü, N. (2015). In vitro/in vivo evaluation of dexamethasone: PAMAM dendrimer complexes for retinal drug delivery, *J. Pharm. Sci.*, **104**, pp. 3814–3823.

29. Selvaraj, K., Gowthamarajan, K., Karri, V. V. S. R., Barauah, U. K., Ravisankar, V. and Jojo, G. M. (2017). Current treatment strategies and nanocarrier based approaches for the treatment and management of diabetic retinopathy, *J. Drug Target.*, **25**, pp. 386–405.

30. Kamaleddin, M. A. (2017). Nano-ophthalmology: applications and considerations, *Nanomed. Nanotechnol. Biol. Med.*, **13**, pp. 1459–1472.

31. Agarwal, R., Iezhitsa, I., Agarwal, P., Abdul Nasir, N. A., Razali, N., Alyautdin, R. and Ismail, N. M. (2016). Liposomes in topical ophthalmic drug delivery: an update, *Drug Deliv.*, **23**, pp. 1075–1091.

32. Souza, J. G., Dias, K., Pereira, T. A., Bernardi, D. S. and Lopez, R. F. V. (2014). Topical delivery of ocular therapeutics: carrier systems and physical methods, *J. Pharm. Pharmacol.*, **66**, pp. 507–530.

33. Tan, G., Yu, S., Pan, H., Li, J., Liu, D., Yuan, K., Yang, X. and Pan, W. (2017). Bioadhesive chitosan-loaded liposomes: a more efficient and higher permeable ocular delivery platform for timolol maleate, *Int. J. Biol. Macromol.*, **94**, Part A, pp. 355–363.

34. Lin, J., Wu, H., Wang, Y., Lin, J., Chen, Q. and Zhu, X. (2016). Preparation and ocular pharmacokinetics of hyaluronan acid-modified mucoadhesive liposomes, *Drug Deliv.*, **23**, pp. 1144–1151.

35. Abdelkader, H., Longman, M. R., Alany, R. G. and Pierscionek, B. (2016). Phytosome-hyaluronic acid systems for ocular delivery of L-carnosine, *Int. J. Nanomed.*, **11**, pp. 2815–2827.

36. Dong, Y., Dong, P., Huang, D., Mei, L., Xia, Y., Wang, Z., Pan, X., Li, G. and Wu, C. (2015). Fabrication and characterization of silk fibroin-coated liposomes for ocular drug delivery, *Eur. J. Pharm. Biopharm.*, **91**, pp. 82–90.

37. Lee, J., Goh, U., Lee, H.-J., Kim, J., Jeong, M. and Park, J.-H. (2017). Effective retinal penetration of lipophilic and lipid-conjugated hydrophilic agents delivered by engineered liposomes, *Mol. Pharmaceutics*, **14**, pp. 423–430.

38. Garg, V., Suri, R., Jain, G. K. and Kohli, K. (2017). Proglycosomes: a novel nano-vesicle for ocular delivery of tacrolimus, *Colloids Surf. B*, **157**, pp. 40–47.

39. Naguib, S. S., Hathout, R. M. and Mansour, S. (2017). Optimizing novel penetration enhancing hybridized vesicles for augmenting the in-vivo effect of an anti-glaucoma drug, *Drug Deliv.*, **24**, pp. 99–108.

40. Chen, H., Pan, H., Li, P., Wang, H., Wang, X., Pan, W. and Yuan, Y. (2016). The potential use of novel chitosan-coated deformable liposomes in an ocular drug delivery system, *Colloids Surf. B*, **143**, pp. 455–462.

41. Nicolosi, D., Cupri, S., Genovese, C., Tempera, G., Mattina, R. and Pignatello, R. (2015). Nanotechnology approaches for antibacterial drug delivery: preparation and microbiological evaluation of fusogenic liposomes carrying fusidic acid, *Int. J. Antimicrob. Agents*, **45**, pp. 622–626.

42. Lajunen, T., Viitala, L., Kontturi, L.-S., Laaksonen, T., Liang, H., Vuorimaa-Laukkanen, E., Viitala, T., Le Guével, X., Yliperttula, M., Murtomäki, L. and Urtti, A. (2015). Light induced cytosolic drug delivery from liposomes with gold nanoparticles, *J. Control. Release*, **203**, pp. 85–98.

43. Salem, H. F., Ahmed, S. M. and Omar, M. M. (2016). Liposomal flucytosine capped with gold nanoparticle formulations for improved ocular delivery, *Drug Des. Dev. Ther.*, **10**, pp. 277–295.

44. Huang, Y., Tao, Q., Hou, D., Hu, S., Tian, S., Chen, Y., Gui, R., Yang, L. and Wang, Y. (2017). A novel ion-exchange carrier based upon liposome-encapsulated montmorillonite for ophthalmic delivery of betaxolol hydrochloride, *Int. J. Nanomed.*, **12**, pp. 1731–1745.

45. Yu, S., Wang, Q.-M., Wang, X., Liu, D., Zhang, W., Ye, T., Yang, X. and Pan, W. (2015). Liposome incorporated ion sensitive in situ gels for opthalmic delivery of timolol maleate, *Int. J. Pharm.*, **480**, pp. 128–136.

46. Faber, K., Zorzi, G. K., Brazil, N. T., Rott, M. B. and Teixeira, H. F. (2017). siRNA-loaded liposomes: inhibition of encystment of Acanthamoeba and toxicity on the eye surface, *Chem. Biol. Drug Des.*, **90**(3), pp. 406–416.

47. Yu-Wai-Man, C., Tagalakis, A. D., Manunta, M. D., Hart, S. L. and Khaw, P. T. (2016). Receptor-targeted liposome-peptide-siRNA nanoparticles represent an efficient delivery system for MRTF silencing in conjunctival fibrosis, *Sci. Rep.*, **6**, p. 21881.

48. Lajunen, T., Hisazumi, K., Kanazawa, T., Okada, H., Seta, Y., Yliperttula, M., Urtti, A. and Takashima, Y. (2014). Topical drug delivery to retinal

pigment epithelium with microfluidizer produced small liposomes, *Eur. J. Pharm. Sci.*, **62**, pp. 23–32.

49. Rajala, A., Wang, Y., Zhu, Y., Ranjo-Bishop, M., Ma, J.-X., Mao, C. and Rajala, R. V. S. (2014). Nanoparticle-assisted targeted delivery of eye-specific genes to eyes significantly improves the vision of blind mice in vivo, *Nano Lett.*, **14**, pp. 5257–5263.

50. Abdelbary, G. A., Amin, M. M. and Zakaria, M. Y. (2017). Ocular ketoconazole-loaded proniosomal gels: formulation, ex vivo corneal permeation and in vivo studies, *Drug Deliv.*, **24**, pp. 309–319.

51. Ojeda, E., Puras, G., Agirre, M., Zarate, J., Grijalvo, S., Eritja, R., DiGiacomo, L., Caracciolo, G. and Pedraz, J.-L. (2016). The role of helper lipids in the intracellular disposition and transfection efficiency of niosome formulations for gene delivery to retinal pigment epithelial cells, *Int. J. Pharm.*, **503**, pp. 115–126.

52. Khalil, R. M., Abdelbary, G. A., Basha, M., Awad, G. E. A. and El-Hashemy, H. A. (2017). Enhancement of lomefloxacin Hcl ocular efficacy via niosomal encapsulation: in vitro characterization and in vivo evaluation, *J. Liposome Res.*, **27**(4), 312–323.

53. Paradkar, M. U. and Parmar, M. (2017). Formulation development and evaluation of Natamycin niosomal in-situ gel for ophthalmic drug delivery, *J. Drug Deliv. Sci. Technol.*, **39**, pp. 113–122.

54. Abdelbary, A., Salem, H. F., Khallaf, R. A. and Ali, A. M. A. (2017). Mucoadhesive niosomal in situ gel for ocular tissue targeting: in vitro and in vivo evaluation of lomefloxacin hydrochloride, *Pharm. Dev. Technol.*, **22**, pp. 409–417.

55. Zeng, W., Li, Q., Wan, T., Liu, C., Pan, W., Wu, Z., Zhang, G., Pan, J., Qin, M., Lin, Y., Wu, C. and Xu, Y. (2016). Hyaluronic acid-coated niosomes facilitate tacrolimus ocular delivery: mucoadhesion, precorneal retention, aqueous humor pharmacokinetics, and transcorneal permeability, *Colloids Surf. B*, **141**, pp. 28–35.

56. El-Sayed, M. M., Hussein, A. K., Sarhan, H. A. and Mansour, H. F. (2017). Flurbiprofen-loaded niosomes-in-gel system improves the ocular bioavailability of flurbiprofen in the aqueous humor, *Drug Dev. Ind. Pharm.*, **43**, pp. 902–910.

57. Khalil, R. M., Abdelbary, G. A., Basha, M., Awad, G. E. and El-Hashemy, H. A. (2017). Design and evaluation of proniosomes as a carrier for ocular delivery of lomefloxacin HCl, *J. Liposome Res.*, **27**, pp. 118–129.

58. Mashal, M., Attia, N., Puras, G., Martínez-Navarrete, G., Fernández, E. and Pedraz, J. L. (2017). Retinal gene delivery enhancement by

lycopene incorporation into cationic niosomes based on DOTMA and polysorbate 60, *J. Control. Release*, **254**, pp. 55–64.

59. Puras, G., Martínez-Navarrete, G., Mashal, M., Zárate, J., Agirre, M., Ojeda, E., Grijalvo, S., Eritja, R., Diaz-Tahoces, A., Avilés-Trigueros, M., Fernández, E. and Pedraz, J. L. (2015). Protamine/DNA/niosome ternary nonviral vectors for gene delivery to the retina: the role of protamine, *Mol. Pharmaceutics*, **12**, pp. 3658–3671.
60. Ojeda, E., Puras, G., Agirre, M., Zarate, J., Grijalvo, S., Eritja, R., Martinez-Navarrete, G., Soto-Sánchez, C., Diaz-Tahoces, A., Aviles-Trigueros, M., Fernández, E. and Pedraz, J. L. (2016). The influence of the polar head-group of synthetic cationic lipids on the transfection efficiency mediated by niosomes in rat retina and brain, *Biomaterials*, **77**, pp. 267–279.
61. Abdelbary, A. A., Abd-Elsalam, W. H. and Al-mahallawi, A. M. (2016). Fabrication of novel ultradeformable bilosomes for enhanced ocular delivery of terconazole: in vitro characterization, ex vivo permeation and in vivo safety assessment, *Int. J. Pharm.*, **513**, pp. 688–696.
62. ElMeshad, A. N. and Mohsen, A. M. (2016). Enhanced corneal permeation and antimycotic activity of itraconazole against Candida albicans via a novel nanosystem vesicle, *Drug Deliv.*, **23**, pp. 2115–2123.
63. Wadhwa, S., Paliwal, R., Paliwal, S. R. and Vyas, S. P. (2009). Nanocarriers in ocular drug delivery: an update review, *Curr. Pharm. Des.*, **15**, pp. 2724–2750.
64. Nagarwal, R. C., Kant, S., Singh, P. N., Maiti, P. and Pandit, J. K. (2009). Polymeric nanoparticulate system: a potential approach for ocular drug delivery, *J. Control. Release*, **136**, pp. 2–13.
65. Diebold, Y. and Calonge, M. (2010). Applications of nanoparticles in ophthalmology, *Prog. Retin. Eye Res.*, **29**, pp. 596–609.
66. Ludwig, A. (2005). The use of mucoadhesive polymers in ocular drug delivery, *Adv. Drug Deliv. Rev.*, **57**, pp. 1595–1639.
67. Kaur, I. P. and Kakkar, S. (2014). Nanotherapy for posterior eye diseases, *J. Control. Release*, **193**, pp. 100–112.
68. Battaglia, L., Serpe, L., Foglietta, F., Muntoni, E., Gallarate, M., Del Pozo Rodriguez, A. and Solinis, M. A. (2016). Application of lipid nanoparticles to ocular drug delivery, *Expert Opin. Drug Deliv.*, **13**, pp. 1743–1757.
69. El-Salamouni, N. S., Farid, R. M., El-Kamel, A. H. and El-Gamal, S. S. (2015). Effect of sterilization on the physical stability of brimonidine-

loaded solid lipid nanoparticles and nanostructured lipid carriers, *Int. J. Pharm.*, **496**, pp. 976–983.

70. Sánchez-López, E., Espina, M., Doktorovova, S., Souto, E. B. and García, M. L. (2017). Lipid nanoparticles (SLN, NLC): overcoming the anatomical and physiological barriers of the eye – Part II - Ocular drug-loaded lipid nanoparticles, *Eur. J. Pharm. Biopharm.*, **110**, pp. 58–69.

71. Seyfoddin, A. and Al-Kassas, R. (2013). Development of solid lipid nanoparticles and nanostructured lipid carriers for improving ocular delivery of acyclovir, *Drug Dev. Ind. Pharm.*, **39**, pp. 508–519.

72. Gan, L., Wang, J., Jiang, M., Bartlett, H., Ouyang, D., Eperjesi, F., Liu, J. and Gan, Y. (2013). Recent advances in topical ophthalmic drug delivery with lipid-based nanocarriers, *Drug Discov. Today*, **18**, pp. 290–297.

73. Li, J., Guo, X., Liu, Z., Okeke, C. I., Li, N., Zhao, H., Aggrey, M. O., Pan, W. and Wu, T. (2014). Preparation and evaluation of charged solid lipid nanoparticles of tetrandrine for ocular drug delivery system: pharmacokinetics, cytotoxicity and cellular uptake studies, *Drug Dev. Ind. Pharm.*, **40**, pp. 980–987.

74. Mohanty, B., Majumdar, D. K., Mishra, S. K., Panda, A. K. and Patnaik, S. (2015). Development and characterization of itraconazole-loaded solid lipid nanoparticles for ocular delivery, *Pharm. Dev. Technol.*, **20**, pp. 458–464.

75. Sharma, A. K., Sahoo, P. K., Majumdar, D. K., Sharma, N., Sharma, R. K. and Kumar, A. (2016). Fabrication and evaluation of lipid nanoparticulates for ocular delivery of a COX-2 inhibitor, *Drug Deliv.*, **23**, pp. 3364–3373.

76. Fangueiro, J. F., Andreani, T., Fernandes, L., Garcia, M. L., Egea, M. A., Silva, A. M. and Souto, E. B. (2014). Physicochemical characterization of epigallocatechin gallate lipid nanoparticles (EGCG-LNs) for ocular instillation, *Colloids Surf. B*, **123**, pp. 452–460.

77. Fangueiro, J. F., Calpena, A. C., Clares, B., Andreani, T., Egea, M. A., Veiga, F. J., Garcia, M. L., Silva, A. M. and Souto, E. B. (2016). Biopharmaceutical evaluation of epigallocatechin gallate-loaded cationic lipid nanoparticles (EGCG-LNs): in vivo, in vitro and ex vivo studies, *Int. J. Pharm.*, **502**, pp. 161–169.

78. Apaolaza, P. S., del Pozo-Rodríguez, A., Solinís, M. A., Rodríguez, J. M., Friedrich, U., Torrecilla, J., Weber, B. H. F. and Rodríguez-Gascón, A. (2016). Structural recovery of the retina in a retinoschisin-deficient mouse after gene replacement therapy by solid lipid nanoparticles, *Biomaterials*, **90**, pp. 40–49.

79. Baig, M. S., Ahad, A., Aslam, M., Imam, S. S., Aqil, M. and Ali, A. (2016). Application of Box–Behnken design for preparation of levofloxacin-loaded stearic acid solid lipid nanoparticles for ocular delivery: optimization, in vitro release, ocular tolerance, and antibacterial activity, *Int. J. Biol. Macromol.*, **85**, pp. 258–270.

80. Kakkar, S., Karuppayil, S. M., Raut, J. S., Giansanti, F., Papucci, L., Schiavone, N. and Kaur, I. P. (2015). Lipid-polyethylene glycol based nano-ocular formulation of ketoconazole, *Int. J. Pharm.*, **495**, pp. 276–289.

81. Araújo, J., Garcia, M. L., Mallandrich, M., Souto, E. B. and Calpena, A. C. (2012). Release profile and transscleral permeation of triamcinolone acetonide loaded nanostructured lipid carriers (TA-NLC): in vitro and ex vivo studies, *Nanomed. Nanotechnol. Biol. Med.*, **8**, pp. 1034–1041.

82. Almeida, H., Lobão, P., Frigerio, C., Fonseca, J., Silva, R., Quaresma, P., Lobo, J. M. S. and Amaral, M. H. (2016). Development of mucoadhesive and thermosensitive eyedrops to improve the ophthalmic bioavailability of ibuprofen, *J. Drug Deliv. Sci. Technol.*, **35**, pp. 69–80.

83. Tan, G., Yu, S., Li, J. and Pan, W. (2017). Development and characterization of nanostructured lipid carriers based chitosan thermosensitive hydrogel for delivery of dexamethasone, *Int. J. Biol. Macromol.*, **103**, pp. 941–947.

84. Liu, R., Liu, Z., Zhang, C. and Zhang, B. (2012). Nanostructured lipid carriers as novel ophthalmic delivery system for mangiferin: improving in vivo ocular bioavailability, *J. Pharm. Sci.*, **101**, pp. 3833–3844.

85. Tan, H., Peng, Z., Li, Q., Xu, X., Guo, S. and Tang, T. (2012). The use of quaternised chitosan-loaded PMMA to inhibit biofilm formation and downregulate the virulence-associated gene expression of antibiotic-resistant staphylococcus, *Biomaterials*, **33**, pp. 365–377.

86. Xu, X., Li, Y., Wang, F., Lv, L., Liu, J., Li, M., Guo, A., Jiang, J., Shen, Y. and Guo, S. (2013). Synthesis, in vitro and in vivo evaluation of new norcantharidin-conjugated hydroxypropyltrimethyl ammonium chloride chitosan derivatives as polymer therapeutics, *Int. J. Pharm.*, **453**, pp. 610–619.

87. Delgado, D., del Pozo-Rodríguez, A., Solinís, M. Á. and Rodríguez-Gascón, A. (2011). Understanding the mechanism of protamine in solid lipid nanoparticle-based lipofection: the importance of the entry pathway, *Eur. J. Pharm. Biopharm.*, **79**, pp. 495–502.

88. Singh, J., Chhabra, G. and Pathak, K. (2014). Development of acetazolamide-loaded, pH-triggered polymeric nanoparticulate in

situ gel for sustained ocular delivery: in vitro. ex vivo evaluation and pharmacodynamic study, *Drug Dev. Ind. Pharm.*, **40**, pp. 1223–1232.

89. Ammar, H. O., Salama, H. A., Ghorab, M. and Mahmoud, A. A. (2010). Development of dorzolamide hydrochloride in situ gel nanoemulsion for ocular delivery, *Drug Dev. Ind. Pharm.*, **36**, pp. 1330–1339.

90. Agrawal, A. K., Das, M. and Jain, S. (2012). In situ gel systems as 'smart' carriers for sustained ocular drug delivery, *Expert Opin. Drug Deliv.*, **9**, pp. 383–402.

91. Gupta, H., Aqil, M., Khar, R. K., Ali, A., Bhatnagar, A. and Mittal, G. (2010). Sparfloxacin-loaded PLGA nanoparticles for sustained ocular drug delivery, *Nanomed. Nanotechnol. Biol. Med.*, **6**, pp. 324–333.

92. Lin, H.-R. and Sung, K. C. (2000). Carbopol/pluronic phase change solutions for ophthalmic drug delivery, *J. Control. Release*, **69**, pp. 379–388.

93. Qi, H., Chen, W., Huang, C., Li, L., Chen, C., Li, W. and Wu, C. (2007). Development of a poloxamer analogs/carbopol-based in situ gelling and mucoadhesive ophthalmic delivery system for puerarin, *Int. J. Pharm.*, **337**, pp. 178–187.

94. Soltani, S., Zakeri-Milani, P., Barzegar-Jalali, M. and Jelvehgari, M. (2016). Design of eudragit RL nanoparticles by nanoemulsion method as carriers for ophthalmic drug delivery of ketotifen fumarate, *Iran. J. Basic Med. Sci.*, **19**, pp. 550–560.

95. Morsi, N., Ghorab, D., Refai, H. and Teba, H. (2016). Ketoroloac tromethamine loaded nanodispersion incorporated into thermosensitive in situ gel for prolonged ocular delivery, *Int. J. Pharm.*, **506**, pp. 57–67.

96. Shi, S., Zhang, Z., Luo, Z., Yu, J., Liang, R., Li, X. and Chen, H. (2015). Chitosan grafted methoxy poly(ethylene glycol)-poly(ε-caprolactone) nanosuspension for ocular delivery of hydrophobic diclofenac, *Sci. Rep.*, **5**, p. 11337.

97. Xu, T., Zhang, J., Chi, H. and Cao, F. (2016). Multifunctional properties of organic-inorganic hybrid nanocomposites based on chitosan derivatives and layered double hydroxides for ocular drug delivery, *Acta Biomater.*, **36**, pp. 152–163.

98. Maged, A., Mahmoud, A. A. and Ghorab, M. M. (2016). Nano spray drying technique as a novel approach to formulate stable econazole nitrate nanosuspension formulations for ocular use, *Mol. Pharmaceutics*, **13**, pp. 2951–2965.

99. Mahor, A., Prajapati, S. K., Verma, A., Gupta, R., Iyer, A. K. and Kesharwani, P. (2016). Moxifloxacin loaded gelatin nanoparticles for ocular delivery: formulation and in-vitro, in-vivo evaluation, *J. Colloid Interface Sci.*, **483**, pp. 132–138.

100. Ambhore, N. P., Dandagi, P. M. and Gadad, A. P. (2016). Formulation and comparative evaluation of HPMC and water soluble chitosan-based sparfloxacin nanosuspension for ophthalmic delivery, *Drug Deliv. Transl. Res.*, **6**, pp. 48–56.

101. Romero, G. B., Keck, C. M., Müller, R. H. and Bou-Chacra, N. A. (2016). Development of cationic nanocrystals for ocular delivery, *Eur. J. Pharm. Biopharm.*, **107**, pp. 215–222.

102. Han, H., Son, S., Son, S., Kim, N., Yhee, J. Y., Lee, J. H., Choi, J. S., Joo, C. K., Lee, H., Lee, D., Kim, W. J., Kim, S. H., Kwon, I. C., Kim, H. and Kim, K. (2016). Reducible polyethylenimine nanoparticles for efficient siRNA delivery in corneal neovascularization therapy, *Macromol. Biosci.*, **16**, pp. 1583–1597.

103. Cavallaro, G., Sardo, C., Craparo, E. F., Porsio, B. and Giammona, G. (2017). Polymeric nanoparticles for siRNA delivery: production and applications, *Int. J. Pharm.*, **525**, pp. 313–333.

104. Couvreur, P., Barratt, G., Fattal, E., Legrand, P. and Vauthier, C. (2002). Nanocapsule technology: a review, *Crit. Rev. Ther. Drug Carrier Syst.*, **19**, pp. 99–134.

105. Mora-Huertas, C. E., Fessi, H. and Elaissari, A. (2010). Polymer-based nanocapsules for drug delivery, *Int. J. Pharm.*, **385**, pp. 113–142.

106. Jager, E., Venturini, C. G., Poletto, F. S., Colome, L. M., Pohlmann, J. P., Bernardi, A., Battastini, A. M., Guterres, S. S. and Pohlmann, A. R. (2009). Sustained release from lipid-core nanocapsules by varying the core viscosity and the particle surface area, *J. Biomed. Nanotechnol.*, **5**, pp. 130–140.

107. Reimondez-Troitino, S., Alcalde, I., Csaba, N., Inigo-Portugues, A., de la Fuente, M., Bech, F., Riestra, A. C., Merayo-Lloves, J. and Alonso, M. J. (2016). Polymeric nanocapsules: a potential new therapy for corneal wound healing, *Drug Deliv. Transl. Res.*, **6**, pp. 708–721.

108. Calvo, P., Vila-Jato, J. L. and Alonso, M. A. J. (1997). Evaluation of cationic polymer-coated nanocapsules as ocular drug carriers, *Int. J. Pharm.*, **153**, pp. 41–50.

109. Cholkar, K., Patel, A., Vadlapudi, A. D. and Mitra, A. K. (2012). Novel nanomicellar formulation approaches for anterior and posterior segment ocular drug delivery, *Recent Pat. Nanomed.*, **2**, pp. 82–95.

110. Liu, S., Jones, L. and Gu, F. X. (2012). Nanomaterials for ocular drug delivery, *Macromol. Biosci.*, **12**, pp. 608–620.

111. Vaishya, R. D., Khurana, V., Patel, S. and Mitra, A. K. (2014). Controlled ocular drug delivery with nanomicelles, *Wiley Interdiscip. Rev. Nanomed. Nanobiotechnol.*, **6**, pp. 422–437.

112. Civiale, C., Licciardi, M., Cavallaro, G., Giammona, G. and Mazzone, M. G. (2009). Polyhydroxyethylaspartamide-based micelles for ocular drug delivery, *Int. J. Pharm.*, **378**, pp. 177–186.

113. Di Prima, G., Saladino, S., Bongiovi, F., Adamo, G., Ghersi, G., Pitarresi, G. and Giammona, G. (2017). Novel inulin-based mucoadhesive micelles loaded with corticosteroids as potential transcorneal permeation enhancers, *Eur. J. Pharm. Biopharm.*, **117**, pp. 385–399.

114. Licciardi, M., Scialabba, C., Sardo, C., Cavallaro, G. and Giammona, G. (2014). Amphiphilic inulin graft co-polymers as self-assembling micelles for doxorubicin delivery, *J. Mater. Chem. B*, **2**, pp. 4262–4271.

115. Sintubin, L., Verstraete, W. and Boon, N. (2012). Biologically produced nanosilver: current state and future perspectives, *Biotechnol. Bioeng.*, **109**, pp. 2422–2436.

116. Kalishwaralal, K., Barathmanikanth, S., Pandian, S. R., Deepak, V. and Gurunathan, S. (2010). Silver nano - a trove for retinal therapies, *J. Control. Release*, **145**, pp. 76–90.

117. Kalishwaralal, K., Banumathi, E., Ram Kumar Pandian, S., Deepak, V., Muniyandi, J., Eom, S. H. and Gurunathan, S. (2009). Silver nanoparticles inhibit VEGF induced cell proliferation and migration in bovine retinal endothelial cells, *Colloids Surf. B*, **73**, pp. 51–57.

118. Natesan, S., Krishnaswami, V., Ponnusamy, C., Madiyalakan, M., Woo, T. and Palanisamy, R. (2017). Hypocrellin B and nano silver loaded polymeric nanoparticles: enhanced generation of singlet oxygen for improved photodynamic therapy, *Mater. Sci. Eng. C*, **77**, pp. 935–946.

119. Anbukkarasi, M., Thomas, P. A., Sheu, J. R. and Geraldine, P. (2017). In vitro antioxidant and anticataractogenic potential of silver nanoparticles biosynthesized using an ethanolic extract of Tabernaemontana divaricata leaves, *Biomed. Pharmacother.*, **91**, pp. 467–475.

120. Jones, B. (2009). Monte Carlo calculations of microscopic dose enhancement for gold nanoparticle-aided radiation therapy, Thesis, Georgia Institute of Technology.

121. Rezaei, H., Zabihzadeh, M., Ghorbani, M., Goli Ahmadabad, F. and Mostaghimi, H. (2017). Evaluation of dose enhancement in presence

of gold nanoparticles in eye brachytherapy by 103Pd source, *Australas. Phys. Eng. Sci. med.*, **40**(3), 545–553.

122. Söderstjerna, E., Bauer, P., Cedervall, T., Abdshill, H., Johansson, F. and Johansson, U. E. (2014). Silver and gold nanoparticles exposure to in vitro cultured retina--studies on nanoparticle internalization, apoptosis, oxidative stress, glial- and microglial activity, *PLoS One*, **9**, pp. e105359.

123. Das, S. and Suresh, P. K. (2011). Nanosuspension: a new vehicle for the improvement of the delivery of drugs to the ocular surface. Application to amphotericin B, *Nanomed. Nanotechnol. Biol. Med.*, **7**, pp. 242–247.

124. Kabanov, A. V. and Vinogradov, S. V. (2009). Nanogels as pharmaceutical carriers: finite networks of infinite capabilities, *Angew. Chem. Int. Ed. Engl.*, **48**, pp. 5418–5429.

125. Neamtu, I., Rusu, A. G., Diaconu, A., Nita, L. E. and Chiriac, A. P. (2017). Basic concepts and recent advances in nanogels as carriers for medical applications, *Drug Deliv.*, **24**, pp. 539–557.

126. Zhang, H., Zhai, Y., Wang, J. and Zhai, G. (2016). New progress and prospects: the application of nanogel in drug delivery, *Mater. Sci. Eng. C*, **60**, pp. 560–568.

127. Jamard, M., Hoare, T. and Sheardown, H. (2016). Nanogels of methylcellulose hydrophobized with N-tert-butylacrylamide for ocular drug delivery, *Drug Deliv. Transl. Res.*, **6**, pp. 648–659.

128. Neamtu, I., Rusu, A. G., Diaconu, A., Nita, L. E. and Chiriac, A. P. (2017). Basic concepts and recent advances in nanogels as carriers for medical applications, *Drug Deliv.*, **24**, pp. 539–557.

129. Soni, K. S., Desale, S. S. and Bronich, T. K. (2016). Nanogels: an overview of properties, biomedical applications and obstacles to clinical translation, *J. Control. Release*, **240**, pp. 109–126.

130. Sivaram, A. J., Rajitha, P., Maya, S., Jayakumar, R. and Sabitha, M. (2015). Nanogels for delivery, imaging and therapy, *Wiley Interdiscip. Rev. Nanomed. Nanobiotechnol.*, **7**, pp. 509–533.

131. Gupta, H., Aqil, M., Khar, R. K., Ali, A., Bhatnagar, A. and Mittal, G. (2013). Nanoparticles laden in situ gel of levofloxacin for enhanced ocular retention, *Drug Deliv.* **20**, pp. 306–309.

132. Mohammed, N., Rejinold, N. S., Mangalathillam, S., Biswas, R., Nair, S. V. and Jayakumar, R. (2013). Fluconazole loaded chitin nanogels as a topical ocular drug delivery agent for corneal fungal infections, *J. Biomed. Nanotechnol.*, **9**, pp. 1521–1531.

133. Wang, G., Nie, Q., Zang, C., Zhang, B., Zhu, Q., Luo, G. and Wang, S. (2016). Self-assembled thermoresponsive nanogels prepared by reverse micelle --> positive micelle method for ophthalmic delivery of muscone, a poorly water-soluble drug, *J. Pharm. Sci.*, **105**, pp. 2752–2759.

134. Nasr, F. H. and Khoee, S. (2015). Design, characterization and in vitro evaluation of novel shell crosslinked poly(butylene adipate)-co-N-succinyl chitosan nanogels containing loteprednol etabonate: a new system for therapeutic effect enhancement via controlled drug delivery, *Eur. J. Med. Chem.*, **102**, pp. 132–142.

135. Brannigan, R. P. and Khutoryanskiy, V. V. (2017). Synthesis and evaluation of mucoadhesive acryloyl-quaternized PDMAEMA nanogels for ocular drug delivery, *Colloids Surf. B*, **155**, pp. 538–543.

136. Davaran, S., Lotfipour, F., Sedghipour, N., Sedghipour, M. R., Alimohammadi, S. and Salehi, R. (2015). Preparation and in vivo evaluation of in situ gel system as dual thermo-/pH-responsive nanocarriers for sustained ocular drug delivery, *J. Microencapsulation*, **32**, pp. 511–519.

137. Liu, R., Sun, L., Fang, S., Wang, S., Chen, J., Xiao, X. and Liu, C. (2016). Thermosensitive in situ nanogel as ophthalmic delivery system of curcumin: development, characterization, in vitro permeation and in vivo pharmacokinetic studies, *Pharm. Dev. Technol.*, **21**, pp. 576–582.

138. Huang, J., Peng, T., Li, Y., Zhan, Z., Zeng, Y., Huang, Y., Pan, X., Wu, C.-Y. and Wu, C. (2017). Ocular cubosome drug delivery system for timolol maleate: preparation, characterization, cytotoxicity, ex vivo, and in vivo evaluation, *AAPS PharmSciTech*, **18**(8), pp. 2919–2926.

139. Verma, P. and Ahuja, M. (2016). Cubic liquid crystalline nanoparticles: optimization and evaluation for ocular delivery of tropicamide, *Drug Deliv.*, **23**, pp. 3043–3054.

140. Lancelot, A., Sierra, T. and Serrano, J. L. (2014). Nanostructured liquid-crystalline particles for drug delivery, *Expert Opin. Drug Deliv.*, **11**, pp. 547–564.

141. Chen, Y., Ma, P. and Gui, S. (2014). Cubic and hexagonal liquid crystals as drug delivery systems, *BioMed Res. Int.*, **2014**, p. 815981.

142. Li, J., Wu, L., Wu, W., Wang, B., Wang, Z., Xin, H. and Xu, Q. (2013). A potential carrier based on liquid crystal nanoparticles for ophthalmic delivery of pilocarpine nitrate, *Int. J. Pharm.*, **455**, pp. 75–84.

143. Karami, Z. and Hamidi, M. (2016). Cubosomes: remarkable drug delivery potential, *Drug Discov. Today*, **21**, pp. 789–801.

144. Hartnett, T. E., O'Connor, A. J. and Ladewig, K. (2015). Cubosomes and other potential ocular drug delivery vehicles for macromolecular therapeutics, *Expert Opin. Drug Deliv.*, **12**, pp. 1513–1526.

145. Gautam, N. and Kesavan, K. (2017). Development of microemulsions for ocular delivery, *Ther. Deliv.*, **8**, pp. 313–330.

146. Ustundag-Okur, N., Gokce, E. H., Egrilmez, S., Ozer, O. and Ertan, G. (2014). Novel ofloxacin-loaded microemulsion formulations for ocular delivery, *J. Ocul. Pharmacol. Ther.*, **30**, pp. 319–332.

147. Kumar, R. and Sinha, V. R. (2014). Preparation and optimization of voriconazole microemulsion for ocular delivery, *Colloids Surf. B*, **117**, pp. 82–88.

148. Kalam, M. A., Alshamsan, A., Aljuffali, I. A., Mishra, A. K. and Sultana, Y. (2016). Delivery of gatifloxacin using microemulsion as vehicle: formulation, evaluation, transcorneal permeation and aqueous humor drug determination, *Drug Deliv.*, **23**, pp. 896–907.

149. Bharti, S. K. and Kesavan, K. (2016). Phase-transition W/O microemulsions for ocular delivery: evaluation of antibacterial activity in the treatment of bacterial keratitis, *Ocul. Immunol. Inflamm.*, **25**(4), pp. 463–474.

150. Singh, Y., Meher, J. G., Raval, K., Khan, F. A., Chaurasia, M., Jain, N. K. and Chourasia, M. K. (2017). Nanoemulsion: concepts, development and applications in drug delivery, *J. Control. Release*, **252**, pp. 28–49.

151. Morsi, N., Ibrahim, M., Refai, H. and El Sorogy, H. (2017). Nanoemulsion-based electrolyte triggered in situ gel for ocular delivery of acetazolamide, *Eur. J. Pharm. Sci.*, **104**, pp. 302–314.

152. Patel, N., Nakrani, H., Raval, M. and Sheth, N. (2016). Development of loteprednol etabonate-loaded cationic nanoemulsified in-situ ophthalmic gel for sustained delivery and enhanced ocular bioavailability, *Drug Deliv.*, **23**, pp. 3712–3723.

153. Akhter, S., Anwar, M., Siddiqui, M. A., Ahmad, I., Ahmad, J., Ahmad, M. Z., Bhatnagar, A. and Ahmad, F. J. (2016). Improving the topical ocular pharmacokinetics of an immunosuppressant agent with mucoadhesive nanoemulsions: formulation development, in-vitro and in-vivo studies, *Colloids Surf. B*, **148**, pp. 19–29.

154. Li, X., Muller, R. H., Keck, C. M. and Bou-Chacra, N. A. (2016). Mucoadhesive dexamethasone acetate-polymyxin B sulfate cationic ocular nanoemulsion--novel combinatorial formulation concept, *Pharmazie*, **71**, pp. 327–333.

155. Liu, C.-H., Lai, K.-Y., Wu, W.-C., Chen, Y.-J., Lee, W.-S. and Hsu, C.-Y. (2015). *In vitro* scleral lutein distribution by cyclodextrin containing nanoemulsions, *Chem. Pharm. Bull.*, **63**, pp. 59–67.

156. Cai, W., Shin, D.-W., Chen, K., Gheysens, O., Cao, Q., Wang, S. X., Gambhir, S. S. and Chen, X. (2006). Peptide-labeled near-infrared quantum dots for imaging tumor vasculature in living subjects *Nano Lett.*, **6**, pp. 669–676.

157. Hauck, T. S., Anderson, R. E., Fischer, H. C., Newbigging, S. and Chan, W. C. (2010). In vivo quantum-dot toxicity assessment, *Small*, **6**, pp. 138–144.

158. Hennig, R., Ohlmann, A., Staffel, J., Pollinger, K., Haunberger, A., Breunig, M., Schweda, F., Tamm, E. R. and Goepferich, A. (2015). Multivalent nanoparticles bind the retinal and choroidal vasculature, *J. Control. Release*, **220**, pp. 265–274.

159. Hild, W. A., Breunig, M. and Goepferich, A. (2008). Quantum dots – nano-sized probes for the exploration of cellular and intracellular targeting, *Eur. J. Pharm. Biopharm.*, **68**, pp. 153–168.

160. Jones, L. W., Chauhan, A., Di Girolamo, N., Sheedy, J. and Smith, E., 3rd (2016). Expert views on innovative future uses for contact lenses, *Optom. Vis. Sci.*, **93**, pp. 328–335.

161. Filipe, H. P., Henriques, J., Reis, P., Silva, P. C., Quadrado, M. J. and Serro, A. P. (2016). Contact lenses as drug controlled release systems: a narrative review, *Rev. Bras. Oftalmol.*, **75**, pp. 241–247.

162. Mosuela, R., Thapa, A., Alany, R. G. and ElShaer, A. (2017). Contact lenses: clinical evaluation, associated challenges and perspectives, *Pharm. Pharmacol. Int. J.*, **5**, pp. 2379–6367.

163. Guzman-Aranguez, A., Fonseca, B., Carracedo, G., Martin-Gil, A., Martinez-Aguila, A. and Pintor, J. (2016). Dry eye treatment based on contact lens drug delivery: a review, *Eye Contact Lens*, **42**, pp. 280–288.

164. Ribeiro, A. M., Figueiras, A. and Veiga, F. (2015). Improvements in topical ocular drug delivery systems: hydrogels and contact lenses, *J. Pharm. Pharm. Sci.*, **18**, pp. 683–695.

165. Huang, J.-F., Zhong, J., Chen, G.-P., Lin, Z.-T., Deng, Y., Liu, Y.-L., Cao, P.-Y., Wang, B., Wei, Y., Wu, T., Yuan, J. and Jiang, G.-B. (2016). A hydrogel-based hybrid theranostic contact lens for fungal keratitis, *ACS Nano*, **10**, pp. 6464–6473.

166. Pimenta, A. F. R., Serro, A. P., Paradiso, P., Saramago, B. and Colaço, R. (2016). Diffusion-based design of multi-layered ophthalmic lenses for controlled drug release, *PLoS One*, **11**, pp. e0167728.

167. Pimenta, A. F. R., Valente, A., Pereira, J. M. C., Pereira, J. C. F., Filipe, H. P., Mata, J. L. G., Colaço, R., Saramago, B. and Serro, A. P. (2016). Simulation of the hydrodynamic conditions of the eye to better reproduce the drug release from hydrogel contact lenses: experiments and modeling, *Drug Deliv. Transl. Res.*, **6**, pp. 755–762.

168. Phan, C. M., Bajgrowicz-Cieslak, M., Subbaraman, L. N. and Jones, L. (2016). Release of moxifloxacin from contact lenses using an in vitro eye model: impact of artificial tear fluid composition and mechanical rubbing, *Transl. Vis. Sci. Technol.*, **5**, p. 3.

169. Mahomed, A., Wolffsohn, J. S. and Tighe, B. J. (2016). Structural design of contact lens-based drug delivery systems; in vitro and in vivo studies of ocular triggering mechanisms, *Cont. Lens Anterior Eye*, **39**, pp. 97–105.

170. Maulvi, F. A., Lakdawala, D. H., Shaikh, A. A., Desai, A. R., Choksi, H. H., Vaidya, R. J., Ranch, K. M., Koli, A. R., Vyas, B. A. and Shah, D. O. (2016). In vitro and in vivo evaluation of novel implantation technology in hydrogel contact lenses for controlled drug delivery, *J. Control. Release*, **226**, pp. 47–56.

171. Ciolino, J. B., Ross, A. E., Tulsan, R., Watts, A. C., Wang, R. F., Zurakowski, D., Serle, J. B. and Kohane, D. S. (2016). Latanoprost-eluting contact lenses in glaucomatous monkeys, *Ophthalmology*, **123**, pp. 2085–2092.

172. Brandt, J. D., DuBiner, H. B., Benza, R., Sall, K. N., Walker, G. A. and Semba, C. P. (2017). Long-term safety and efficacy of a sustained-release bimatoprost ocular ring, *Ophthalmology*, **124**(10), pp. 1565–1566.

173. Lee, D., Cho, S., Park, H. S. and Kwon, I. (2016). Ocular drug delivery through pHEMA-hydrogel contact lenses co-loaded with lipophilic vitamins, *Sci. Rep.*, **6**, p. 34194.

174. Garcia-Millan, E., Quintans-Carballo, M. and Otero-Espinar, F. J. (2017). Improved release of triamcinolone acetonide from medicated soft contact lenses loaded with drug nanosuspensions, *Int. J. Pharm.*, **525**, pp. 226–236.

175. Pescina, S., Sonvico, F., Santi, P. and Nicoli, S. (2015). Therapeutics and carriers: the dual role of proteins in nanoparticles for ocular delivery, *Curr. Top. Med. Chem.*, **15**, pp. 369–385.

176. Sun, Q. and Xu, X. (2015). A promising future for peptides in ophthalmology: work effectively and smartly, *Curr. Med. Chem.*, **22**, pp. 1030–1040.

177. Johnson, L. N., Cashman, S. M. and Kumar-Singh, R. (2008). Cell-penetrating peptide for enhanced delivery of nucleic acids and drugs

to ocular tissues including retina and cornea, *Mol. Ther.*, **16**, pp. 107–114.

178. Johnson, L. N., Cashman, S. M., Read, S. P. and Kumar-Singh, R. (2010). Cell penetrating peptide POD mediates delivery of recombinant proteins to retina, cornea and skin, *Vis. Res.*, **50**, pp. 686–697.

179. Wang, Y., Lin, H., Lin, S., Qu, J., Xiao, J., Huang, Y., Xiao, Y., Fu, X., Yang, Y. and Li, X. (2010). Cell-penetrating peptide TAT-mediated delivery of acidic FGF to retina and protection against ischemia–reperfusion injury in rats, *J. Cell. Mol. Med.*, **14**, pp. 1998–2005.

180. Jayaraman, M. S., Bharali, D. J., Sudha, T. and Mousa, S. A. (2012). Nano chitosan peptide as a potential therapeutic carrier for retinal delivery to treat age-related macular degeneration, *Mol. Vis.*, **18**, pp. 2300–2308.

181. Liu, C., Tai, L., Zhang, W., Wei, G., Pan, W. and Lu, W. (2014). Penetratin, a potentially powerful absorption enhancer for noninvasive intraocular drug delivery, *Mol. Pharmaceutics*, **11**, pp. 1218–1227.

182. Pescina, S., Sala, M., Padula, C., Scala, M. C., Spensiero, A., Belletti, S., Gatti, R., Novellino, E., Campiglia, P., Santi, P., Nicoli, S. and Ostacolo, C. (2016). Design and synthesis of new cell penetrating peptides: diffusion and distribution inside the cornea, *Mol. Pharmaceutics*, **13**, pp. 3876–3883.

183. de Cogan, F., Hill, L. J., Lynch, A., Morgan-Warren, P. J., Lechner, J., Berwick, M. R., Peacock, A. F. A., Chen, M., Scott, R. A. H., Xu, H. and Logan, A. (2017). Topical delivery of anti-VEGF drugs to the ocular posterior segment using cell-penetrating peptides, *Invest. Ophthalmol. Vis. Sci.*, **58**, pp. 2578–2590.

184. Tai, W. and Gao, X. (2017). Functional peptides for siRNA delivery, *Adv. Drug Deliv. Rev.*, **110–111**, pp. 157–168.

185. Eskandari, S., Guerin, T., Toth, I. and Stephenson, R. J. (2017). Recent advances in self-assembled peptides: implications for targeted drug delivery and vaccine engineering, *Adv. Drug Deliv. Rev.*, **110–111**, pp. 169–187.

186. Liang, R., Luo, Z., Pu, G., Wu, W., Shi, S., Yu, J., Zhang, Z., Chen, H. and Li, X. (2016). Self-assembled peptide-based supramolecular hydrogel for ophthalmic drug delivery, *RSC Adv.*, **6**, pp. 76093–76098.

187. Senturk, B., Cubuk, M. O., Ozmen, M. C., Aydin, B., Guler, M. O. and Tekinay, A. B. (2016). Inhibition of VEGF mediated corneal neovascularization by anti-angiogenic peptide nanofibers, *Biomaterials*, **107**, pp. 124–132.

188. Lovett, M. L., Wang, X., Yucel, T., York, L., Keirstead, M., Haggerty, L. and Kaplan, D. L. (2015). Silk hydrogels for sustained ocular delivery of anti-vascular endothelial growth factor (anti-VEGF) therapeutics, *Eur. J. Pharm. Biopharm.*, **95**, pp. 271–278.

Chapter 5

Dendrimers as a Candidate for Microbicide in Prevention of HIV-1 Infection in Women: Steps toward Their Clinical Evaluation

Daniel Sepúlveda-Crespo, Jose Luis Jiménez-Fuentes, and María Angeles Muñoz-Fernández
Hospital General Universitario Gregorio Marañón,
Instituto de Investigación Sanitaria Gregorio Marañón,
Spanish HIV HGM BioBank, CIBER BBN
C/Dr. Esquerdo 27, 28007 Madrid, Spain
mmunoz.hgugm@salud.madrid.org; mmunoz.hgugm@gmail.com

5.1 Introduction

Nanotechnology is a multidisciplinary field requiring an integration of physical, chemical, and biological sciences with the field of engineering. Nanotechnology is defined as the intentional design, synthesis, characterization, and applications of materials and devices by controlling their size in the 1–100 nm range [1]. Nanotechnology is considered as an emerging, exponential, and

Drug Delivery Nanosystems: From Bioinspiration and Biomimetics to Clinical Applications
Edited by Costas Demetzos, Stergios Pispas, and Natassa Pippa

ISBN 978-981-4774-92-5 (Hardcover), 978-0-429-49054-5 (eBook)
www.panstanford.com

cutting-edge technology due to the possibility to create novel products with new features and enormous potential in a wide range of applications that will promise scientific advancements and will impact our everyday life. Some of these applications lie on the fields of medicine, cosmetics, pharmaceutics, electronics, chemical engineering, energy production, optics, environment, and food [2–5]. Interestingly enough, nanotechnology is potentially useful for medical applications because nanomaterials are similar in size to biological structures. The aim of nanotechnology-enabled medicine, nanomedicine, is to use properties and physicochemical characteristics of these nanomaterials, opening up a wide field of research for the diagnosis and treatment of diseases at the molecular level.

According to the European Science Foundation, the aim of nanomedicine may be broadly defined as follows: the process of diagnosing, treating, and preventing disease and traumatic injury; relieving pain; and preserving and improving human health by using molecular tools and molecular knowledge of the human body [6–8]. The main applications of nanomedicine are the delivery of pharmaceuticals; in vitro and in vivo diagnostics, including imaging; regenerative medicine; and implanted devices. Examples of nanomaterials with diagnostic applications in biology and medicine are liposomes, dendrimers, polymeric micelles, gold nanoparticles, quantum dots, and iron oxide crystals or fullerenes [9]. In particular, dendrimers are emerging as promising candidates for many applications in nanomedicine and deserve attention as they are used as solubility enhancers; anticancer, anti-inflammatory, and antiviral drugs; drug delivery carriers; and diagnosis and imaging agents [10–14]. In this context, the human immunodeficiency virus type 1 (HIV-1) remains a growing and evolving epidemic, but new developments and enhanced models offer promising outcomes. Nanotechnology and especially dendrimers are considered as emerging and exponential technologies with great potential in the development of novel therapeutic and preventive strategies against HIV-1 infection because they are similar in size to biological structures.

Dendritic structures are widely accepted as the fourth class of polymers, after linear, branched, and cross-linked molecular structures. This fourth architectural class is subdivided into four dendritic subclasses, namely random hyperbranched polymers, dendrigraft polymers, dendrons, and dendrimers. These dendritic architectures differ by the degree of structural control present in each of subsets [15]. Dendrons, particularly dendrimers, are the most widely researched subsets of dendritic polymers. Dendrimers are formed of three components: an initiator core, scaffold layers or generations, and functional groups at the outer surface. The nucleus molecule is demonstrated by generation 0 (G0), while successive addition of branching units leads to higher generations: G1, G2, G3, and so on. Generations are defined as the number of repeated layers with branching [16].

HIV-1 is a retrovirus that belongs to the *Lentivirus* genus in the family *Retroviridae* [17]. The HIV-1 life cycle is a multistep process that depends on sequential interactions between viral and host cell factors. After virus adsorption, HIV-1 enters the cell by virus-cell fusion. Entry of HIV-1 involves binding of gp120 to CD4, followed by binding to the coreceptor. This sequential binding leads to the release of gp41, with the subsequent fusion of the viral the host membranes [18]. Replication of the genome occurs after reverse transcription and integration into the host cell, followed by translation, proteolytic processing of the precursor polypeptide, viral proteins assembly at the cell membrane, and budding.

Unprotected heterosexual intercourse is the first route sustaining the global spread of HIV-1, being responsible for 80% of new HIV-1 infections in the world. Women are more susceptible to HIV-1 due to hormonal changes, vaginal microbial ecology and physiology, and a higher prevalence of sexually transmitted infections (STIs). Due to limited economy, lack of education, gender disparity, and violence, women cannot negotiate sexual encounters, leaving them vulnerable to unwanted pregnancy [19]. Women acquire the HIV-1 infection at least five to seven years earlier than men [20]. In the absence of an approved and effective vaccine, there is an urgent need to develop other alternative methods of pre-exposure prophylaxis. Although topical microbicides stand out as promising candidates in reducing annual HIV-1 transmission, after numerous unsuccessful clinical trials [21, 22] the failure of these microbicides turned out to be due to the presence of inflammation in either the female reproductive tract or in the semen, increasing the risk of heterosexual HIV-1 transmission [23]. Contact with amyloid fibrils present in the semen may transiently increase susceptibility to HIV-1 by perturbing mucosal barrier function and triggering localized inflammation. Therefore, HIV infection is not yet a prophylactic or curable disease.

5.2 Dendritic Structures: Dendrimers as New Tools in HIV Microbicide Strategies

Dendrimers are highly branched, star-shaped, and nanosized molecules consisting of tree-like arms or branches constructed through the sequential addition of branching units from an initiator. A dendrimer is divided into three architectural components: nucleus, interior layers with repeating units or generations, and an exterior with functional end-groups [24].

Most of the dendrimers have diameters ranging from 1 to 20 nm. The diameter of dendrimers increases linearly at a rate of around 1 nm/generation, while the surface groups increase exponentially at each generation [25]. The core and the number of the interior branching units affect the dendrimer morphology. The core affects the 3D shape of dendrimers, the interior affects the host-guest properties of dendrimers, and the charge of end-groups determines a large number of potentially reactive sites [26, 27]. The core, and especially generation number, is relevant to the 3D shape of the dendrimer. Lower generations of dendrimers are more flexible and tend to be open and amorphous structures than dendrimers of higher generations, which can adopt spherical conformations [28].

5.2.1 Synthesis

Most dendrimers are synthesized following a divergent or convergent route. The divergent method involves two stages: the activation of end-groups and the addition of branching monomer units [29]. Some advantages of this method are that it provides the ability to modify the end-groups at the outermost layer and that the physicochemical properties of dendrimers can be adjusted to specific needs. The convergent approach comprises two steps: reiterative coupling of protected/unprotected branches to produce a dendron with a functional core and the core anchoring to produce several dendrons that form the dendrimer [30]. The main advantages of this method are the control over molecular weight and the functionality in exact positions, whereas the main limitation is the difficulty in synthesizing dendrimers in large amounts because of the need to protect active sites in successive reactions. Other technologies, such as hypercores' and branched monomers' growth, double exponential growth, lego chemistry, and click chemistry are also used [28]. However, further studies are needed to select the most cost-effective synthesis strategies for their successful and correct commercialization [31].

5.2.1.1 Polyanionic carbosilane dendrimers

Most of the reported carbosilane dendrimers have been synthesized via the divergent approach. From tetraallylsilane or tetravinylsilane as core, a hydrosilylation reaction with trichlorosilane and a nucleophilic displacement of chloride by allylmagnesium bromide complete the formation of the first generation. Subsequent generations are added by repetition of the hydrosilylation and Grignard steps, and carbosilane dendrimers up to the fifth generation can be synthesized [32, 33]. The strength of carbosilane dendrimers is related to the high energy of the C–Si bond and the low polarity, endowing them with high hydrophobicity. This can be modified by functionalization of the periphery with polar moieties, turning them hydrophilic. Because of the reproducibility of this approach, additional research is focused on modifications of these dendrimers, including the change of the core and the functionalization of the dendrimer surface and interior.

The presence of the 1,3,5-trihydroxybenzene core leads to carbosilane dendrimers less congested than related dendrimers with silicon atom cores [34]. Other synthetic strategies are based on the use of thiol-ene chemistry. Allyl-terminated carbosilane dendrimers are treated with commercially available thiols under UV light to provide the functionalized dendrimers in short reaction times. The resulting solution is purified by nanofiltration through appropriate molecular weight cut-off membrane, and the solvent is eliminated by evaporation [33]. Overall, the main features of the synthetic routes to carbosilane dendrimers are their simplicity, versatility, flexibility, reproducibility, high quantitative yields of reaction, mild reaction conditions, and easy availability of reagents.

Both synthetically and economically for utilization in biomedical applications, and more specifically as microbicides against HIV, the use of carbosilane dendrimers at low generations (G0, G1, and G2) is more profitable than at high generations. As reported previously, the reaction time for the synthesis of the G3 allyl carbosilane dendrimers is too long (over 20 days) compared with G1 and G2 (2–6 days) [34]. Moreover, from a biological perspective, as antivirals, higher doses of dendrimers at low generations (<G3) are used and lower doses of dendrimers at high generations (>G3) are needed to achieve the same antiviral efficacy. This is because we should take into account other associated factors, such as cytotoxicity.

5.2.2 Characterization of Dendrimers

Due to various applications of dendrimers, there is a critical need for their physicochemical characterization by employing a wide range of analytical techniques. Several thousands of publications are related to the characterization of dendrimers, but only a few selected typical examples are illustrated (Fig. 5.1) [35]. It is essential that the researcher clearly defines the purpose and knows the limitations of analytical tools, not only to determine chemical composition of dendrimers, but also to determine their morphology, size/shape, purity, and homogeneity, among other properties.

5.2.3 Nomenclature and Types of Dendrimers

Dendrimer size is classified by generations, layers, or repetitive units. The generation count does not follow a fixed rule and is not always consistent, although it must be specified which nomenclature is followed when a dendrimer is selected. The generation can be defined taking into account the number of repeated layers forming the dendrimer, where G0 describes the dendrimer after the first reaction cycle and successive addition of repeated layers leads to higher generations. However, the most widely used nomenclature considers that each generation corresponds to the number of repeated layers with branching units, where G0 refers to the core and successive addition of branching units leads to higher generations.

To date, dendrimers with diverse functionalities and architectures have been designed: carbon/oxygen-based dendrimers (polyether, polyester, glycodendrimers), chiral dendrimers, metallodendrimers, PAMAM (polyamidoamine) dendrimers, PAMAMOS (polyamidoamine-organosilicon) dendrimers, peptide dendrimers, phosphorus-based dendrimers, PLL (polylysine) dendrimers, hybrid dendrimers, porphyrin-based dendrimer, PPI (polypropylene-imine) dendrimers, silicon-based dendrimers (silane, carbosilane, carbosiloxane, siloxane) and triazine dendrimers [28, 36].

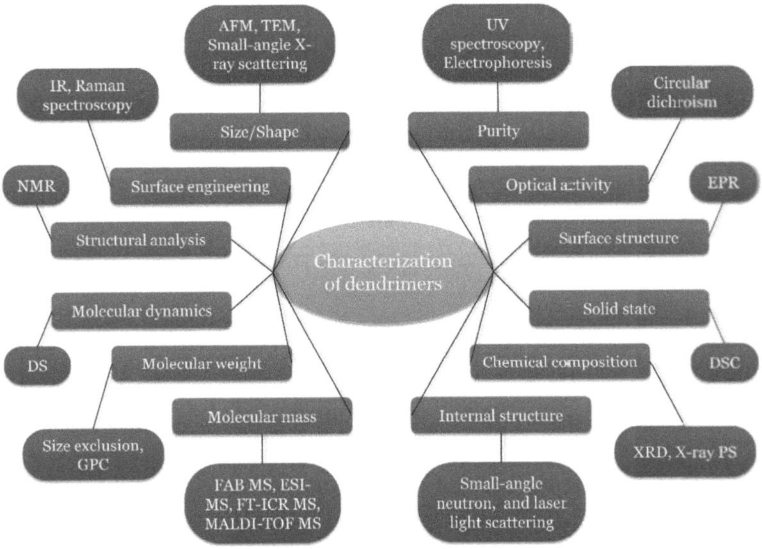

Figure 5.1 Methods for the characterization of dendrimers. AFM, atomic force microscopy; DS, dielectric spectroscopy; DSC, differential scanning calorimetry; EPR, electron paramagnetic resonance; ESI MS, electrospray ionization mass spectrometry; FAB MS, fast atom bombardment mass spectrometry; FT-ICR MS, Fourier-transform ion cyclotron resonance mass spectrometry; GPC, gel permeation chromatography; IR, infrared; MALDI-TOF MS, matrix-assisted laser desorption/ionization time-of-flight mass spectrometry; NMR, nuclear magnetic resonance; PS, photoelectron spectroscopy; TEM, transmission electron microscopy; UV, ultraviolet; XRD, X-ray diffraction.

5.2.4 Anionic and Cationic Dendrimers: Biological Applications

Dendrimers offer unique opportunities for biological applications in the synthesis of agents with antiviral activity [12, 37–44] and use as delivery agents [45–48], against both gram-positive and gram-negative bacteria [49], and potential in Alzheimer's disease [50, 51] and cancer [13, 52, 53]. The nature of the charge on the surface of dendrimer affects the distribution, and the cationic disposition of the dendrimer generates a significant impact. Surface functionality has an important effect on absorption, distribution, metabolism, and elimination properties of dendrimers [26]. Dendrimers with cationic surface groups tend to interact with negative lipid bilayer, enhancing the permeability and decreasing the integrity of the membrane, which finally causes its destabilization and cell lysis. In contrast, anionic dendrimers are less toxic due to charge repulsion, which prevents close contact between negative charges of cell membranes and dendrimers [54].

5.3 The Human Immunodeficiency Virus Type I

5.3.1 The HIV-1 Morphology and Genome

HIV-1 is a retrovirus that belongs to the *Lentivirus* genus in the family *Retroviridae*. HIV-1 are spherical particles 80–150 nm in diameter enveloped by a lipid bilayer derived from host cell membranes. The matrix shell is composed by p17 matrix proteins that internally coat the viral envelope. The innermost structural layer is the conical capsid, which is made of p24 capsid proteins. The capsid encloses two copies of noncovalently linked, unspliced, positive-sense single-stranded RNA that are stabilized with p7 nucleocapsid proteins, and it contains the enzymatic machinery required for the early steps of viral replication. The HIV-1 genome is approximately 9.8 kb and encodes 15 proteins: 9 structural, 2 essential regulatory, and 4 accessory regulatory proteins. From the 5' end to the 3'end of the genome are found gag, pol, and env genes. The gag gene encodes p17, p24, p7, and p6 proteins; the pol gene encodes reverse transcriptase (RT), integrase (IN), and protease (PR); and the env gene encodes the surface envelope glycoprotein (gp120) and the transmembrane envelope glycoprotein (gp41). Tat and Rev provide gene regulatory functions; Vif, Vpr, and Nef contribute to efficient virus spread and disease induction; and Vpu assists in the assembly of the virion [17, 55].

5.3.2 The HIV-1 Life Cycle

The HIV-1 life cycle is a multistep process that depends on sequential interactions between viral and host cell factors that can be divided into six stages, as follows:

1. Virus entry into the host cells: The first steps in the HIV-1 entry are the binding of HIV-1 gp120 to CD4 on the surface of T-helper lymphocytes or macrophages and a series of conformational changes in gp120. Initially, the D1 domain of CD4 joins the CD4-binding site of gp120, a highly conserved carbohydrate-free region. Then, the V1/V2 domain of gp120 modifies its position and its flexibility and the V3 loop extends away from the virion spike and is positioned toward the cell membrane to interact with CCR5 or CXCR4 coreceptors. Therefore, the V3 loop is the main domain involved in this interaction and V3 amino sequences determine the coreceptors used by HIV-1 for entry into the host cell [56]. The binding of gp120 to coreceptors, which involves two sequential interactions: The N-terminus of CCR5 or CXCR4 binds to the V3 loop, altering its conformation and facilitating the second interaction, with the extracellular loops of coreceptors that are critical for HIV-1 entry. These conformational changes allow the heptad repeat regions HR1 and HR2 to undergo an energetically favorable arrangement into a six-helix bundle where the HR1 domains form a central coiled-coil and the HR2 domains wrap around in an antiparallel direction. The proximity between cellular and viral membranes allows gp41 fusion and the entry of the viral capsid into host cells [56]. Finally, the location of the viral entry may or may not require the endocytosis of viral particles for full fusion [57]. In summary, the entry of HIV-1 involves binding of gp120 to CD4, followed by its binding to the coreceptor. This sequential binding leads to the release of gp41, with the subsequent fusion of the viral and host membranes [58, 59].
2. Reverse transcription: The RT catalyzes the formation of a double-stranded viral DNA using the viral RNA as a template [60]. The newly synthesized proviral DNA is the substrate for the integration process.

3. Integration: The viral DNA moves into the nucleus, and the IN catalyzes its integration into the host's genomic DNA [61]. The integrated viral DNA can reversibly remain latent in an unproductive infection or can undergo active virus production.
4. Transcription and translation: The integrated DNA is transcribed into a viral RNA, and it is translated into a long-chain polypeptide. The long polypeptide is then dissected into smaller individual proteins by the PR and undergoes further modifications to become functional [62].
5. Viral assembly, budding, and maturation: Viral proteins and two single-stranded viral RNAs are assembled, and new virions are released out of host cells, which convert the immature virion into mature infectious HIV-1 [63].

5.3.3 The HIV-1 Pandemic and the Impact of HIV-1 on Women

According to the Joint United Nations Programme on HIV and AIDS (UNAIDS) estimates, in 2015 more than 36.7 million people were living with HIV-1 globally, and women account for nearly 50% of the infected people (of these, 80% live in sub-Saharan Africa), who acquire HIV-1 mostly by heterosexual contact [64]. In the last 15 years reductions in new HIV infections and acquired immunodeficiency syndrome (AIDS)-related deaths have been generated. However, in order to reach the vision of zero new HIV infections, zero discrimination, and zero AIDS-related deaths, new targets need to be set [65]. The most common way to be infected with HIV-1 is through sexual exposure [66]. Women are more susceptible to HIV-1 than men due to hormonal changes, vaginal microbial ecology, and physiology, and a higher prevalence of STIs. The female genital tract is divided into three major parts: the vaginal mucosa, the ectocervix, and the endocervix [67]. The vaginal mucosa and the ectocervix are composed of a multilayered nonkeratinized stratified squamous epithelium, while the endocervix consists of a single-layered columnar epithelium. The intact vaginal epithelial cells have a limited permeability to particles larger than 30 nm. Cell-free HIV-1 enters vaginal epithelium by diffusing across a concentration gradient (transcytosis) and is recruited on the surface of epithelial cells until HIV-1 can be uptaken by intraepithelial Langerhans cells [68]. Successful transfer of HIV-1 results in HIV-1 uptake by dendritic cells (DCs) at the subepithelium and subsequent dissemination to draining lymph nodes. HIV-1-infected cells can also cross the epithelial barrier by physical abrasion or by transmigration [69, 70].

The transition area between ectocervix and endocervix and the endocervix are the most common sites for HIV-1 transmission, probably due to an abundance of HIV-1 target cells [71]. Epithelial disruption due to traumatic sex, dry sex, bacterial vaginosis, or STI [72] enhances the chances of HIV-1 transmission by recruiting a pool of target cells for local expansion and interfering with innate antimicrobial activity. Moreover, high levels of progesterone during the luteal phase of the menstrual cycle lead to a thinning of epithelium, increasing the risk of HIV-1 spread [73].

The first step of male-to-female heterosexual transmission of HIV-1 is the transfer of infectious HIV-1 in semen onto the female mucosal surface. Features of cervicovaginal secretions, such as the acidic pH, hydrogen peroxide, and normal vaginal microflora, protect women from HIV proliferation and acquisition [74, 75]. However, a high concentration of HIV-1 during the acute infection period increases the probability of men-to-women heterosexual transmission by up to ninefold [76]. During ejaculation, semen-borne virus exists in a cell-free form and within infected CD4+ T-cells for several hours, although the cell-free HIV-1 is more infectious [68]. Semen contains amyloid fibrils, which promote HIV-1 infection by up to 10^5-fold by facilitating virion attachment to target cells, in particular, semen-derived enhancer of viral infection (SEVI) fibrils. SEVI fibrils act as cationic bridges that simultaneously agglutinate the virus onto the cell surface and decrease the electrostatic repulsion between the negatively charged surfaces of viruses and host cells [77, 78].

5.3.4 Microbicides for the Prevention of HIV-1

Efforts to prevent the heterosexual transmission of HIV-1 are based on three approaches: behavioral change (safer sex), development of vaccines, and development of microbicides. Abstinence and use of condoms to reduce the risk of cross-sex transmission have not been successful for reasons of financial insecurity, fear of retaliation, desire for pregnancy, or avoidance of sex. Advances in vaccines have been disappointing [79–81], and topical microbicides provide excellent potential for a female-controlled preventive option that does not require negotiation, consent, or even the partners' knowledge. Thus, a microbicide is likely to become available more quickly than a vaccine, also because its use is bidirectional [21].

An ideal vaginal microbicide will:

- Display activity against most HIV-1 strains and other sexually transmitted pathogens.
- Act as a direct virucidal agent.
- Retain the activity for several hours in the presence of vaginal fluids and semen and over a broad pH range.
- Not disrupt the normal vaginal flora or the structural integrity of the vaginal (or rectal) mucosal epithelium
- Be odorless, colorless, tasteless, and stable at higher temperatures.
- Be easy to use, have a long shelf-life, be inexpensive, be readily accessible, and be compatible for use with latex, among other [22, 82].

Polyanionic carbosilane dendrimers are potential candidates for the development of new microbicides for the prevention of HIV transmission.

5.3.4.1 Formulation

The formulation of the delivery system of microbicides plays an important role in developing dosage forms with safety, acceptability, and efficacy in clinical trials. The microbicide vehicle is important because it allows the active pharmaceutical ingredients (APIs) to reach the proper site of activity, get distributed throughout the vaginal surface, and remain there for a sufficient period of time. Liquid formulations (as suspensions or solutions) are inappropriate due to their short retention/contact time on the surface vaginal. Thus, diverse formulations for the vaginal delivery of microbicides are classified as semisolid (gels, cream ointments) and solid (films, tablets, suppositories, intravaginal rings) [82–84].

For all formulations, it is important that APIs be stable in the vehicle where they are formulated and uniformly distributed, to allow distribution in the vaginal compartment [85, 86]. Physicochemical characteristics of gel vehicles to optimize are volume, viscosity, yields stress, sheer rate, pH, and osmolarity [84].

5.3.4.2 Brief evolution of clinical vaginal microbicides

The earliest compounds clinically developed as vaginal microbicides were surfactants, or detergents. These agents destroy surface-active pathogens by disrupting membranes. Three surfactants were tested clinically as microbicides: nonoxynol 9 (N-9), SAVVY® or C31G, and sodium lauryl sulfate as an invisible condom. N-9 and C31G increased the risk of HIV-1 infection [87, 88]. Although the invisible condom gel formulation was well tolerated and acceptable [89], nonspecific surfactants are no longer considered a viable option as a microbicide.

The second class of microbicides was vaginal milieu protectors, or acidic buffers. These agents act as direct acidifying agents or as enhancers of lactobacilli production, maintaining, restoring, or enhancing natural protective mechanisms within the vaginal epithelium. Carbopol® 974P (BufferGel) was well tolerated but not effective in preventing HIV-1 vaginal transmission [90]. The acid form was well tolerated during intercourse, but mild to moderate vulvar irritation was shown [91]. Moreover, natural acidic compounds based on lime juice that were effective in vitro against HIV infection showed toxicity in clinical trial formulations [92].

The next microbicide candidates evaluated were linear polyanions that block the binding of HIV-1 to target cells. These agents include carrageenan (Carraguard®) gel, cellulose sulfate (Ushercell) gel, naphthalene sulfonate (PRO2000) gel, and cellulose and acetate phthalate (CAP) gel. Carraguard, Ushercell, and PRO2000 were not effective against heterosexual HIV-1 spread and in the case of PRO2000 also showed an increased risk of HIV-1 infection [93]. Due to heavy vaginal discharge in all recipients of CAP-based microbicide, this clinical trial was declined [94].

Given the disappointing clinical trial results of early microbicides, the progress pathway of microbicides was based on the use of antiretrovirals (ARVs) that specifically act against the HIV-1 life cycle. Most of ARV-based microbicides are entry and RT inhibitors, although IN inhibitors begin to gain strength. The most studied microbicides for topical vaginal delivery are tenofovir and maraviroc. Their last results in clinic are explained in detail in the scientific literature [82, 95]. Dapivirine and UC781 have also been evaluated as vaginal microbicides in clinic studies. However, further research on UC781 has been stopped due to difficulties encountered with formulating UC781 in diverse dosage forms and in combination [96].

Owing to the lack of efficacy and adherence of linear polymers and ARVs, significant attempts have been focused on the application of nanotechnology for HIV/AIDS prevention. The only topical nanomicrobicide to enter clinic is SPL7013 dendrimer, the active product of VivaGel™. SPL7013 provided antiviral activity against HIV-1 and herpes simplex virus type 2 (HSV-2) in healthy women [97]. The lack of anti-HIV activity against R5-HIV-1 isolates [98] and evidence of mild irritation after repeated vaginal use [99] are the main limits of VivaGel. However, VivaGel is currently in a phase II trial against bacterial vaginosis [12, 95].

5.4 Biocompatibility and Toxicity

The terms "biocompatibility" and "toxicity" when we discuss dendrimers are very difficult to generalize because there are many factors to consider. Dendrimer cytotoxicity is relevant to the following features: surface charge, chemical composition, size and surface-to-volume ratio, and hydrophilicity/hydrophobicity of nanoarchitectures [100–103].

Surface characteristics have an important effect on efficacy, cellular uptake, and toxicity of dendrimers. It is well known that cationic dendrimers interact with negative biological membranes, enhancing the permeability and decreasing the integrity of membrane, which finally causes its destabilization and cell lysis [104, 105]. Moreover, various studies have shown that neutral and anionic dendrimers do not interact with biological membranes, are, consequently, less toxic than cationic dendrimers, and are mostly compatible for clinical application [105].

To discuss and to justify the use of anionic dendrimers in terms of toxicity and safety, we have to consider other factors, such as pharmacokinetics, biodistribution, and the route and frequency of administration. Polyanionic dendrimers can modulate cytokine/chemokine release. It is also important to define whether these dendrimers are biodegradable and the amount of time they need to degrade, because incorrect use can produce unacceptable toxicity in clinical trials.

5.4.1 Polyanionic Carbosilane Dendrimers: Cells and Viruses

First, it is important to choose suitable cells and viral strains to do the in vitro assays. Suitable cell lines could be human epithelial cells derived from vaginal mucosa (VK2/E6E7), uterus mucosa (HEC-1A), and colorectal epithelium (Caco-2). These three cell lines can be infected by HIV-1, but it is good to use more types of cells. For example, it would be good to use the TZM.bl cell line because it contains integrated copies of luciferase gen under control of the HIV-1 promoter [106], and HIV infection can be analyzed with the use of a luminometer, and not with a $p24^{gag}$ enzyme-linked immunosorbent assay (ELISA), which is more complicated and expensive.

The viral strains that would be good to use would be R5-tropic viral strains, because the majority of the infections during sexual intercourse are via R5-tropic. T-cells CD4+ are along the lamina propria in the human vagina (endo- and ectocervix), often under the basal membrane [107]. Most are memory T-cells, which have increased expression of CCR5 compared to T-cells circulating in peripheral blood [108]. But as it was explained before, it is important not to forget the X4 viral strains because they are present in vaginal fluids and semen. In this way, every compound should be tested using R5- and X4-tropic viral strains. Due to the difficulty that involves the use of primary viral strains, working with established laboratory viral strains would be the easier and quick method. In that case, the most common X4-tropic viral strain is the HIV-$1_{NL4.3}$ (B subtype) and in the case of R5-tropic viral strains, the more common are HIV-1_{BaL}, HIV-$1_{NL(AD8)}$ and HIV-$1_{JR\text{-}CSF}$ (B subtype). All of them can productively infect human epithelial cells.

5.4.2 Cell Viability and Stability of Dendrimers in an Acid Medium

To determine the working concentrations for the different dendrimers, cell viability and 50% toxic concentration (TC_{50}) will be measured using commercial assays. Two commercial reagents that use a colorimetric method for determining cell viability can be utilized. MTT and MTS assays require active mitochondria. Moreover, these assays measure the mitochondrial activity changing the yellow substrate that is cleaved by living cells to yield a dark-blue formazan product, not changing in case of cell toxicity. A second method to study the toxicity of the compound in the cells is using the 7-aminoactinomycin D (7-AAD) assay. 7-AAD is a fluorescent compound with a strong affinity for DNA that intercalates in double-stranded DNA. Such cells with compromised membranes will stain with 7-AAD, while in live cells with intact cell membranes the 7-AAD will not intercalate into the DNA. Another important point in the use of a vaginal microbicide is that the compound should not alter the normal vaginal flora or have spermicidal activity. Normal vaginal flora consists of different *Lactobacillus* species and other bacteria associated with fungal or bacterial vaginosis, like *Candida albicans*, *Neisseria gonorrhoeae*, or *Gardnerella vaginalis* [109]. It is important that the normal sperm survival is not altered by the use of the microbicide. The progressive motility of the sperm has to be measured using the sperm survival index, calculated from changes in progressive motility compared with a control condition. Finally, to the stability of the compounds, it is important that they can maintain their antiviral characteristics in an acidic medium, like that present in the human vagina (pH ≈ 4–5.8). An acid pH is necessary for natural protection in the vagina against pathogens. Thereby, it is important to dissolve the compounds in an acidic medium and treat different cell lines with it to probe its stability.

5.4.3 In Vitro Assays to Study the Anti-HIV Activity of Dendrimers

For a quick screening of the different dendrimers, infection assays could be conducted in the TZM.bl cell line. Following this, infection assays in human epithelial cell lines would be performed. Pretreating the cells before the infection to study the preventive activity of the compounds could determine whether the compounds could be used as potential microbicides [12, 31, 95]. To study whether the compounds are involved during HIV-1 attachment or entry steps, peripheral blood mononuclear cells (PBMCs) will be treated in the presence of the compounds and then infected at 4°C, a temperature that does not allow Env-induced membrane fusion, thus arresting the virus at the attachment step (attachment), or at 37°C, a permissive temperature for membrane fusion and consequently for viral entry (entry) [110].

One of the main paths of HIV transmission is sexual, mediated by exposure to infected cells or seminal fluid secretions in the mucosa [77]. Currently, it is not well understood whether the transmissibility is due to cell-free viruses or via cell-associated viruses. The risks of transmitting or contracting the infection are varied. Epidemiological studies indicate that the transmission is connected to the amount of infectious virus present in the genitalia. Approximately 30%–40% of new HIV infections in women occur in the vaginal epithelium, with less probability of exposure via parenteral or anal routes. During sexual intercourse, viral transmission from men to women is more efficient than the other way around, so women are more susceptible to HIV infection [20]. The vaginal or rectal epithelia are the first places where the semen containing cell-free or cell-associated viruses will be deposited. The use of trans well–permeable supports as microbicides simulating in vivo conditions for studying potential candidates has been described [111]. This type of support can be used to see whether treatment with the compounds of the epithelial cells prevents transmission of the virus through a monolayer of epithelial cells. This assay could be conducted using cell-free or cell-associated virus, simulating the natural viral transmission in the vaginal/rectal epithelia. In the case of cell-associated transmission, indicator cells such as PBMCs in the lower chamber of the trans-well can be used [112]. Once the monolayer of epithelial cells has formed, trans-epithelial electrical resistance ($\Omega \cdot cm^2$) across the monolayer of epithelial cells can be monitored using a voltmeter and an electrode to analyze that there are no alterations of the tight junction dynamics in cell culture, caused by the treatment with the compounds. This type of assay could be conducted in vitro as well as ex vivo. Different studies have shown the importance of the use of human vaginal or rectal explants to test the antiviral characteristics of the compounds in a more physiological way [113].

Unfortunately, the majority of microbicides have proved inactive or even increased the risk of HIV infection in clinical trials, most probably due to the fact that these compounds failed to prevent semen-exposed HIV infection [37, 39]. We demonstrated that a polyanionic carbosilane dendrimer, G2-S16, is active against mock and semen exposed HIV-1 and could be a promising microbicide against HIV infection [37].

5.4.4 Mechanism of Action of Dendrimers

Once the potential microbicide and its biosafety are known, the mechanism of action can be studied to better understand how the dendrimers acts. Using molecular modeling it is easy to hypothesize about the mechanism of action and determine the step of the viral cycle in which the dendrimer can act. Furthermore, in case the nanocompound fails during the clinical phase, molecular modeling could be carried out to better understand why it failed and what can be improved in order to develop a new and better nanocompound that acts against HIV infection. To complete these studies, a time-of-addition experiment could be carried out to study the stage of the HIV life cycle where the compounds act. Using a variety of ARVs that act at different steps of the viral life cycle as controls, it can be determined where the dendrimer is acting. It is important to use the microbicide at the onset of HIV infection, inhibiting viral attachment to the host cell or membrane fusion. These results could be confirmed with a gp120 capture ELISA to study the inhibitory activity of compounds on the gp120-CD4 binding. It is known that the combination of at least two families of ARVs is more effective than the use of monotherapy for HIV treatment. Therefore, the combination of different compounds is a strategy to consider in the design of new microbicides.

5.4.5 In Vivo Infection Assays to Study the Anti-HIV Activity of Dendrimers

Transmission of HIV-1 through the mucosal epithelium plays a critical role in the onset of systemic HIV-1 infection and the development of AIDS. Adult cervical and foreskin epithelia serve as an entry site for sexual transmission of HIV-1 [114]. The activity of the dendrimers should be limited to these regions. For this, we needed to have dendrimers labeled with fluorescein or another probe. The labeled dendrimer must penetrate the vaginal epithelium in BALB/c mice, detecting the bioluminescence in the vagina and in the whole animal by using the IVIS Lumina Image System and confocal microscopy [47, 115].

The EpiVaginal™ (VEC-100) ectocervical tissue model (Carl-Bertelsmann-Strasse, Gütersloh, Germany) is used to evaluate the safety of dendrimers for vaginal application. The EpiVaginal in vitro test is gradually replacing the traditional in vivo models to study vaginal irritation, due to its high reliability and reproducibility. The 3D full-thickness VEC-100 FT EpiVaginal tissue is a highly differentiated structure, which parallels in vivo tissue and is ideal for toxicity studies of feminine hygiene, vaginal care, and microbicide products. Also, the results of histopathological vaginal studies do not induce vaginal irritation, inflammation, lesions, or damage in the vaginal mucosa after dendrimer vaginal administration at different concentrations and even when repeatedly treated with high doses in rabbits, female CD1(ICR) mice [116], and female BALB/c mice [41, 43].

Finally, although rodents are the standard animal models for toxic drugs, zebrafish embryo (Daniorerio) is emerging as an important tool for toxicity testing for the opportunity to carry out fast reproducible tests [117]. The zebrafish genome has approximately 70% homology with human genome. The small size, rapid external development, optical transparency, less space and husbandry care, and easy manipulation are a few of the added advantages that play in its favor. A wide range of substances that exhibit different modes of action, solubility, volatility, and hydrophobicity have been successfully studied by this test. With this animal model we can study the embryonic mean death time, the LC50 and teratogenicity, the minimum concentration with observed effect of dendrimers, and the maximum concentration without observed effect.

5.4.6 Animal Models for HIV-1 Research

The absence of a validated animal model has been the major obstacle for selecting and evaluating compounds that will advance to human clinical trials, in particular vaccines and preventive therapies, such as vaginal microbicide candidates. Macaque models have long been used for HIV-1 microbicide testing due to the many similarities between macaques and humans with respect to genital tract anatomy and physiology [118]. However, this model has the following drawbacks: a high cost; a limited supply, preventing large-scale screening of several compounds; and the inability to employ HIV-1 for challenge studies and to test against drug-resistant HIV-1 isolates. Due to substantial differences between humans and macaques, it is unclear whether the nonhuman primate model exactly predicts what would occur in humans. Thus, a small animal model that overcomes these limitations will facilitate rapid evaluation of potential microbicide candidates.

The small animals infected in the initial attempts included mice, rats, rabbits, and cats. Although cats are not susceptible to HIV-1, the feline immunodeficiency virus (FIV) infection served as a surrogate model for HIV-1 infection in humans due to similarities in the pathogenesis with HIV-1. However, this model has many limitations and is not used: FIV lacks certain accessory genes present in HIV-1, uses CD134 rather than CD4 as a primary receptor, and can also infect B cells and CD8+ T-cells [119]. Mice, rats, and rabbits express the needed proteins for HIV-1 replication. However, none of these models supports robust viral replication or the development of the disease because the cells from these animals do not provide essential cofactors for HIV-1 replication and can express proteins that inhibit the HIV-1 infection. Although these small-animal models offer evident advantages in terms of high reproductive rates, low maintenance costs, and providing the ability to conduct studies using inbred, genetically identical animals, they are distantly related to humans. Thus, the best small-animal models for HIV-1 are based on humanized mice, genetically immune-compromised mice, and mice engrafted with human tissues to reconstitute their immune system [120].

Humanized mice are systemically reconstituted with human lymphoid cells, offering rapid, reliable, and reproducible features for HIV-1 research. NODscid and NSG (NOD/scid/gamma) mice implanted with human fetal thymus/liver cells followed by bone marrow transplantation with human CD34+ cells from the same donor lead to humanized BLT (bone marrow–liver-thymus) mice. Compared with other humanized mice models, this model shows the highest levels of human engraftment, mimics T-cells development in humans, and can be infected with HIV-1 by mucosal routes of inoculation [121–123].

5.4.7 Polyanionic Carbosilane Dendrimers as Microbicides

An effective, potent, and safe broad-spectrum topical vaginal microbicide against HIV infection activity in vitro and in vivo and against other sexually transmitted diseases must:

- Present high anti-HIV activity in urogenital epithelial cells against HIV-1-R5-tropic, HIV-1-X4-tropic, and HIV-1-dual-tropic (R5X4), various subtypes, and T/F HIV-1 strains.
- Be stable over a broad pH range (pH vagina: 4–5.8) and seminal fluid (pH: 8–8.5), maintaining the anti-HIV-1 activity.
- Be active against mock- and semen exposed HIV-1.
- Decrease HIV-1 infection when pretreatment of cells is done for short periods of time and its inhibitory effect is prolonged over time, protecting the monolayer against tight junction disruption induced by HIV-1, impeding HIV-1 partial transmission through the epithelial monolayer, and blocking subsequent HIV-1 infection of PBMC.
- Not induce cell proliferation; not modify the expression of CD4, CD8, CCR5, and CXCR4; and not alter markers of activation in subsets of PBMC.
- Not alter vaginal microbiota.
- Retain its antiviral activity for up to 2–3 h after HIV-1 inoculation.
- Block an early step in the HIV-1 infection cycle.
- Act nonspecifically toward Env- and CD4-expressing cells in a dose-dependent manner though specifically so toward the host CD4 cells (being involved in HIV-1 attachment and HIV-1 entry steps on activated PBMCs, the dendrimer treatment against HIV-1 decreases the infectivity of the viral particles in a dose-dependent and tropism-independent manner, indicating that the dendrimer acts strongly on the virion, inactivating it).
- Not alter the sperm motility and not affect other sperm functions.
- Not produce detected irritation and vaginal lesions in rabbits after two weeks of intravaginal application or in female CD1(ICR) or BALB/c mice after vaginal administration. The application of one dose of 1.5%, 3%, and 4.5% of the

dendrimer HEC gel–treated BALB/c at various consecutive times must not cause disruption of the epithelial cells and must not produce damage in the vaginal mucosa. Adult cervical and foreskin epithelia serve as an entry site for sexual transmission of HIV-1. The activity of the dendrimer should be limited to these regions.

- Penetrate the vaginal epithelium in BALB/c mice, detecting the bioluminescence in the vagina and in the whole animal with the help of IVIS Lumina Image System and confocal microscopy.
- Demonstrate that the dendrimer does not cause vaginal irritation, with the use of the EpiVaginal in vitro test.
- Must inhibit HIV-1 infection by more than 85% in humanized BLT mice without symptoms, including inflammation and vaginal irritation.

A dendrimer with these characteristics stands up as an ideal candidate for the development of a topical microbicide against HIV-1 infection. This dendrimer will be ready to step into the clinical trials.

References

1. Sahoo, S. K., Parveen, S. and Panda, J. J. (2007). The present and future of nanotechnology in human health care, *Nanomedicine*, **3**, pp. 20–31.
2. Chan, W. C. W., Khademhosseini, A., Mohwald, H., Parak, W. J., Miller, J. F., Ozcan, A. and Weiss, P. S. (2017). Accelerating advances in science, engineering, and medicine through nanoscience and nanotechnology, *ACS Nano*, **11**, pp. 3423–3424.
3. Chan, W. W., Chhowalla, M., Glotzer, S., Gogotsi, Y., Hafner, J. H., Hammond, P. T., Hersam, M. C., Javey, A., Kagan, C. R., Khademhosseini, A., Kotov, N. A., Lee, S. T., Li, Y., Mohwald, H., Mulvaney, P. A., Nel, A. E., Nordlander, P. J., Parak, W. J., Penner, R. M., Rogach, A. L., Schaak, R. E., Stevens, M. M., Wee, A. T., Willson, C. G., Fernandez, L. E. and Weiss, P. S. (2016). Nanoscience and nanotechnology impacting diverse fields of science, engineering, and medicine, *ACS Nano*, **10**, pp. 10615–10617.
4. Formoso, P., Muzzalupo, R., Tavano, L., De Filpo, G. and Nicoletta, F. P. (2016). Nanotechnology for the environment and medicine, *Mini Rev. Med. Chem.*, **16**, pp. 668–675.
5. Jahangirian, H., Lemraski, E. G., Webster, T. J., Rafiee-Moghaddam, R. and Abdollahi, Y. (2017). A review of drug delivery systems based

on nanotechnology and green chemistry: green nanomedicine, *Int. J. Nanomed.*, **12**, pp. 2957–2978.

6. Alakhova, D. Y. and Kabanov, A. V. (2015). Nanomedicine and nanotechnology are rapidly developing fields across the nation and worldwide, *J. Control. Release*, **208**, p. 1.
7. Londono, M. E. (2015). [Nanotechnology and nanomedicine: advances and promises for human health], *Biomedica*, **35**, pp. 451–453.
8. Satalkar, P., Elger, B. S. and Shaw, D. M. (2015). Defining nano, nanotechnology and nanomedicine: why should it matter?, *Sci. Eng. Ethics*, **22**, pp. 1255–1276.
9. Berkner, S., Schwirn, K. and Voelker, D. (2016). Nanopharmaceuticals: tiny challenges for the environmental risk assessment of pharmaceuticals, *Environ. Toxicol. Chem.*, **35**, pp. 780–787.
10. Hsu, H. J., Bugno, J., Lee, S. R. and Hong, S. (2017). Dendrimer-based nanocarriers: a versatile platform for drug delivery, *Wiley Interdiscip. Rev. Nanomed. Nanobiotechnol.*, **9**, doi: 10.1002/wnan.1409.
11. Li, D., Wen, S. and Shi, X. (2015). Dendrimer-entrapped metal colloids as imaging agents, *Wiley Interdiscip. Rev. Nanomed. Nanobiotechnol.*, **7**, pp. 678–690.
12. Sepulveda-Crespo, D., Gomez, R., de la Mata, F. J., Jimenez, J. L. and Munoz-Fernandez, M. A. (2015). Polyanionic carbosilane dendrimer-conjugated antiviral drugs as efficient microbicides: recent trends and developments in HIV treatment/therapy, *Nanomedicine*, **11**, pp. 1481–1498.
13. Sharma, A. K., Gothwal, A., Kesharwani, P., Alsaab, H., Iyer, A. K. and Gupta, U. (2017). Dendrimer nanoarchitectures for cancer diagnosis and anticancer drug delivery, *Drug Discov. Today*, **22**, pp. 314–326.
14. Svenson, S. (2015). The dendrimer paradox--high medical expectations but poor clinical translation, *Chem. Soc. Rev.*, **44**, pp. 4131–4144.
15. Abbasi, E., Aval, S. F., Akbarzadeh, A., Milani, M., Nasrabadi, H. T., Joo, S. W., Hanifehpour, Y., Nejati-Koshki, K. and Pashaei-Asl, R. (2014). Dendrimers: synthesis, applications, and properties, *Nanoscale Res. Lett.*, **9**, p. 247.
16. Carlmark, A., Hawker, C., Hult, A. and Malkoch, M. (2009). New methodologies in the construction of dendritic materials, *Chem. Soc. Rev.*, **38**, pp. 352–362.
17. Goodsell, D. S. (2015). Illustrations of the HIV life cycle, *Curr. Top. Microbiol. Immunol.*, **389**, pp. 243–252.

18. Lu, L., Yu, F., Cai, L., Debnath, A. K. and Jiang, S. (2016). Development of small-molecule HIV entry inhibitors specifically targeting gp120 or gp41, *Curr. Top. Med. Chem.*, **16**, pp. 1074–1090.

19. Quinn, T. C. and Overbaugh, J. (2005). HIV/AIDS in women: an expanding epidemic, *Science*, **308**, pp. 1582–1583.

20. UNAIDS (2015). How AIDS changed everything: MDG6; 15 years, 15 lessons of hope from the AIDS response.

21. Alexandre, K. B., Mufhandu, H. T., London, G. M., Chakauya, E. and Khati, M. (2016). Progress and Perspectives on HIV-1 microbicide development, *Virology*, **497**, pp. 69–80.

22. Fernandez-Romero, J. A., Teleshova, N., Zydowsky, T. M. and Robbiani, M. (2015). Preclinical assessments of vaginal microbicide candidate safety and efficacy, *Adv. Drug Deliv. Rev.*, **92**, pp. 27–38.

23. Southern, P. J. (2013). Missing out on the biology of heterosexual HIV-1 transmission, *Trends Microbiol.*, **21**, pp. 245–252.

24. Tomalia, D. A. (1996). Starburst dendrimers: nanoscopic supermolecules according to dendritic rules and principles, *Macromol. Symp.*, **101**, pp. 243–255.

25. Svenson, S. and Tomalia, D. A. (2005). Dendrimers in biomedical applications--reflections on the field, *Adv. Drug Deliv. Rev.*, **57**, pp. 2106–2129.

26. Kaminskas, L. M., Boyd, B. J. and Porter, C. J. (2011). Dendrimer pharmacokinetics: the effect of size, structure and surface characteristics on ADME properties, *Nanomedicine (Lond)*, **6**, pp. 1063–1084.

27. Kannan, R. M., Nance, E., Kannan, S. and Tomalia, D. A. (2014). Emerging concepts in dendrimer-based nanomedicine: from design principles to clinical applications, *J. Intern. Med.*, **276**, pp. 579–617.

28. Kesharwani, P., Jain, K. and Jain, N. K. (2014). Dendrimer as nanocarrier for drug delivery, *Prog. Polym. Sci.*, **39**, pp. 268–307.

29. Tomalia, D. A., Baker, H., Dewald, J., Hall, M., Kallos, S., Roeck, J., Ryder, J. and Smith, P. (1985). A new class of polymers: starburst-dendritic macromolecules, *Polym. J.*, **17**, pp. 117–132.

30. Hawker, C. J. and Fréchet, J. M. J. (1990). Preparation of polymers with controlled molecular architecture. A new convergent approach to dendritic macromolecules, *J. Am. Chem. Soc.*, **112**, pp. 7638–7647.

31. Sepulveda-Crespo, D., Cena-Diez, R., Jimenez, J. L. and Angeles Munoz-Fernandez, M. (2017). Mechanistic studies of viral entry: an overview

of dendrimer-based microbicides as entry inhibitors against both HIV and HSV-2 overlapped infections, *Med. Res. Rev.*, **37**, pp. 149–179.

32. Galan, M., Sanchez-Rodriguez, J., Cangiotti, M., Garcia-Gallego, S., Jimenez, J. L., Gomez, R., Ottaviani, M. F., Munoz-Fernandez, M. A. and de la Mata, F. J. (2012). Antiviral properties against HIV of water soluble copper carbosilane dendrimers and their EPR characterization, *Curr. Med. Chem.*, **19**, pp. 4984–4994.
33. Galan, M., Sanchez Rodriguez, J., Jimenez, J. L., Relloso, M., Maly, M., de la Mata, F. J., Munoz-Fernandez, M. A. and Gomez, R. (2014). Synthesis of new anionic carbosilane dendrimers via thiol-ene chemistry and their antiviral behaviour, *Org. Biomol. Chem.*, **12**, pp. 3222–3237.
34. Sánchez-Nieves, J., Ortega, P., Muñoz-Fernandez, M. A., Gomez, R. and de la Mata, F. J. (2010). Synthesis of carbosilane dendrons and dendrimers derived from 1,3,5-trihydroxybenzene, *Tetrahedron*, **66**, pp. 9203–9213.
35. Cho, E. J., Holback, H., Liu, K. C., Abouelmagd, S. A., Park, J. and Yeo, Y. (2013). Nanoparticle characterization: state of the art, challenges, and emerging technologies, *Mol. Pharmaceutics*, **10**, pp. 2093–2110.
36. Vögtle, F., Richardt, G. and Werner, N. (2009). Types of dendrimers and their syntheses, in *Dendrimer Chemistry: Concepts, Syntheses, Properties, Applications*, Wiley-VCH Verlag GmbH and Co. KGaA, Weinham, Germany, pp. 81–167.
37. Cena-Diez, R., Garcia-Broncano, P., de la Mata, F. J., Gomez, R. and Munoz-Fernandez, M. A. (2016). Efficacy of HIV antiviral polyanionic carbosilane dendrimer G2-S16 in the presence of semen, *Int. J. Nanomed.*, **11**, pp. 2443–2450.
38. Cena-Diez, R., Vacas-Cordoba, E., Garcia-Broncano, P., de la Mata, F. J., Gomez, R., Maly, M. and Munoz-Fernandez, M. A. (2016). Prevention of vaginal and rectal herpes simplex virus type 2 transmission in mice: mechanism of antiviral action, *Int. J. Nanomed.*, **11**, pp. 2147–2162.
39. Garcia-Broncano, P., Cena-Diez, R., de la Mata, F. J., Gomez, R., Resino, S. and Munoz-Fernandez, M. A. (2017). Efficacy of carbosilane dendrimers with an antiretroviral combination against HIV-1 in the presence of semen-derived enhancer of viral infection, *Eur. J. Pharmacol.*, **811**, pp. 155–163.
40. Parboosing, R., Chonco, L., de la Mata, F. J., Govender, T., Maguire, G. E. and Kruger, H. G. (2017). Potential inhibition of HIV-1 encapsidation by oligoribonucleotide-dendrimer nanoparticle complexes, *Int. J. Nanomed.*, **12**, pp. 317–325.

41. Sanchez-Rodriguez, J., Diaz, L., Galan, M., Maly, M., Gomez, R., de la Mata F. J., Jimenez, J. L. and Munoz-Fernandez, M. A. (2015). Anti-human immunodeficiency virus activity of thiol-ene carbosilane dendrimers and their potential development as a topical microbicide, *J. Biomed. Nanotechnol.*, **11**, pp. 1783–1798.

42. Sepulveda-Crespo, D., Jimenez, J. L., Gomez, R., de la Mata, F. J., Majano, P. L., Munoz-Fernandez, M. A. and Gastaminza, P. (2017). Polyanionic carbosilane dendrimers prevent hepatitis C virus infection in cell culture, *Nanomedicine*, **13**, pp. 49–58.

43. Sepulveda-Crespo, D., Serramia, M. J., Tager, A. M., Vrbanac, V., Gomez, R., de la Mata, F. J., Jimenez, J. L. and Munoz-Fernandez, M. A. (2015). Prevention vaginally of HIV-1 transmission in humanized BLT mice and mode of antiviral action of polyanionic carbosilane dendrimer G2-S16, *Nanomedicine*, **11**, pp. 1299–1308.

44. Vacas-Cordoba, E., Maly, M., de la Mata, F. J., Gomez, R., Pion, M. and Munoz-Fernandez, M. A. (2016). Antiviral mechanism of polyanionic carbosilane dendrimers against HIV-1, *Int. J. Nanomed.*, **11**, pp. 1281–1294.

45. Melikishvili, S., Poturnayova, A., Ionov, M., Bryszewska, M., Vary, T., Cirak, J., Munoz-Fernandez, M. A., Gomez-Ramirez, R., de la Mata, F. J. and Hianik, T. (2016). The effect of polyethylene glycol-modified lipids on the interaction of HIV-1 derived peptide-dendrimer complexes with lipid membranes, *Biochim. Biophys. Acta*, **1858**, pp. 3005–3016.

46. Sepulveda-Crespo, D., Vacas-Cordoba, E., Marquez-Miranda, V., Araya-Duran, I., Gomez, R., Mata, F. J., Gonzalez-Nilo, F. D. and Munoz-Fernandez, M. A. (2016). Effect of several HIV antigens simultaneously loaded with G2-NN16 carbosilane dendrimer in the cell uptake and functionality of human dendritic cells, *Bioconjugate Chem.*, **27**, pp. 2844–2849.

47. Serramia, M. J., Alvarez, S., Fuentes-Paniagua, E., Clemente, M. I., Sanchez-Nieves, J., Gomez, R., de la Mata, J. and Munoz-Fernandez, M. A. (2015). In vivo delivery of siRNA to the brain by carbosilane dendrimer, *J. Control. Release*, **200**, pp. 60–70.

48. Shcharbin, D., Shcharbina, N., Dzmitruk, V., Pedziwiatr-Werbicka, E., Ionov, M., Mignani, S., de la Mata, F. J., Gomez, R., Munoz-Fernandez, M. A., Majoral, J. P. and Bryszewska, M. (2017). Dendrimer-protein interactions versus dendrimer-based nanomedicine, *Colloids Surf. B*, **152**, pp. 414–422.

49. Leire, E., Amaral, S. P., Louzao, I., Winzer, K., Alexander, C., Fernandez-Megia, E. and Fernandez-Trillo, F. (2016). Dendrimer mediated

clustering of bacteria: improved aggregation and evaluation of bacterial response and viability, *Biomater. Sci.*, **4**, pp. 998–1006.

50. Klajnert, B., Cangiotti, M., Calici, S., Majoral, J. P., Caminade, A. M., Cladera, J., Bryszewska, M. and Ottaviani, M. F. (2007). EPR study of the interactions between dendrimers and peptides involved in Alzheimer's and prion diseases, *Macromol. Biosci.*, **7**, pp. 1065–1074.

51. Wasiak, T., Ionov, M., Nieznanski, K., Nieznanska, H., Klementieva, O., Granell, M., Cladera, J., Majoral, J. P., Caminade, A. M. and Klajnert, B. (2012). Phosphorus dendrimers affect Alzheimer's (Abeta1-28) peptide and MAP-Tau protein aggregation, *Mol. Pharmaceutics*, **9**, pp. 458–469.

52. Nigam, S. and Bahadur, D. (2017). Dendrimer-conjugated iron oxide nanoparticles as stimuli-responsive drug carriers for thermally-activated chemotherapy of cancer, *Colloids Surf. B*, **155**, pp. 182–192.

53. Perise-Barrios, A. J., Gomez, R., Corbi, A. L., de la Mata, J., Dominguez-Soto, A. and Munoz-Fernandez, M. A. (2015). Use of carbosilane dendrimer to switch macrophage polarization for the acquisition of antitumor functions, *Nanoscale*, **7**, pp. 3857–3866.

54. Mecke, A., Majoros, I. J., Patri, A. K., Baker, J. R., Jr., Holl, M. M. and Orr, B. G. (2005). Lipid bilayer disruption by polycationic polymers: the roles of size and chemical functional group, *Langmuir*, **21**, pp. 10348–10354.

55. Gomez, C. and Hope T. J. (2005). The ins and outs of HIV replication, *Cell Microbiol.*, **7**, pp. 621–626.

56. Wilen, C. B., Tilton, J. C. and Doms, R. W. (2012). HIV: cell binding and entry, *Cold Spring Harb. Perspect. Med.*, **2**, pp. a006866.

57. Permanyer, M., Ballana, E., Badia, R., Pauls, E., Clotet, B. and Este, J. A. (2012). Trans-infection but not infection from within endosomal compartments after cell-to-cell HIV-1 transfer to CD4+ T cells, *J. Biol. Chem.*, **287**, pp. 32017–32026.

58. De Clercq, E. (2002). Strategies in the design of antiviral drugs, *Nat. Rev. Drug Discov.*, **1**, pp. 13–25.

59. Matthews, T., Salgo, M., Greenberg, M., Chung, J., DeMasi, R. and Bolognesi, D. (2004). Enfuvirtide: the first therapy to inhibit the entry of HIV-1 into host CD4 lymphocytes, *Nat. Rev. Drug Discov.*, **3**, pp. 215–225.

60. Hu, W. S. and Hughes, S. H. (2012). HIV-1 reverse transcription, *Cold Spring Harb. Perspect. Med.*, **2**, pp. a006882.

61. Craigie, R. and Bushman, F. D. (2012). HIV DNA integration, *Cold Spring Harb. Perspect. Med.*, **2**, pp. a006890.
62. Karn, J. and Stoltzfus, C. M. (2012). Transcriptional and posttranscriptional regulation of HIV-1 gene expression, *Cold Spring Harb. Perspect. Med.*, **2**, pp. a006916.
63. Sundquist, W. I. and Krausslich, H. G. (2012). HIV-1 assembly, budding, and maturation, *Cold Spring Harb. Perspect. Med.*, **2**, pp. a006924.
64. UNAIDS (2016). Global AIDS Update 2016.
65. UNAIDS (2017). Getting to Zero: global social work responds to HIV.
66. UNAIDS (2016). Condoms: the prevention of HIV, other sexually transmitted infections and unintended pregnancies.
67. Lee, S. K., Kim, C. J., Kim, D. J. and Kang, J. H. (2015). Immune cells in the female reproductive tract, *Immune Netw.*, **15**, pp. 16–26.
68. Barreto-de-Souza, V., Arakelyan, A., Margolis, L. and Vanpouille, C. (2014). HIV-1 vaginal transmission: cell-free or cell-associated virus?, *Am. J. Reprod. Immunol.*, **71**, pp. 589–599.
69. Iwasaki, A. (2010). Antiviral immune responses in the genital tract: clues for vaccines, *Nat. Rev. Immunol.*, **10**, pp. 699–711.
70. Lederman, M. M., Offord, R. E. and Hartley, O. (2006). Microbicides and other topical strategies to prevent vaginal transmission of HIV, *Nat. Rev. Immunol.*, **6**, pp. 371–382.
71. Kariuki, S. M., Selhorst, P., Arien, K. K. and Dorfman, J. R. (2017). The HIV-1 transmission bottleneck, *Retrovirology*, **14**, p. 22.
72. Alcaide, M. L., Chisembele, M., Malupande, E., Arheart, K., Fischl, M. and Jones, D. L. (2015). A cross-sectional study of bacterial vaginosis, intravaginal practices and HIV genital shedding; implications for HIV transmission and women's health, *BMJ Open*, **5**, pp. e009036.
73. Brawner, B. M., Sommers, M. S., Moore, K., Aka-James, R., Zink, T., Brown, K. M. and Fargo, J. D. (2016). Exploring genitoanal injury and HIV risk among women: menstrual phase, hormonal birth control, and injury frequency and prevalence, *J. Acquir. Immune Defic. Syndr.*, **71**, pp. 207–212.
74. Miller, E. A., Beasley, D. E., Dunn, R. R. and Archie, E. A. (2016). Lactobacilli dominance and vaginal pH: why is the human vaginal microbiome unique?, *Front. Microbiol.*, **7**, p. 1936.
75. Mitchell, C., Fredricks, D., Agnew, K. and Hitti, J. (2015). Hydrogen peroxide-producing lactobacilli are associated with lower levels of vaginal interleukin-1beta, independent of bacterial vaginosis, *Sex. Transm. Dis.*, **42**, pp. 358–363.

76. Pilcher, C. D., Tien, H. C., Eron, J. J., Jr., Vernazza, P. L., Leu, S. Y., Stewart, P. W., Goh, L. E. and Cohen, M. S. (2004). Brief but efficient: acute HIV infection and the sexual transmission of HIV, *J. Infect. Dis.*, **189**, pp. 1785–1792.

77. Allen, S. A., Carias, A. M., Anderson, M. R., Okocha, E. A., Benning, L., McRaven, M. D., Kelley, Z. L., Lurain, J., Veazey, R. S. and Hope, T. J. (2015). Characterization of the influence of semen-derived enhancer of virus infection on the interaction of HIV-1 with female reproductive tract tissues, *J. Virol.*, **89**, pp. 5569–5580.

78. Sheik, D. A., Brooks, L., Frantzen, K., Dewhurst, S. and Yang, J. (2015). Inhibition of the enhancement of infection of human immunodeficiency virus by semen-derived enhancer of virus infection using amyloid-targeting polymeric nanoparticles, *ACS Nano*, **9**, pp. 1829–1836.

79. Pollara, J., Easterhoff, D. and Fouda, G. G. (2017). Lessons learned from human HIV vaccine trials, *Curr. Opin. HIV AIDS*, **12**, pp. 216–221.

80. Shin, S. Y. (2016). Recent update in HIV vaccine development, *Clin. Exp. Vaccine Res.*, **5**, pp. 6–11.

81. van Haaren, M. M., van den Kerkhof, T. L. and van Gils, M. J. (2017). Natural infection as a blueprint for rational HIV vaccine design, *Hum. Vaccin. Immunother.*, **13**, pp. 229–236.

82. Antimisiaris, S. G. and Mourtas, S. (2015). Recent advances on anti-HIV vaginal delivery systems development, *Adv. Drug Deliv. Rev.*, **92**, pp. 123–145.

83. Malcolm, R. K., Boyd, P. J., McCoy, C. F. and Murphy, D. J. (2016). Microbicide vaginal rings: technological challenges and clinical development, *Adv. Drug Deliv. Rev.*, **103**, pp. 33–56.

84. Shattock, R. J. and Moore, J. P. (2003). Inhibiting sexual transmission of HIV-1 infection, *Nat. Rev. Microbiol.*, **1**, pp. 25–34.

85. D'Cruz, O. J. and Uckun, F. M. (2014). Vaginal microbicides and their delivery platforms, *Expert Opin. Drug Deliv.*, **11**, pp. 723–740.

86. Rohan, L. C., Devlin, B. and Yang, H. (2014). Microbicide dosage forms, *Curr. Top. Microbiol. Immunol.*, **383**, pp. 27–54.

87. Peterson, L., Nanda, K., Opoku, B. K., Ampofo, W. K., Owusu-Amoako, M., Boakye, A. Y., Rountree, W., Troxler, A., Dominik, R., Roddy, R. and Dorflinger, L. (2007). SAVVY (C31G) gel for prevention of HIV infection in women: a Phase 3, double-blind, randomized, placebo-controlled trial in Ghana, *PLoS One*, **2**, pp. e1312.

88. Roddy, R. E., Zekeng, L., Ryan, K. A., Tamoufe, U., Weir, S. S. and Wong, E. L. (1998). A controlled trial of nonoxynol 9 film to reduce male-to-

female transmission of sexually transmitted diseases, *N. Engl. J. Med.*, **339**, pp. 504–510.

89. Mbopi-Keou, F. X., Trottier, S., Omar, R. F., Nkele, N. N., Fokoua, S., Mbu, E. R., Domingo, M. C., Giguere, J. F., Piret, J., Mwatha, A., Masse, B. and Bergeron, M. G. (2010). A randomized, double-blind, placebo-controlled Phase II extended safety study of two Invisible Condom formulations in Cameroonian women, *Contraception*, **81**, pp. 79–85.
90. Abdool Karim, S. S., Richardson, B. A., Ramjee, G., Hoffman, I. F., Chirenje, Z. M., Taha, T., Kapina, M., Maslankowski, L., Coletti, A., Profy, A., Moench, T. R., Piwowar-Manning, E., Masse, B., Hillier, S. L. and Soto-Torres, L. (2011). Safety and effectiveness of BufferGel and 0.5% PRO2000 gel for the prevention of HIV infection in women, *AIDS*, **25**, pp. 957–966.
91. Amaral, E., Perdigao, A., Souza, M. H., Mauck, C., Waller, D., Zaneveld, L. and Faundes, A. (2006). Vaginal safety after use of a bioadhesive, acid-buffering, microbicidal contraceptive gel (ACIDFORM) and a 2% nonoxynol-9 product, *Contraception*, **73**, pp. 542–547.
92. Hemmerling, A., Potts, M., Walsh, J., Young-Holt, B., Whaley, K. and Stefanski, D. A. (2007). Lime juice as a candidate microbicide? An open-label safety trial of 10% and 20% lime juice used vaginally, *J. Womens Health (Larchmt)*, **16**, pp. 1041–1051.
93. Pirrone, V., Wigdahl, B. and Krebs, F. C. (2011). The rise and fall of polyanionic inhibitors of the human immunodeficiency virus type 1, *Antiviral Res.*, **90**, pp. 168–182.
94. Lacey, C. J., Woodhall, S., Qi, Z., Sawant, S., Cowen M., McCormack, S. and Jiang, S. (2010). Unacceptable side-effects associated with a hyperosmolar vaginal microbicide in a phase 1 trial, *Int. J. STD AIDS*, **21**, pp. 714–717.
95. Sanchez-Rodriguez, J., Vacas-Cordoba, E., Gomez, R., de la Mata, F. J. and Munoz-Fernandez, M. A. (2015). Nanotech-derived topical microbicides for HIV prevention: the road to clinical development, *Antiviral Res.*, **113**, pp. 33–48.
96. Abdool Karim, S. S. and Baxter, C. (2014). Microbicides for prevention of HIV infection: clinical efficacy trials, *Curr. Top. Microbiol. Immunol.*, **383**, pp. 97–115.
97. Price, C. F., Tyssen, D., Sonza, S., Davie, A., Evans, S., Lewis, G. R., Xia, S., Spelman, T., Hodsman, P., Moench, T. R., Humberstone, A., Paull, J. R. and Tachedjian, G. (2011). SPL7013 Gel (VivaGel(R)) retains potent HIV-1 and HSV-2 inhibitory activity following vaginal administration in humans, *PLoS One*, **6**, pp. e24095.

98. Telwatte, S., Moore, K., Johnson, A., Tyssen, D., Sterjovski, J., Aldunate, M., Gorry, P. R., Ramsland, P. A., Lewis, G. R., Paull, J. R., Sonza, S. and Tachedjian, G. (2011). Virucidal activity of the dendrimer microbicide SPL7013 against HIV-1, *Antiviral Res.*, **90**, pp. 195–199.

99. Moscicki, A. B., Kaul, R., Ma, Y., Scott, M. E., Daud, II, Bukusi, E. A., Shiboski, S., Rebbapragada, A., Huibner, S. and Cohen, C. R. (2012). Measurement of mucosal biomarkers in a phase 1 trial of intravaginal 3% StarPharma LTD 7013 gel (VivaGel) to assess expanded safety, *J. Acquir. Immune Defic. Syndr.*, **59**, pp. 134–140.

100. Dobrovolskaia, M. A. (2017). Dendrimers effects on the immune system: insights into toxicity and therapeutic utility, *Curr. Pharm. Des.*, **23**(21), pp. 3134–3141.

101. Gurbuz, M. U., Ozturk, K., Erturk, A. S., Yoyen-Ermis, D., Esendagli, G., Calis, S. and Tulu, M. (2016). Cytotoxicity and biodistribution studies on PEGylated EDA and PEG cored PAMAM dendrimers, *J. Biomater. Sci. Polym. Ed.*, **27**, pp. 1645–1658.

102. Wang, H., Chang, H., Zhang, Q. and Cheng, Y. (2017). Fabrication of low-generation dendrimers into nanostructures for efficient and nontoxic gene delivery, *Top. Curr. Chem.*, **375**, p. 62.

103. Zeng, Y., Kurokawa, Y., Win-Shwe, T. T., Zeng, Q., Hirano, S., Zhang, Z. and Sone, H. (2016). Effects of PAMAM dendrimers with various surface functional groups and multiple generations on cytotoxicity and neuronal differentiation using human neural progenitor cells, *J. Toxicol. Sci.*, **41**, pp. 351–370.

104. Bodewein, L., Schmelter, F., Di Fiore, S., Hollert, H., Fischer, R. and Fenske, M. (2016). Differences in toxicity of anionic and cationic PAMAM and PPI dendrimers in zebrafish embryos and cancer cell lines, *Toxicol. Appl. Pharmacol.*, **305**, pp. 83–92.

105. Madaan, K., Kumar, S., Poonia, N., Lather, V. and Pandita, D. (2014). Dendrimers in drug delivery and targeting: drug-dendrimer interactions and toxicity issues, *J. Pharm. Bioallied Sci.*, **6**, pp. 139–150.

106. Trotard, M., Tsopoulidis, N., Tibroni, N., Willemsen, J., Binder, M., Ruggieri, A. and Fackler, O. T. (2015). Sensing of HIV-1 infection in Tzm-bl cells with reconstituted expression of STING, *J. Virol.*, **90**, pp. 2064–2076.

107. Grivel, J. C., Shattock, R. J. and Margolis, L. B. (2011). Selective transmission of R5 HIV-1 variants: where is the gatekeeper?, *J. Transl. Med.*, **9**(Suppl 1), p. S6.

108. Zaunders, J., Xu, Y., Kent, S. J., Koelsch, K. K. and Kelleher, A. D. (2017). Divergent expression of CXCR5 and CCR5 on CD4+ T cells and the

paradoxical accumulation of T follicular helper cells during HIV infection, *Front. Immunol.*, **8**, p. 495.

109. Brubaker, L. and Wolfe, A. J. (2017). The female urinary microbiota, urinary health and common urinary disorders, *Ann. Transl. Med.*, **5**, p. 34.

110. Gordon-Alonso, M., Rocha-Perugini, V., Alvarez, S., Moreno-Gonzalo, O., Ursa, A., Lopez-Martin, S., Izquierdo-Useros, N., Martinez-Picado, J., Munoz-Fernandez, M. A., Yanez-Mo, M. and Sanchez-Madrid, F. (2012). The PDZ-adaptor protein syntenin-1 regulates HIV-1 entry, *Mol. Biol. Cell*, **23**, pp. 2253–2263.

111. Ham, A. S., Nugent, S. T., Peters, J. J., Katz, D. F., Shelter, C. M., Dezzutti, C. S., Boczar, A. D., Buckheit, K. W. and Buckheit, R. W., Jr. (2015). The rational design and development of a dual chamber vaginal/rectal microbicide gel formulation for HIV prevention, *Antiviral Res.*, **120**, pp. 153–164.

112. Vacas Cordoba, E., Arnaiz, E., Relloso, M., Sanchez-Torres, C., Garcia, F., Perez-Alvarez, L., Gomez, R., de la Mata, F. J., Pion, M. and Munoz-Fernandez, M. A. (2013). Development of sulphated and naphthylsulphonated carbosilane dendrimers as topical microbicides to prevent HIV-1 sexual transmission, *AIDS*, **27**, pp. 1219–1229.

113. Dezzutti, C. S., Else, L. J., Yandura, S. E., Shetler, C., Russo, J., Back, D. J. and McGowan, I. (2016). Distinct pharmacodynamic activity of rilpivirine in ectocervical and colonic explant tissue, *Antimicrob. Agents Chemother.*, **60**, pp. 2765–2770.

114. Dinh, M. H., Anderson, M. R., McRaven, M. D., Cianci, G. C., McCoombe, S. G., Kelley, Z. L., Gioia, C. J., Fought, A. J., Rademaker, A. W., Veazey, R. S. and Hope, T. J. (2015). Visualization of HIV-1 interactions with penile and foreskin epithelia: clues for female-to-male HIV transmission, *PLoS Pathog.*, **11**, pp. e1004729.

115. Portal, C., Gouyer, V., Magnien, M., Plet, S., Gottrand, F. and Desseyn, J. L. (2017). In vivo imaging of the Muc5b gel-forming mucin, *Sci. Rep.*, **7**, p. 44591.

116. Chonco, L., Pion, M., Vacas, E., Rasines, B., Maly, M., Serramia, M. J., Lopez-Fernandez, L., de la Mata, J., Alvarez, S., Gomez, R. and Munoz-Fernandez, M. A. (2012). Carbosilane dendrimer nanotechnology outlines of the broad HIV blocker profile, *J. Control. Release*, **161**, pp. 949–958.

117. Katz, D. F., Yuan, A. and Gao Y. (2015). Vaginal drug distribution modeling, *Adv. Drug Deliv. Rev.*, **92**, pp. 2–13.

118. Henning, T. R., McNicholl, J. M., Vishwanathan, S. A. and Kersh, E. N. (2015). Macaque models of enhanced susceptibility to HIV, *Virol. J.*, **12**, p. 90.

119. Hatziioannou, T. and Evans, D. T. (2012). Animal models for HIV/AIDS research, *Nat. Rev. Microbiol.*, **10**, pp. 852–867.

120. Roan, N. R. and Munch, J. (2015). Improving preclinical models of HIV microbicide efficacy, *Trends Microbiol.*, **23**, pp. 445–447.

121. Deruaz, M. and Luster, A. D. (2013). BLT humanized mice as model to study HIV vaginal transmission, *J. Infect. Dis.*, **208**(Suppl 2), pp. S131–136.

122. Gruell, H. and Klein, F. (2017). Progress in HIV-1 antibody research using humanized mice, *Curr. Opin. HIV AIDS*, **12**(3), 285–293.

123. Marsden, M. D. and Zack, J. A. (2015). Studies of retroviral infection in humanized mice, *Virology*, **479–480**, pp. 297–309

Chapter 6

Insights into Adsorption of Serum Albumin onto Carbon Nanotubes by Molecular Modeling

Marco Agostino Deriu, Gianvito Grasso, Ginevra Licandro, and Andrea Danani
Dalle Molle Institute for Artificial Intelligence Research (IDSIA), Department of Innovative Technologies, University of Applied Sciences and Arts of Southern Switzerland (SUPSI), University of Italian Switzerland (USI), SUPSI, Centro Galleria 2, Manno, CH-6928, Switzerland
marco.deriu@idsia.ch; andrea.danani@idsia.ch

In recent years, carbon nanotubes (CNTs) have attracted the attention of many researchers owing to their superior structural, mechanical, and electrical properties. However, focusing on biomedical applications, a number of studies in the past decade have demonstrated CNTs to be highly hydrophobic and insoluble both in aqueous environment and organic media, being in general, highly toxic. Nevertheless, in a physiological environment, the formation of a protein corona might affect the toxicity of the organic/inorganic material. Although experiments greatly enhanced the understanding of the interaction between proteins and CNT surfaces, a whole

Drug Delivery Nanosystems: From Bioinspiration and Biomimetics to Clinical Applications
Edited by Costas Demetzos, Stergios Pispas, and Natassa Pippa

ISBN 978-981-4774-92-5 (Hardcover), 978-0-429-49054-5 (eBook)
www.panstanford.com

comprehension of the molecular mechanism driving the protein corona formation is still far from being reached. Molecular dynamics represents a powerful approach to investigating the adsorption of proteins onto organic/inorganic surfaces. Secondary and tertiary structure changes, orientation and reorientation of the protein on the interacting interface, hydrogen bonds, characteristics of adsorbed amino acids, and binding affinity are essential data to properly understand protein adsorption, thus helping in a better rationalization of experimental data. In this work we have investigated the adsorption of human serum albumin onto CNTs with specific geometries. We have characterized albumin adsorption in terms of protein orientation, interacting residues, binding affinity, and protein conformational rearrangements due to its interaction with CNTs.

6.1 Introduction

In recent years, carbon nanotubes (CNTs) have attracted attention owing to their superior structural, mechanical, and electrical properties. Great achievements have been made in physical, biotechnological, and biomaterial fields since their discovery [1]. Biomolecule-CNT complexes have shown great potential for applications in the fields of biosensors, tissue engineering, and biomedical devices [2–4]. For instance, CNTs serve as biocompatible transporters for drug delivery [5]. However, a number of investigations carried out by various researchers in the past decade have suggested single-walled carbon nanotubes (SWCNTs) to be highly hydrophobic and insoluble both in aqueous environment and organic media [2, 3]. SWCNTs generally organize into nonsoluble aggregates, mostly highly toxic. In view of this problem, functionalization, which is normally classified as covalent chemical modification [6] and noncovalent decoration [7], has been employed to improve the original characteristics of CNTs, especially making them soluble in a variety of solvents by combining biological macromolecules with nanotubes. Functionalization has greatly enhanced the possibilities in applications, not only improving the solubility, but also reducing toxicity [8], and hence facilitating the development of novel biotechnology, biomedicine, and bioengineering. Biocompatibility properties may be improved by adsorption of specific proteins or peptides onto CNTs. Also, the covalent binding method has been considered as a more stable solution. However, it involves chemical reactions that impair structural and electronic properties of CNTs [1]. Therefore, noncovalent functionalization strategies have caught the attention of researchers, also in the field of nanoparticles [9–11]. It has been proved that biological molecules, including polymers, proteins, nucleic acids, and carbohydrates, can smoothly wrap around or be inserted inside the tube, and finally achieve the goal of CNT functionalization [1]. Instead of chemical modification, the wrapping and encapsulation phenomena occur primarily owing to the combined effect of hydrophobic forces, van der Waals (vdW) attraction, and electrostatic and π-stacking interactions between biological molecules and the tube [2, 3, 12]. However, the atomistic details of the interactions taking place at the molecular level and the dynamic mechanisms of the biomolecule-CNT complexes are not completely understood, yet. Hence, of great interest is a better understanding of both molecular interaction features (what kind of amino acids are more adsorbed, the interaction force between a peptide and the nanotube, etc.) and the dynamics of the process (i.e., the conformational changes induced on the molecules involved that could directly impact their biological functions). Although this interaction mechanism is not completely understood until now, it was reported in experimental studies that the affinity of a peptide for a CNT is sequence dependent and that hydrophobic amino acids, especially aromatic ones, have stronger affinities for CNTs than nonaromatic ones [12].

It was also established that the vdW interaction contributes dominantly to the interaction binding energy between a peptide and a SWCNT, suggesting that the vdW energy could be used to describe the binding affinity of a peptide for the SWCNT [13, 14]. Although experiments greatly enhanced the understanding of the interaction between the peptide and the CNT surfaces, the atomic details of the interactions taking place at the molecular level are still debated, due to the limitation of the experimental methods. The details of function, conformation, and spatial orientation of proteins that are noncovalently adsorbed onto the CNTs cannot be always deeply explored by experiments. Moreover, the dynamics of the adsorption process, which is fundamental in the biological applications of CNTs, is poorly understood via these techniques. Nevertheless, these branches of knowledge are of great importance in understanding the environmental and biological activity of CNTs as well as their potential applications in nanostructure fabrication. Atomistic molecular simulations present one of the most direct approaches to investigating the atomic details of the surface interaction mechanisms, investigating the dynamics at the molecular level. Secondary and tertiary structure changes, orientation and reorientation of the protein on the interface, hydrogen bonds, characteristics of adsorbed amino acids, etc., are relevant to properly understand protein adsorption on materials, and these behaviors are accounted for by atomistic simulations [9, 15–21].

For example, the vdW energy between 20 peptides with different sequences adsorbed onto the same SWCNT has been calculated to explore the variations in sequence-dependent affinity. The estimation was based on simulations of molecular dynamics (MD). Results showed that the interaction affinity varies with different sequences of peptides. Among the tested 20 peptides, those consisting of aromatic amino acids (PHE, TRP, and TYR) showed stronger vdW interactions with the SWCNT, in agreement with experimental observations [13, 14].

In this work, in order to better understand the above-mentioned interaction phenomena, MD simulations were performed on protein-nanotube systems. Here, human serum albumin (HSA) has been considered as the model to explore the adsorption behavior and protein dynamics on the CNT surface, given that albumin is one of the key proteins that may regulate material biocompatibility [22] and, thus, is a target for CNT functionalization.

6.2 Materials and Methods

The molecular system was composed of an armchair (6,6) SWCNT and the chain A of HSA protein in a water environment. The tube length was about 5 nm. The initial coordinates of the protein were taken from the protein data bank (ID code 3BL9), whereas the SWCNT atomic structure was built by using visual molecular dynamics (VMD).

The HSA and SWCNT were placed in a cubic box of about $12 \times 12 \times 12$ nm^3 with an initial distance of about 3 nm between the outer surface of the protein and the SWCNT wall. To increase the simulation statistics six intial configuration were considered, each characterized by the protein exposing a different face toward the SWCNT wall (the protein was rotated with respect to a fixed SWCNT according to the faces of a cube). The box was fully solvated in explicitly modeled water, and the total charge was neutralized by the addition of Cl– and Na+ ions. (Fig. 6.1). As a term of comparison also HSA alone in water has been simulated.

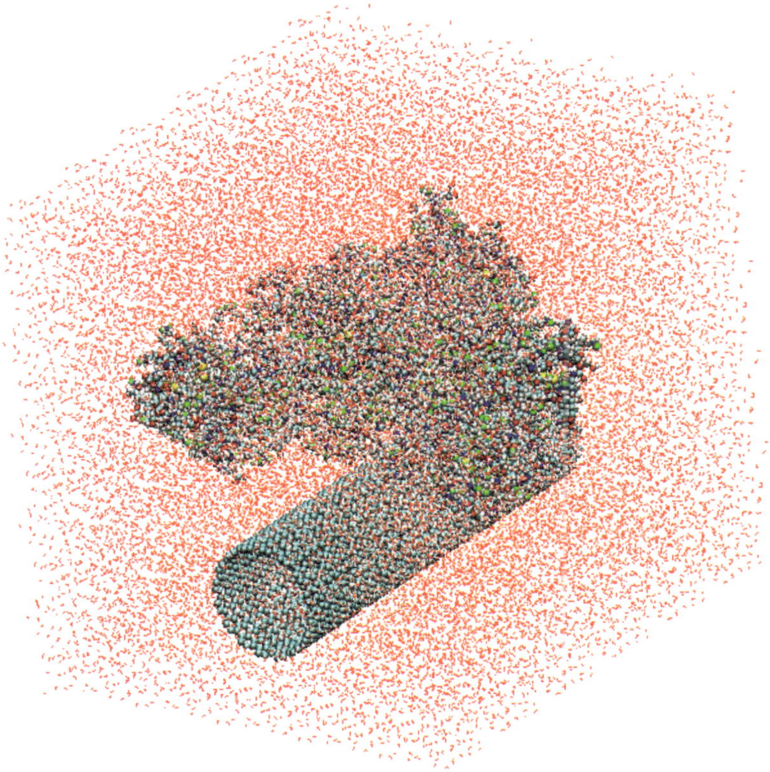

Figure 6.1 Human serum albumin and carbon nanotube in a water box.

Each system in water consisted of about 120,000 interacting particles. Simulation steps followed a procedure widely adopted in our recent studies [11, 17–20, 23–32]. In greater detail, following an initial energy minimization of 1000 steps of steepest descent, two preliminary position restraint MD simulations (each one 100 ps in duration) were carried out in a constant number of particles, temperature, and volume (NVT) ensemble and a constant number of particles, temperature, and pressure (NPT) ensemble, respectively, where the heavy atoms of the proteins were restrained using a force constant of 1000 kJ $mol^{-1}nm^{-2}$. During the first restrained MD simulation, involving MD in the NVT ensemble, protein and nonprotein atoms were coupled separately to temperature baths using a v-rescale coupling algorithm [33] with a coupling time of 1 ps. Subsequently, the second restrained MD simulation was performed keeping the pressure at 1 bar by applying Berendsen's weak coupling method [34] with a time constant of 5 ps. Finally, for each configuration, 100 ns of production MD was simulated in the NPT ensemble. The v-rescale coupling algorithm [33] was applied again to maintain the system's temperature at 310 K (time constant of τ_T = 0.1 ps), and the pressure was maintained at 1 bar using the Parrinello–Rahman [35, 36] barostat (time constant of τ_P = 2 ps) in the isobaric-isochoric ensemble with long-range dispersion correction applied for both energy and pressure terms. The all-atom optimized potentials for liquid simulations (OPLS-AA) force field [37–39] and the TIP3P model [40] were employed to define the protein topology and water molecules, respectively. The Groningen machine for chemical simulations (GROMACS) [41–44] was employed for MD simulations and data analysis. A VMD [45] package was employed for the visual inspection of the simulated systems. The residue mainly responsible for HSA-CNT interaction was identified by contact probability plots following a procedure explained and successfully employed in our previous works [9, 15].

6.3 Results and Discussion

Conformational changes of the HSA protein are shown in terms of root mean square deviation (RMSD) throughtout the overal simulation (Fig. 6.2a). In the absence or presence of the CNT, the HSA moved toward a conformational equilibrium reached around 80 ns or before. The protein gyration radius did not show any relevant deviation when interacting with the CNT with respect to the one calculated for the protein alone in water (data not shown). This result indicates that the protein underwent conformational changes only close to the CNT wall.

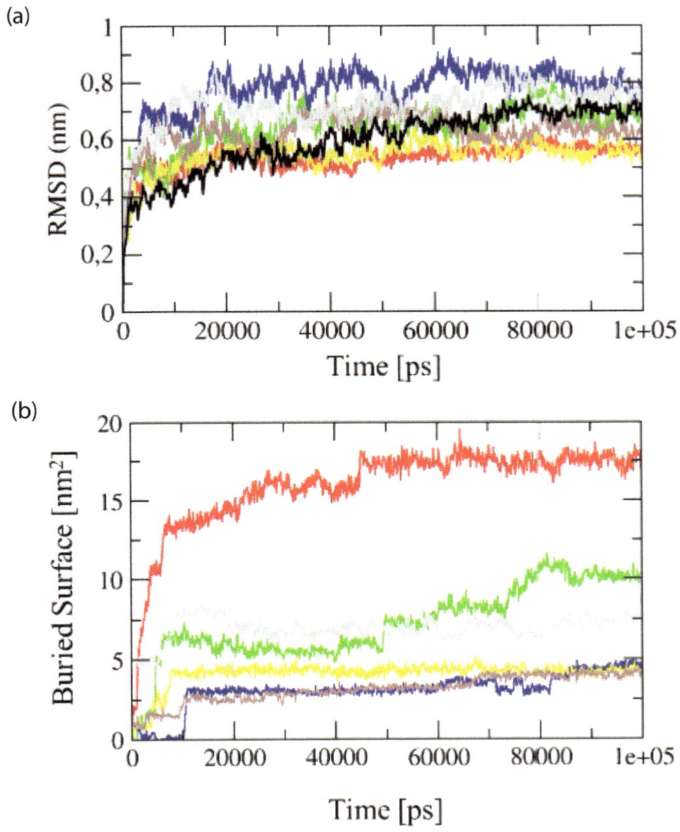

Figure 6.2 (a) HSA backbone RMSD for systems: HSA alone in water (black curve) and an albumin-CNT complex in water (other curves) throughout 100 ns of molecular dynamics. (b) HSA-CNT contact surface throughout 100 ns of molecular dynamics.

All the simulated configurations result in a stable HSA-CNT interaction in the last 20 ns of the simulation (Fig. 6.2b). The last 20 ns of each simulation are then considered as structural equilibrium for further analysis.

In Fig. 6.3 an example (Conf1) of the final conformations of the adsorbed protein system after 100 ns of MD simulation is shown. The water molecules are omitted for clarity. It could be observed how the protein rearranges its structural conformation to fit the curving surface of the SWCNT, as already indicated by recent studies [46].

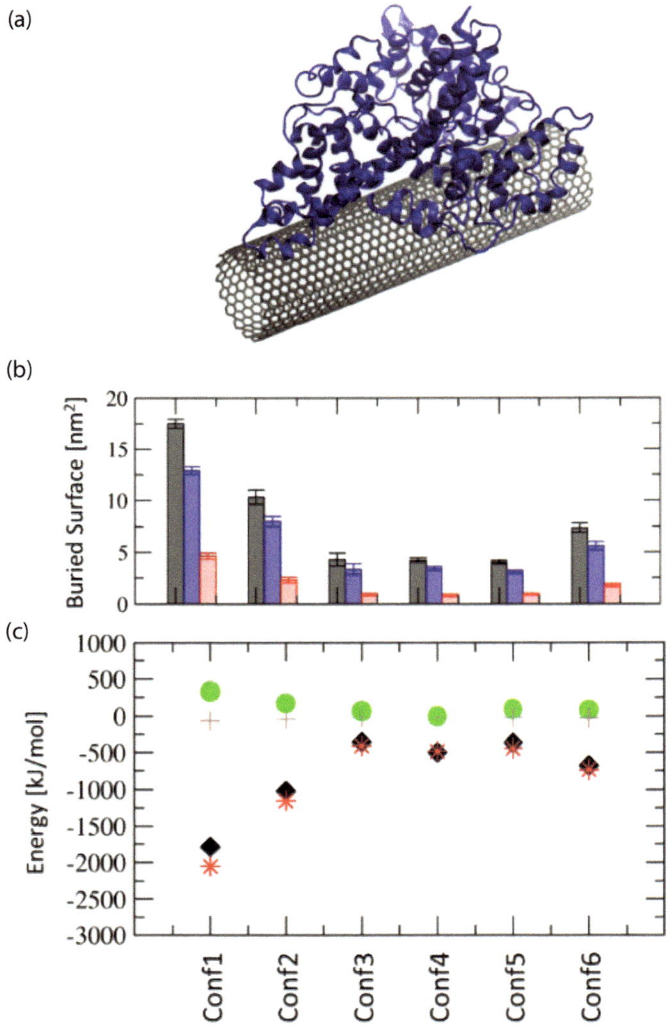

Figure 6.3 (a) Example of HSS-CNT interaction mode. (b) Average HSA-CNT contact surface in the last 20 ns of MD simulation. (c) HSA-CNT interaction binding (black), vdW (red), polar (green), and nonpolar (pink) energy for each configuration calculated as an average over the last 20 ns of the MD simulations. Standard deviations are always less than 1 order of magnitude with respect to the corresponding average.

Interestingly, Conf1 and Conf2 showed an interaction characterized by a much higher contact surface with respect to the other configurations (Fig. 6.3b). Moreover, enhanced binding energy is observed in the case of Conf1 and Conf2 (Fig. 6.3c). The results allow us to consider Conf1 and Conf2 as the most stable interacting configurations. In agreement with previous literature [13, 14], we found the vdW energy to contribute dominantly to the binding energy (Fig. 6.3c).

Concerning interacting residues (Figs. 6.4a and 6.4b), simulation data indicate a tendency for the protein to protrude and interact with the wall with several protein domains in an nonspecific manner. Nevertheless, on considering all the simulations as an ensemble, the following residues have been found as the ones most likely involved in the HSA-CNT contact surface: ARG81-ASP89, GLU100-ASP107, HIS128, GLN204-ARG209, CYS316-PHE325, GLU354-ALA362, and HIS463-SER480. Mostly hydrophobic residues are involved in the contact surface. This is intuitive since the CNT does not contribute to any electrostatic interactions. In greater detail, aromatic rings tend to move parallel to the wall, as HIS463, TYR83, HIS128, and PHE325. Interestingly, also several more polar residues were found as part of the contact surface.

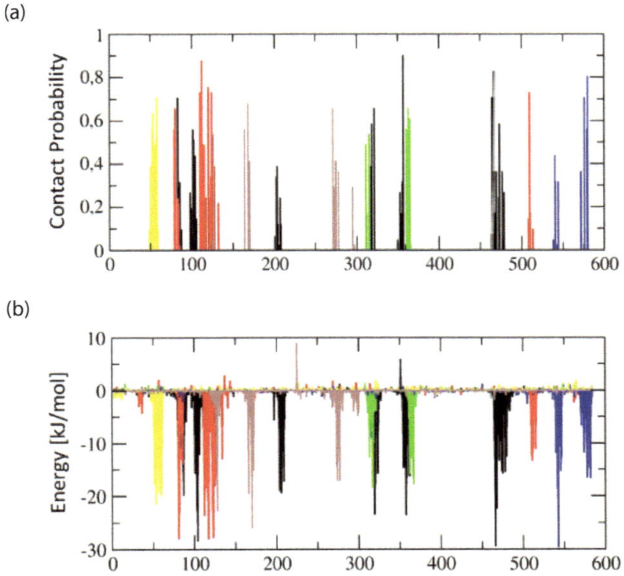

Figure 6.4 (a) HSA-CNT per residue probability contact. (b) HSA-CNT per residue binding energy (vdW + polar + nonpolar).

A secondary structure analysis (Fig. 6.5) was carried out by DSSP (define secondary structure of proteins) [47, 48]. Concerning secondary structure analysis, the HSA-CNT interaction drives toward a very slight decrease in the α-helix content, with a simultaneous increase of Turn regions, in all the simulations and consequently the biological functions might not be affected.

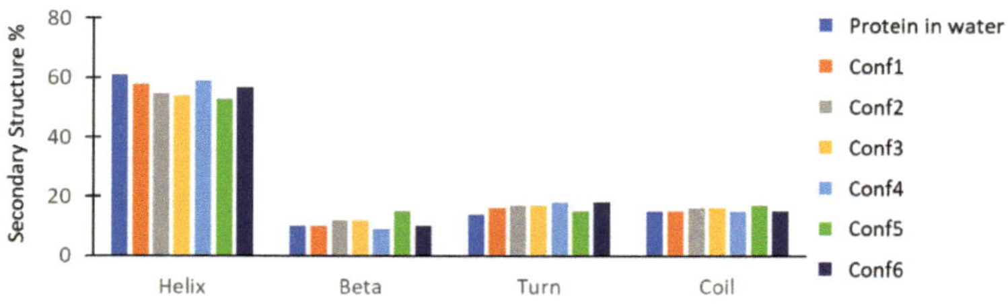

Figure 6.5 HSA secondary structure percentage for each simulated system. Standard deviations are not shown since they are always at least 1 order of magnitude lower than the average value.

6.4 Conclusions

Proteins have been conjugated with CNTs for applications in biosensing, biorecognition, delivery, and functional composites. Despite the growing interest in these CNT/protein hybrids, very little is known about how CNTs affect the structure and function of bound proteins.

In literature, not many studies focused on albumin MD [22, 46, 49–52] and rarer are the computational investigations focusing on the HSA-CNT interactions at the molecular level [22, 46]. The classical MD simulation approach has been applied in this work to investigate the structure, the dynamics, and the adsorption properties of the HSA-CNT complex. To study the effect of CNT on the dynamics of HSA several protein orientations with respect to the CNT were analyzed, via MD simulations. Among all the configurations, Conf1 and Conf2 were characterized by a much higher contact surface and binding energy. Nevertheless, in an MD simulation of 100 ns, the protein tends to wrap around the tube for every configuration, indicating an effective affinity of HSA for the CNT and a consequent adsorption on the surface. Protein residues within 0.35 nm around the nanotube wall were considered as the adsorbed ones in some related works [22, 51]. Nevertheless, the adsorption process, on the whole, has shown to be not specific. It has been widely reported that hydrophobic groups show great affinity to CNTs, particularly for the groups with aromatic rings, because of the π-π stacking [22, 53–55]. Here, it has been found that the aromatic rings tend to move parallel to the wall, confirming the above-mentioned literature evidence. Moreover, we have observed that vdW interaction between biomacromolecules and CNT is the dominant factor, as already suggested [22].

It is worth mentioning that during the adsorption, changes in the conformational arrangement of the protein are not relevant in the simulated time. The loss of the α-helix is minor, with a partial unfolding of the α-helix content. On the whole, the secondary structure is preserved throughout the simulation. The outcome suggests that the protein's biological function might not be affected by the interaction with the nanotube as in the context of a noncovalent functionalization strategy. In this connection, a further prospective simulation study could consider a covalent functionalization of SWCNTs with HSA, to evaluate how this specific binding may affect properties of protein and nanotube.

References

1. Xie, Y. H. and Soh, A. K. (2005). Investigation of non-covalent association of single-walled carbon nanotube with amylose by molecular dynamics simulation, *Mater. Lett.*, **59**, pp. 971–975.
2. Katz, E. and Willner, I. (2004). Biomolecule-functionalized carbon nanotubes: applications in nanobioelectronics, *ChemPhysChem*, **5**, pp. 1084–1104.
3. Yang, W., Thordarson, P., Gooding, J. J., Ringer, S. P. and Braet, F. (2007). Carbon nanotubes for biological and biomedical applications, *Nanotechnology*, **18**, p. 412001.
4. Chen, X., Tam, U. C., Czlapinski, J. L., Lee, G. S., Rabuka, D., Zettl, A. and Bertozzi, C. R. (2006). Interfacing carbon nanotubes with living cells, *J. Am. Chem. Soc.*, **128**, pp. 6292–6293.
5. Shi Kam, N. W., O'Connell, M., Wisdom, J. A. and Dai, H. (2005). Carbon nanotubes as multifunctional biological transporters and near-infrared agents for selective cancer cell destruction, *Proc. Natl. Acad. Sci.*, **102**, pp. 11600–11605.

6. Hirsch, A. (2002). Functionalization of single-walled carbon nanotubes, *Angew. Chem. Int. Ed. Engl.*, **41**, pp. 1853–1859.
7. Chen, S., Berthelier, V., Yang, W. and Wetzel, R. (2001). Polyglutamine aggregation behavior in vitro supports a recruitment mechanism of cytotoxicity, *J. Mol. Biol.*, **311**, pp. 173–182.
8. Kang, Y., Liu, Y.-C., Wang, Q., Shen, J.-W., Wu, T. and Guan, W.-J. (2009). On the spontaneous encapsulation of proteins in carbon nanotubes, *Biomaterials*, **30**, pp. 2807–2815.
9. Grasso, G., Deriu, M. A., Prat, M., Rimondini, L., Vernè, E., Follenzi, A. and Danani, A. (2015). Cell penetrating peptide adsorption on magnetite and silica surfaces: a computational investigation, *J. Phys. Chem. B*, **119**, pp. 8239–8246.
10. Apicella, A., Soncini, M., Deriu, M. A., Natalello, A., Bonanomi, M., Dellasega, D., Tortora, P., Regonesi, M. E. and Casari, C. S. (2013). A hydrophobic gold surface triggers misfolding and aggregation of the amyloidogenic Josephin domain in monomeric form, while leaving the oligomers unaffected, *PLoS One*, **8**, pp. e58794.
11. Deriu, M. A., Popescu, L. M., Ottaviani, M. F., Danani, A. and Piticescu, R. M. (2016). Iron oxide/PAMAM nanostructured hybrids: combined computational and experimental studies, *J. Mater. Sci.*, **51**, pp. 1996–2007.
12. Wang, S., Humphreys, E. S., Chung, S.-Y., Delduco, D. F., Lustig, S. R., Wang, H., Parker, K. N., Rizzo, N. W., Subramoney, S., Chiang, Y.-M. and Jagota, A. (2003). Peptides with selective affinity for carbon nanotubes, *Nat. Mater.*, **2**, pp. 196–200.
13. Tallury, S. S. (2009). Molecular dynamics simulations of single-walled carbon nanotubes wrapped by various polymers, http://www.lib.ncsu.edu/resolver/1840.16/2238.
14. Trzaskowski, B., Jalbout, A. F. and Adamowicz, L. (2006). Molecular dynamics studies of protein-fragment models encapsulated into carbon nanotubes, *Chem. Phys. Lett.*, **430**, pp. 97–100.
15. Deriu, M. A., Grasso, G., Licandro, G., Danani, A., Gallo, D., Tuszynski, J. A. and Morbiducci, U. (2014). Investigation of the Josephin Domain protein-protein interaction by molecular dynamics, *PLoS One*, **9**, pp. e108677.
16. Lepre, M., Omar, S., Grasso, G., Morbiducci, U., Deriu, M. and Tuszynski, J. (2017). Insights into the effect of the G245S single point mutation on the structure of p53 and the binding of the protein to DNA, *Molecules*, **22**, p. 1358.

17. Deriu, M. A., Grasso, G., Tuszynski, J. A., Gallo, D., Morbiducci, U. and Danani, A. (2016). Josephin Domain structural conformations explored by metadynamics in essential coordinates, *PLoS Comput. Biol.*, **12**, pp. e1004699.

18. Grasso, G., Deriu, M. A., Tuszynski, J. A., Gallo, D., Morbiducci, U. and Danani, A. (2016). Conformational fluctuations of the AXH monomer of Ataxin-1, *Proteins Struct. Funct. Bioinforma.*, **84**, pp. 52–59.

19. Grasso, G., Tuszynski, J. A., Morbiducci, U., Licandro, G., Danani, A. and Deriu, M. A. (2017). Thermodynamic and kinetic stability of the Josephin Domain closed arrangement: evidences from replica exchange molecular dynamics, *Biol. Direct*, **12**, p. 2

20. Deriu, M. A., Grasso, G., Tuszynski, J. A., Massai, D., Gallo, D., Morbiducci, U. and Danani, A. (2016). Characterization of the AXH domain of Ataxin-1 using enhanced sampling and functional mode analysis, *Proteins Struct. Funct. Bioinforma.*, **84**, pp. 666–673.

21. Janaszewska, A., Klajnert-Maculewicz, B., Marcinkowska, M., Duchnowicz, P., Appelhans, D., Grasso, G., Deriu, M. A., Danani, A., Cangiotti, M. and Ottaviani, M. F. (2018). Multivalent interacting glycodendrimer to prevent amyloid-peptide fibril formation induced by Cu(II): a multidisciplinary approach, *Nano Res.*, **11**(3), pp. 1204–1226.

22. Shen, J.-W., Wu, T., Wang, Q. and Kang, Y. (2008). Induced stepwise conformational change of human serum albumin on carbon nanotube surfaces, *Biomaterials*, **29**, pp. 3847–3855.

23. Enemark, S., Deriu, M. A., Soncini, M. and Redaelli, A. (2008). Mechanical model of the tubulin dimer based on molecular dynamics simulations, *J. Biomech. Eng.*, **130**, p. 41008.

24. Bidone, T. C., Kim, T., Deriu, M. A., Morbiducci, U. and Kamm, R. D. (2015). Multiscale impact of nucleotides and cations on the conformational equilibrium, elasticity and rheology of actin filaments and crosslinked networks, *Biomech. Model. Mechanobiol.*, **14**, pp. 1143–1155.

25. Deriu, M. A., Shkurti, A., Paciello, G., Bidone, T. C., Morbiducci, U., Ficarra, E., Audenino, A. and Acquaviva, A. (2012). Multiscale modeling of cellular actin filaments: from atomistic molecular to coarse-grained dynamics, *Proteins*, **80**, pp. 1598–1609.

26. Deriu, M. A., Shkurti, A., Paciello, G., Bidone, T. C., Morbiducci, U., Ficarra, E., Audenino, A. and Acquaviva, A. (2012). Multiscale modelling of cellular actin filaments: from atomistic molecular to coarse grained dynamics, *Proteins Struct. Funct. Bioinforma.*, **80**, pp. 1598–1609.

27. Paciello, G., Acquaviva, A., Ficarra, E., Deriu, M. A. and Macii, E. (2011). A molecular dynamics study of a miRNA:mRNA interaction, *J. Mol. Model.*, **17**, pp. 2895–2906.
28. Enemark, S., Deriu, M. A. and Soncini, M. (2006). Mechanical properties of tubulin molecules by molecular dynamics simulations, in *Proceedings of 8th Biennial ASME Conference on Engineering Systems Design and Analysis*, ESDA2006.
29. Soncini, M., Vesentini, S., Ruffoni, D., Orsi, M., Deriu, M. A. and Redaelli, A. (2007). Mechanical response and conformational changes of alpha-actinin domains during unfolding: a molecular dynamics study, *Biomech. Model. Mechanobiol.*, **6**, pp. 399–407.
30. Havelka, D., Kučera, O., Deriu, M. A. and Cifra, M. (2014). Electro-acoustic behavior of the mitotic spindle: a semi-classical coarse-grained model, *PLoS One*, **9**, pp. e86501.
31. Gentile, F., Deriu, M., Licandro, G., Prunotto, A., Danani, A. and Tuszynski, J. (2015). Structure based modeling of small molecules binding to the TLR7 by atomistic level simulations, *Molecules*, **20**, pp. 8316–8340.
32. Deriu, M. A., Enemark, S., Soncini, M., Montevecchi, F. M. and Redaelli, A. (2007). Tubulin: from atomistic structure to supramolecular mechanical properties, *J. Mater. Sci.*, **42**, pp. 8864–8872.
33. Bussi, G., Donadio, D. and Parrinello, M. (2007). Canonical sampling through velocity rescaling, *J. Chem. Phys.*, **126**, p. 14101.
34. Berendsen, H. J. C., Postma, J. P. M., Van Gunsteren, W. F., DiNola, A. and Haak, J. R. (1984). Molecular dynamics with coupling to an external bath, *J. Chem. Phys.*, **81**, pp. 3684–3690.
35. Nosé, S. and Klein, M. L. (1983). Constant pressure molecular dynamics for molecular systems, *Mol. Phys.*, **50**, pp. 1055–1076.
36. Parrinello, M. and Rahman, A. (1981). Polymorphic transitions in single crystals: a new molecular dynamics method, *J. Appl. Phys.*, **52**, pp. 7182–7190.
37. Jorgensen, W. L., Maxwell, D. S. and Tirado-Rives, J. (1996). Development and testing of the OPLS all-atom force field on conformational energetics and properties of organic liquids, *J. Am. Chem. Soc.*, **118**, pp. 11225–11236.
38. Jorgensen, W. L. and Tirado-Rives, J. (1988). The OPLS [optimized potentials for liquid simulations] potential functions for proteins, energy minimizations for crystals of cyclic peptides and crambin, *J. Am. Chem. Soc.*, **110**, pp. 1657–1666.

39. Kahn, K. and Bruice, T. C. (2002). Parameterization of OPLS-AA force field for the conformational analysis of macrocyclic polyketides, *J. Comput. Chem.*, **23**, pp. 977–996.

40. Jorgensen, W. L., Chandrasekhar, J., Madura, J. D., Impey, R. W. and Klein, M. L. (1983). Comparison of simple potential functions for simulating liquid water, *J. Chem. Phys.*, **79**, p. 926.

41. Abraham, M. J., Murtola, T., Schulz, R., Páll, S., Smith, J. C., Hess, B. and Lindah, E. (2015). Gromacs: high performance molecular simulations through multi-level parallelism from laptops to supercomputers, *SoftwareX*, **1–2**, pp. 19–25.

42. Berendsen, H. J. C., van der Spoel, D. and van Drunen, R. (1995). GROMACS: a message-passing parallel molecular dynamics implementation, *Comput. Phys. Commun.*, **91**, pp. 43–56.

43. van der Spoel, D., Lindahl, E., Hess, B., Groenhof, G., Mark, A. E. and Berendsen, H. J. C. (2005). GROMACS: fast, flexible, and free, *J. Comput. Chem.*, **26**, pp. 1701–1718.

44. Hess, B., Kutzner, C., van der Spoel, D. and Lindahl, E. (2008). GROMACS 4: algorithms for highly efficient, load-balanced, and scalable molecular simulation, *J. Chem. Theory Comput.*, **4**, pp. 435–447.

45. Humphrey, W., Dalke, A. and Schulten, K. (1996). VMD: visual molecular dynamics, *J. Mol. Graph.*, **14**, pp. 33–8, 27–8.

46. Gu, Z., Yang, Z., Chong, Y., Ge, C., Weber, J. K., Bell, D. R. and Zhou, R. (2015). Surface curvature relation to protein adsorption for carbon-based nanomaterials, *Sci. Rep.*, **5**, p. 10886.

47. Frishman, D. and Argos, P. (1995). Knowledge-based protein secondary structure assignment, *Proteins*, **23**, pp. 566–579.

48. Joosten, R. R. P., te Beek, T. A. H., Krieger, E., Hekkelman, M. L., Hooft, R. W. W., Schneider, R., Sander, C. and Vriend, G. (2011). A series of PDB related databases for everyday needs, *Nucleic Acids Res.*, **39**, pp. D411–D419.

49. Artali, R., Del Pra, A., Foresti, E., Lesci, I. G., Roveri, N. and Sabatino, P. (2008). Adsorption of human serum albumin on the chrysotile surface: a molecular dynamics and spectroscopic investigation, *J. R. Soc. Interface*, **5**, pp. 273–283.

50. Castellanos, M. M. and Colina, C. M. (2013). Molecular dynamics simulations of human serum albumin and role of disulfide bonds, *J. Phys. Chem. B*, **117**, pp. 11895–11905.

51. Raffaini, G. and Ganazzoli, F. (2003). Simulation study of the interaction of some albumin subdomains with a flat graphite surface, *Langmuir*, **19**, pp. 3403–3412.

52. Lehtinen, J., Magarkar, A., Stepniewski, M., Hakola, S., Bergman, M., Róg, T., Yliperttula, M., Urtti, A. and Bunker, A. (2012). Analysis of cause of failure of new targeting peptide in PEGylated liposome: molecular modeling as rational design tool for nanomedicine, *Eur. J. Pharm. Sci.*, **46**, pp. 121–130.

53. Kang, Y., Wang, Q., Liu, Y.-C., Wu, T., Chen, Q. and Guan, W.-J. (2008). Dynamic mechanism of collagen-like peptide encapsulated into carbon nanotubes, *J. Phys. Chem. B*, **112**, pp. 4801–4807.

54. Matsuura, K., Saito, T., Okazaki, T., Ohshima, S., Yumura, M. and Iijima, S. (2006). Selectivity of water-soluble proteins in single-walled carbon nanotube dispersions, *Chem. Phys. Lett.*, **429**, pp. 497–502.

55. Wang, X.-L., Lu, Z.-Y., Li, Z.-S. and Sun, C.-C. (2007). Molecular dynamics simulation study on controlling the adsorption behavior of polyethylene by fine tuning the surface nanodecoration of graphite, *Langmuir*, **23**, pp. 802–808.

Chapter 7

Metal Nanoclusters for Biosensing and Drug Delivery Applications

Malamatenia Koklioti and Nikos Tagmatarchis
Theoretical and Physical Chemistry Institute,
National Hellenic Research Foundation,
48 Vassileos Constantinou Avenue,
11635 Athens, Greece
mkoklioti@eie.gr

7.1 Introduction

With the advent of nanotechnology, materials with sizes in the nanoscale have proved to be excellent platforms in biomedical applications. Different kinds of nanomaterials, such as iron oxide nanoparticles, quantum dots, metal nanoparticles (such as Au and Ag), carbon nanotubes, and silica nanoparticles, have all spurred tremendous interest as theranostic species [1]. Particularly metal nanoclusters (MNCs) have been lately exploited in biorelated applications as an outcome of their ultrasmall size and extraordinary physicochemical properties and present encouraging results promoting their utility over conventional nanoparticles.

Drug Delivery Nanosystems: From Bioinspiration and Biomimetics to Clinical Applications
Edited by Costas Demetzos, Stergios Pispas, and Natassa Pippa

ISBN 978-981-4774-92-5 (Hardcover), 978-0-429-49054-5 (eBook)
www.panstanford.com

The objective of this chapter is to summarize recent research progress in the application of MNCs in biological systems, namely selective targeting of specific bio-oriented species and drug delivery, especially regarding cancer treatment. Moreover, a brief outlook regarding, current challenges in, and limitations in MNCs research are also provided.

7.2 Definition of Metal Nanoclusters

In the past decades, considerable scientific progress has been made in the exploration of the attractive properties of metal nanoparticles, which has manifested great application potential in catalysis [2], sensing [3], and drug delivery [4]. At the same time, particles that are a few nanometers or less in diameter, named MNCs [5, 6], bridge the gap between metal atoms and nanoparticles. Significantly, MNCs have triggered a heightened scientific interest due to their unique optical and electronic and physical properties, along with good biocompatibility and low toxicity, as opposed to their corresponding large nanoparticle counterparts. Briefly, MNCs are composed of several to roughly a hundred atoms and possess dimensions comparable to the Fermi wavelength of electrons, exhibiting semiconducting molecule-like properties and strong size-dependent photoluminescence [7, 8]. Although materials in the dimension range from 0.1 nm to 100 nm are termed nanoparticles, it is lately revealed that a core size of 2 nm is the limit for ultrafine nanoparticle to be considered nanoclusters [9, 10].

Remarkably, due to the ultrasmall size of MNCs, their novel features are of particular interest, rendering them promising candidates in multiple applications, such as sensing, bioimaging, optoelectronics, catalysis, energy conversion, and storage [10–12]. One of the most stimulating hallmarks of MNCs is their photoluminescence, as they exhibit distinct and size-tunable electronic transitions. However, discovering ways to controllably govern their size, composition, crystal structure, and surface properties without using sophisticated synthesis protocols is still a daunting challenge [10, 13]. Minor modifications regarding size and composition, such as the addition or removal of a single atom within MNCs, can notably influence their properties. Because MNCs are tiny in size, many of their functionalities are completely altered, since MNCs display discrete electronic energy levels compared to traditional metal nanoparticles, in which the surface plasmon resonance property is dominant. Specifically, in bulk metals, the conduction band has no energy gap separating it from the valence band, permitting electrons moving freely without facing any barrier. On the contrary, concerning MNCs, the band structure becomes discontinuous, divided into energy levels. Therefore, interaction with light still exists, similar to organic dyes, via electronic transitions between the energy levels, resulting in light absorption and emission [14].

Recent progress has enabled simple protocols for the synthesis of water-soluble MNCs with tunable fluorescence emission in a variety of bio-oriented applications, establishing them as the next generation of biocompatible fluorophores for applications. In particular, MNC-based ensembles are purported to be promising candidates as theranostic platforms. This is because the excellent physicochemical properties of the metal core can be harnessed for fluorescence imaging and sensing of pathogens [15]. To incorporate MNCs into rational applications, they need to be functionalized because bare nanoclusters are thermodynamically labile as the excess surface energy leads to agglomeration phenomena. The stabilization of MNCs through protective ligands surrounding their metal core is necessary. Extensionally, MNCs can be easily functionalized with biorecognition modules for selective sensing and targeted drug delivery (Fig. 7.1). Due to the large surface-to-volume ratio of MNCs, they can also serve as a reservoir sink to

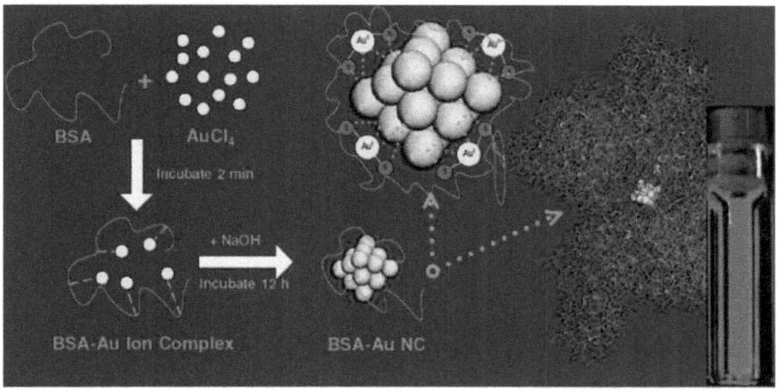

Figure 7.1 Schematic representation of bovine serum albumin (BSA)-stabilized Au NCs. Reprinted with permission from Ref. [15]. Copyright (2009) with permission by American Chemical Society.

load numerous drugs/genes and be modified with sensing/imaging species to be imbued with both therapeutic and diagnostic functions. Particularly, for in vivo applications, a small hydrodynamic diameter is preferred for efficient transmembrane permeation and urinary excretion. Additionally, high biocompatibility along with prolonged circulation time and exceptional activity to target the desired tumor tissues, while killing only cancerous cells, without affecting healthy ones, are a prerequisite.

7.3 Metal Nanoclusters for Biosensing

MNCs stabilized with thiol-based ligands (e.g., glutathione, or GSH), amines, biomolecules, DNA, and bovine serum albumin (BSA) [16] display a unique core-shell configuration [9, 17], which can serve as the recognition site that will tether to a target molecule, leading to a change in the optical properties of MNCs. Hence, the fluorescence of MNCs can be exploited as an optical probe to witness interactions with biologically oriented species. Additionally, the detection of specific molecules is important when separation-free probes are involved, especially in the case of intracellular studies, where removal of unbound probes is difficult. In general, there are three types of detection elements for biological sensing, namely nuclei acid sequences, proteins, and cell receptor ligands. To this end, silver nanoclusters (Ag NCs) have been predominantly developed for the selective detection of DNA via the fabrication of the so-called nanocluster beacon (NCB). For instance, specific DNA-templated Ag NCs were developed via a facile strategy and it was found that their fluorescence was significantly enhanced when they were placed near guanine-rich DNA sequences [18]. Astonishingly, a five hundred–fold fluorescence enhancement was detected upon addition of Ag NCs and their hybridization with a complementary DNA strand bearing also a guanine-rich tail, as observed in a 3D contour plot of the excitation/emission spectra. To further prove these findings, a "turn-on" DNA assay to detect an influenza target (a sequence from H1N1 virus) was designed. Indeed, an extraordinarily high signal-to-background ratio upon employment of Ag NCs was achieved, as compared with another conventional probe. Furthermore, in a pioneering study DNA-capped Ag NCs were served as a chameleon

NCB and the ability to respond to different stimuli, that is, to light up according to the environment surrounding the clusters, was demonstrated [19]. More precisely, those Ag NCs were templated on single-stranded (ss) DNA with a guanine-rich sequence acting as a fluorescence enhancer. A 60–70 nm shift in the emission was detected because different target nucleotides can establish their own conformation between Ag NCs and the enhancer, producing a color change in Ag NCs. Furthermore, their protocol was exploited not only qualitatively but also quantitatively via examination of targets associated with Werner's syndrome and type 2 diabetes. An identical scenario was also applied for the selective detection of N^6-methyladenine at single-base level, whose recognition is importance as it is related to human disease [20, 21]. The same signal transduction approach was also adopted for the detection of *Homo sapiens*' hemoglobin beta chain gene [22]. In particular, a "turn-on" DNA probe was designed by shuttling dark Ag NCs to a bright scaffold through DNA hybridization. A seventyfold emission enhancement was recorded when double-stranded (ds) DNA was functionalized with two templates on its opposite sides, whereas increased emission intensity was also observed when templates were placed at other positions (Fig. 7.2).

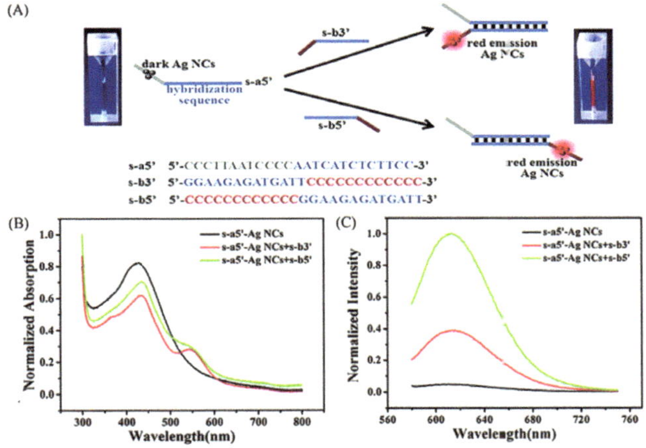

Figure 7.2 Schematic representation of NCB based on DNA-templated Ag NCs depicting the generation of Ag NC photoluminescence upon hybridization with complementary DNA strands irrespective of the position of the two DNA templates. Reproduced from Ref. [22] with permission of The Royal Society of Chemistry.

Fluorescence increment is not the only means for sensitive DNA targeting, but an optical property switch accompanied by color change is also reported. In this regard, DNA-bound violet-absorbing Ag NCs composed of 11 silver atoms were reported to exhibit a 330 nm red-shift in the absorption spectrum and recovery of their near-infrared (NIR) emission upon dimerization with target DNA strands [23]. More recently, it was demonstrated that violet-emissive Ag NCs consisting of 10 silver atoms capped with single-stranded (ss) DNA can be converted into a new species with highly green emissive ones due to hybridization with the target's complementary oligonucleotides [24]. The photoluminescence alteration was attributable to various DNA structural changes and their effect on interactions with silver atoms as well as alterations in nucleobase conformation.

On a different note, MNCs can be combined with aptamers, which are synthetic nucleic acids fitting snugly to a specific target molecule. Such aptamer- Ag NCs with cytosine-rich DNA sequences that promote photoluminescence have been applied for the selective detection of human a-thrombin as a target protein [25]. Upon anchoring of aptamer–Ag NCs on thrombin, their corresponding emission peak at 700 nm was quenched, signaling successful detection, as no photoluminescence change was detected when other proteins of varied structures and charge states were examined. The sensing of two types of cancer cells (acute lymphoblastic leukemia human and Burkitt's lymphoma) was also achieved with Ag NCs after the selection of the appropriate binding probe for each case in terms of optical property from among a series of aptamers and linkers [26]. Confocal laser scanning microscopy confirmed that the properly functionalized Ag NCs could effectively recognize the malignant growth. More recently, hairpin-labeled Ag NCs conjugated with the appropriate segments for hepatitis B virus (HBV) recognition were tested [27]. In the presence of the target, the conformation of the target with the recognition sequence changed, freeing up the nucleation sequence, where fluorescent Ag NCs can be formed, providing a readout signal for successful sensing. To further demonstrate the feasibility of the latter findings, a thrombin aptamer was put in lieu of the hairpin, proving that careful design of the recognition sequences is a prerequisite for the specific detection of diverse targets. The same protocol, that is, to construct photoluminescence enhancement assays using guanine-rich DNA sequences and functionalized Ag NCs, which boast photoluminescence upon recognition-induced hybridization, was also followed for targeting proteins [28] and cancerous cells (Fig. 7.3) [29].

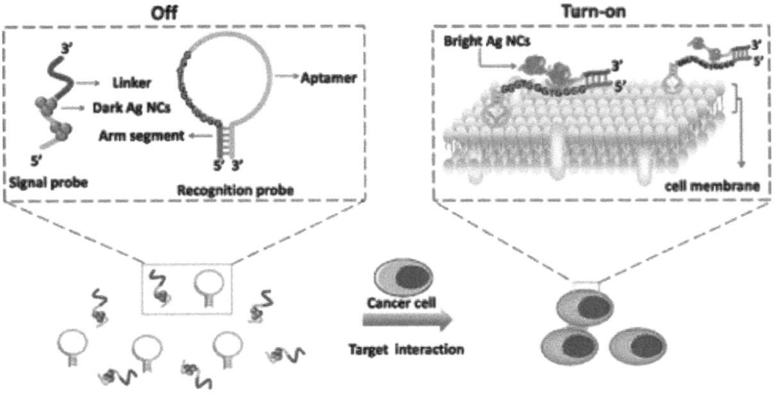

Figure 7.3 Typical schematic demonstration of the "turn-on" aptamer strategy for cancer cell detection based on DNA–Ag NC photoluminescence recognition-induced hybridization. Reprinted with permission from Ref. [29]{Yin, 2013 #4164}. Copyright (2017) American Chemical Society.

Apart from being modified by nucleic acids, MNCs can also be conjugated with proteins and peptides in order to develop a robust bionanosensor. For example, blue-emitting collagen-protected gold nanoclusters (Au NCs) and macerozyme R-10–labeled Au NCs have been synthesized as a visual sensor array for the discrimination of eight proteins [30]. Different emission wavelength shifts were generated and observed even by the naked eye under an ultraviolet (UV) lamp when a different target protein was introduced. The color change is strongly associated with the interactions between target proteins and the Au NC surface, which form unique target protein–Au NC complexes emitting light of different wavelengths. Furthermore, the proposed method was applied in real samples to distinguish the protein profiles found in serums from hepatoma and thalassemia patients from those from healthy people. In another work, BSA-stabilized Au NCs were applied to detect proteases, specifically trypsin [31]. A significant enhancement of photoluminescence was detected upon trypsin digestion, highlighting the ability of MNCs to serve also as substrates for target enzymes. Fluorescence quenching is also reported to be a valuable biosensor platform to target specific proteins. Hence, Au NCs stabilized with the proper peptide were employed for label-free sensing of two post-translational modification (PTM) enzymes (i.e., kinase A and histone deacetylase 1), which are closely related to cycle regulation, cell proliferation, and cancer development [32]. The PTM enzymes were capable of causing chemical modifications, which altered the protecting environment of the clusters, resulting in their oxidation and fluorescence quenching and a drop in their lifetime. Alternatively, MNCs can be designed with different targeting components to endow them with multiple functionalities. In this regard, Au NCs were functionalized with bifunctional peptide antigens to stimulate precise immunological responses. Moreover, cytosine-phosphate-guanine (CpG) oligodeoxynucleotides (ODNs) were also coupled, since they exhibit substantial immunostimulatory activities against invading pathogens [33]. The peptide–Au NC–CpG showed strong immunostimulatory activity in both in vitro and in vivo assays as opposed to the performance of peptide or CpG ODN alone, thus underlining the promising potential of MNCs to serve as self-vaccines for immunotherapy.

In addition to selectively detecting proteins, protein-capped MNCs have been found to exhibit excellent enzyme mimetic activity, which is essential for targeting biologically related structures. In this context, BSA-stabilized Au NCs could catalyze the oxidation of the peroxidase substrate 3,3,5,5-tetramethylbenzidine in the presence of H_2O_2, while the color change to blue implied a colorimetric method for the detection of H_2O_2 (Fig. 7.4). An extensive study of the catalytic activity of BSA-stabilized Au NCs showed that the optimal conditions to determine xanthine in urine and human serum samples were pH 3–4 at 35°C–40°C. An identical concept was also applied for the detection of dopamine, which plays a key role in the central nervous, renal, hormonal, and cardiovascular systems [34].

As pointed out previously, MNCs can also be bound to cell receptor ligands to function as identification sites for pathogenic species. In this regard, mannose-capped Au NCs were utilized for the identification of *Escherichia coli* J96 bacteria commonly associated with urinary tract infections. These Au NCs were capable of interacting with target bacteria containing mannose-binding receptors via the selective expression of mannose-binding protein FimH, which was subsequently recognized by Au NCs. On addition of the *E. coli* J96 sample to the mannose-protected Au NCs, a precipitate was generated giving a concentration-dependent red fluorescence, which could be observed with the naked eye [35].

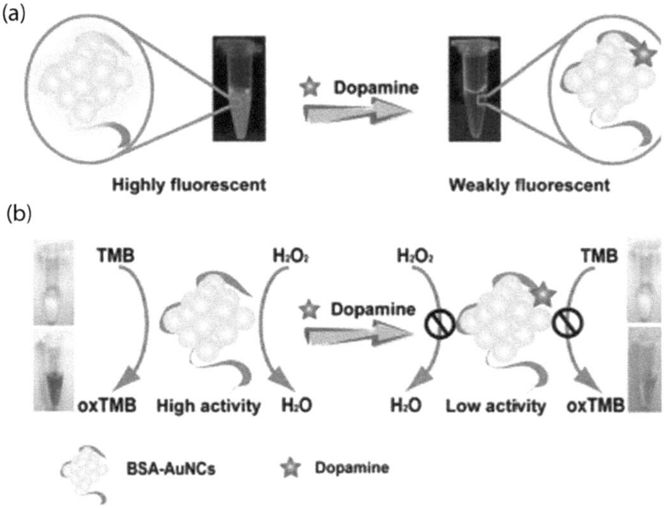

Figure 7.4 (a) Schematic illustration of the fluorescence response of the BSA-stabilized Au NCs to dopamine. (b) Schematic representation of peroxidase-like catalytic color reaction for sensitive sensing of dopamine Reprinted from Ref. [34], Copyright (2013), with permission from Elsevier.

However, biological species with a detrimental impact on human health can be detected by using a donor (MNCs)-acceptor (carbon nanomaterial) system, which causes fluorescence resonance energy transfer (FRET) phenomena. Consequently, a hybrid consisting of Ag NCs and single-walled carbon nanotubes (SWCNTs) was developed for screening folate receptors (FRs), which are mostly found and overexpressed in many cancerous cell types in humans (Fig. 7.5a) [36]. The approach was based on the functionalization of Ag NCs with such an oligonucleotide, which presents complementarity with that conjugated with a folic acid molecule. Notably, modified SWCNTs showed a great affinity for Ag NCs, causing fluorescence quenching due to FRET. However, upon the addition of the target, a double-helix DNA is formed by the ssDNA of the probe and Ag

NCs, resulting in breakage of the Ag NC/SWCNT ensemble. Hence, the electronic interactions between Ag NCs and SWCNTs are absent, thereby facilitating the photoluminescence recovery of Ag NCs and acting as a "turn on" signal. Indeed, the decreased proximity of Ag NCs and SWCNTs is further justified as the sp^2 network of SWCNTs binds more weakly with double-stranded DNA, since the hydrophobic bases of the DNA can be efficiently protected from SWCNTs and weaken the π-π stacking interactions. Through this protocol, the quantification of the target molecule was successfully achieved with a low detection limit, while the findings were applied to detect cancer cells (HeLa) that contained FRs directly. Similarly, a transferrin-functionalized Au NC/graphene oxide (GO) hybrid was prepared and employed as a detection probe for imaging of cancer cells and small animals [37]. Fluorescence restoration was again the driving force to selectively sense HeLa cells even in tumor-bearing mice. The HBV gene, the human immunodeficiency virus (HIV) gene, and the syphilis (*Treponema pallidum*) gene were also targeted via the Ag NC/GO hybrid material (Fig. 7.5b) [38].

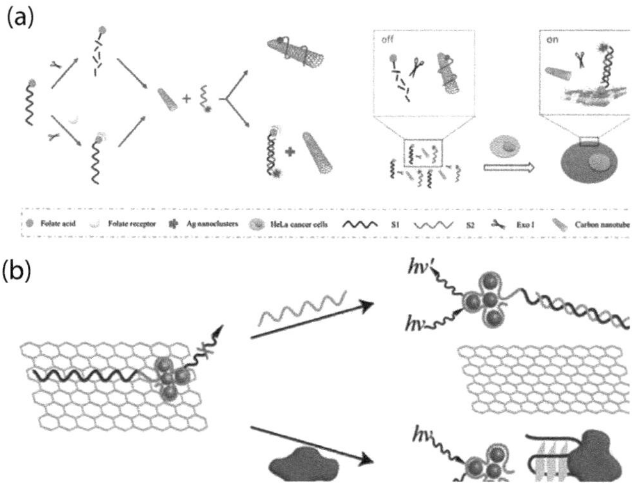

Figure 7.5 (a) Design of the label-free and turn-on fluorescent sensor based on Ag NCs for FR detection (left) and its application in cancer cell detection (right). Reproduced from Ref. [36] with permission of The Royal Society of Chemistry. (b) Multiplexed detection of the HBV and HIV gene using a Ag NC/GO hybrid. Reprinted with permission from Ref. [38]. Copyright (2013) American Chemical Society.

7.4 Metal Nanoclusters for Drug Delivery

In addition to specifically targeting, MNCs can also harness their capabilities as effective delivery nanocarriers in biological systems due to several attractive features, such as their tiny size, helping them to penetrate effectively into cells. BSA-capped Au NCs embedded in BSA nanoparticles were employed as fluorescent probes and delivery systems of doxorubicin hydrochloride (DOX), which is widely used against several forms of cancer [39] The hydrophilic and hydrophobic parts of BSA favored the fabrication of the DOX–Au NC complex, since electrostatic and hydrogen bonding interactions with several amino acids of BSA assisted in the facile preparation of the composite. It was found that the DOX-loaded Au NC composite was effectively delivered in vitro to the malignant growth, as compared with standalone DOX, while Au NCs retained their NIR fluorescence in the human blood serum. In another similar study, GSH-capped Au NCs were combined with a polyacylic acid (PAA)/ calcium phosphate (CaP) shell loaded with DOX to function as pH-sensitive drug delivery carriers. Interestingly, it was demonstrated that DOX-loaded Au NC-assembly@PAA/CaP nanoparticles displayed a smaller tumor volume after 11 days of treatment as compared with free DOX and empty nanoparticles. Furthermore, it was revealed that the developed complex can simultaneously function as a computed tomography and fluorescence imaging nanoprobe for liver cancer chemotherapy in vivo [40].

More recently, Au NCs were self-assembled into nanoparticles of 120 nm diameter after anchoring with poly(allylamine hydrochloride) (PAH), to serve as a successful drug delivery agent in human monocytic cells (THP1 cell line). The working principle was based on the fabrication of GSH-stabilized Au NCs, in which PAH was added under certain pH conditions, forming positively charged nanoparticles. An aggregation-induced emission phenomenon was observed due to electrostatic interactions between PAH and Au NC–stabilizing surface ligands. The drug delivery potential was verified upon conjugation with suitable peptides and antibodies, and it was found that there was better accumulation of Au-GSH-PAH-peptide onto the cell membrane due to the smaller size of the peptide [41]. A more facile methodology employing directly a pH and thermoresponsive stabilizer for Au NCs was introduced by Zhang et al. [42]. Briefly, short-chain polyethylene glycol–Au NCs were conjugated with DOX to investigate their drug delivery potential against A549 lung adenocarcinoma cells and imaging. It was demonstrated that the particular Au NC architecture presents negligible toxicity and was able to enter into cells and even nuclei. Interestingly, it was found that DOX-loaded Au NCs displayed increased drug circulation time and considerable cell-killing effects, underlining the significance of the application of DOX complexes as safer formulations toward anticancer therapy compared to free DOX molecules, which may cause severe toxicity to cells. Analogously, encouraging results were also provided upon camptothecin delivery to uterine cervix carcinoma (HeLa) and A549 cell line based on a complex formulation of Au NCs as core and folate, poly(L-lactide), and sulfated polysaccharide as shell [43]. Additionally, BSA-capped Au NCs conjugated with herceptin (Au NC–Her) were utilized for targeting and treatment of ErbB2-overexpressing breast cancer cells (Fig. 7.6) [44]. More precisely, strong specific binding was observed in the case of malignant cells due to the presence of the corresponding receptors on their surface, while no special uptake was evident for normal cells, as revealed from confocal laser scanning microscopic examination. Importantly, Au NC–Her were able to penetrate the chromosomal region of the nucleus, whereas free Her failed or standalone Au NCs presented limited uptake, rendering their applicability very ambitious toward drug delivery. Indeed, it was proved that Au NC–Her could cause apoptosis due to DNA damage in up to 95% of the treated cells, rather than Her alone, with a 35% success rate, highlighting the significance of the functionalization of Her with Au NCs.

Other breast cancer cells, namely the highly aggressive 4T1 cell line, underwent anticancer therapy with the aid of BSA-templated Au NCs conjugated with a cisplatin prodrug, (*cis,cis,trans*-[Pt(NH3)2Cl2(OH) (O2CCH2CH2CO2H)]) (MDDP), and folic acid as the recognizing moiety for specific breast cancer targeting (Fig. 7.7) [45]. It was shown that the specific Au NC complex could selectively inhibit the cancerous growth by up to 80%, as was clear from fluorescence imaging in tumor-bearing mouse. Also, lung metastasis was averted to a large extent due to the successful treatment of the primary tumor, which restrained the cancerous cells against further accumulation, as examined by bioluminance imaging.

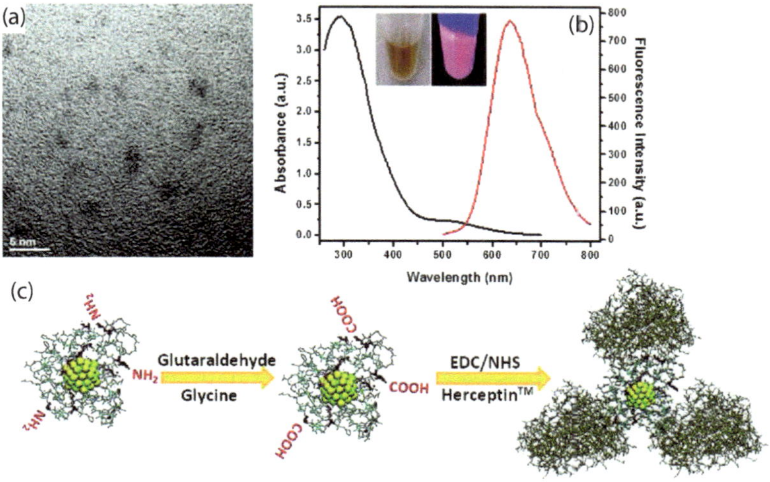

Figure 7.6 (a) Transmission electron microscopy image of the as-prepared Au NCs, (b) UV-vis absorbance and fluorescent spectrum of Au NCs, and (c) schematic of Au NC–Her conjugation. Reprinted with permission from Ref. [44]. Copyright (2011) American Chemical Society.

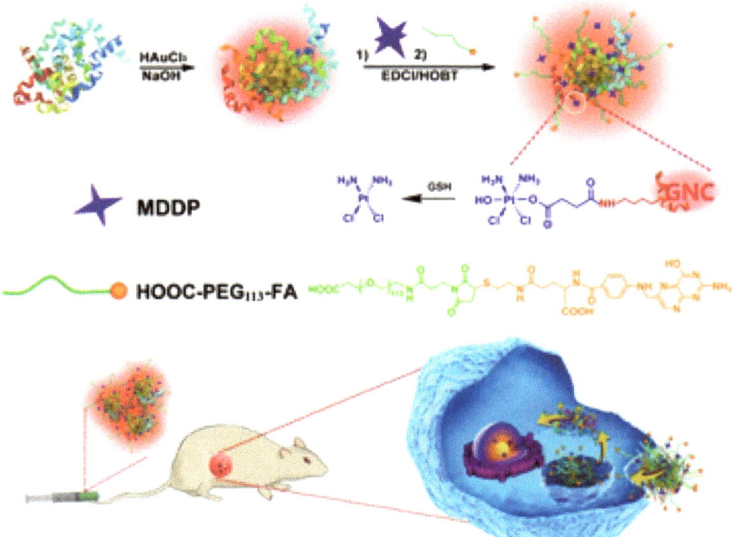

Figure 7.7 Schematic representation of Au NC-based theranostic nanoplatform for tumor-targeted chemotherapy and fluorescence imaging [45].

The utility of gold as a drug vehicle is undoubtedly in the center of researchers' attention covering a major part of the bibliography. Nonetheless, the application of other metal-based nanoclusters is also reported in tandem. To this end, cadmium nanoclusters (Cd NCs) are another example dealing with cell imaging and selective drug delivery of anticancer drugs. More precisely, pH-responsive BSA-harbored Cd NCs were conjugated with hyaluronic acid (HA), which is a cell surface receptor in specific tumor cells (MCF-7 breast cancer cells), and loaded with DOX. Surprisingly, the results revealed that Cd NCs presented high biocompatibility even at a relatively high concentration of 1 mg/mL, while they evidenced lower toxicity upon combination with HA due to its high biocompatibility. Additionally, they demonstrated that the DOX-loaded HA–Cd NCs attained the same cytotoxicity to malignant cells at a lower dose of DOX, thereby diminishing the harmful effects on normal tissues (Fig. 7.8) [46].

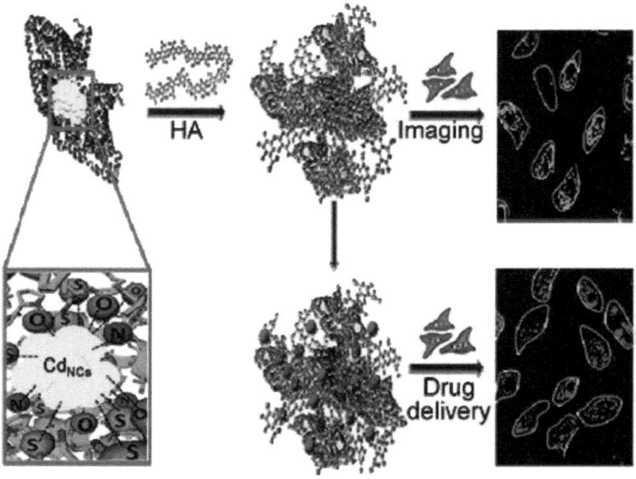

Figure 7.8 Schematic illustration of the BSA-protected Cd NCs, conjugation of HA to Cd NCs (HA–Cd NCs), and imaging. DOX loading into the HA–Cd NC nanocarrier (DOX–HA–Cd NCs) and HA receptor–mediated targeted drug delivery. Reprinted from Ref. [46]. © Tsinghua University Press and Springer-Verlag Berlin Heidelberg 2016. With permission of Springer.

Finally, copper nanoclusters (Cu NCs) were synthesized using lipoic acid in combination with the biocompatible polymer poly(vinylpyrrolidone) as the stabilizer. Also, poly(vinyl alcohol) was added, as a cross-linker, to construct a hydrogel nanocarrier with a cellular uptake potential. This Cu NC–based formulation encapsulated cisplatin for antitumor treatment of HeLa cells. Fluorescence microscopy images confirmed the high uptake of the drug-loaded complex, as evidenced by the emission due to red color under blue light excitation. Importantly, it was deduced that the addition of the Cu NC–hydrogel composite to malignant cells was able to improve drug efficacy, since cell viability was doubled in comparison with the same drug concentration employed in free form [47].

7.5 Conclusions

The intention of this chapter is to provide examples of application of MNCs in different aspects of theranostics, namely targeting of specific bio-oriented species (such as nuclei acid sequences, proteins, and cell receptor ligands) and drug delivery, especially regarding cancer treatment and imaging, accentuating their advantageous properties that are vital in practical applications. The benefits of utilizing MNCs in biorelated applications in lieu of traditional metal nanoparticles or other organic fluorophores are the following: (i) the passivation of ultrasmall MNCs by ligands not only facilitates their growth together with the formation of tunable luminescent markers but also provides facile pathways to tether them to specific probes, promoting the construction of selective sensing platforms, (ii) the good photostability and luminescence unveil essential merits over conventional organic dyes, which suffer from photobleaching, and (iii) the ultrasmall size of MNCs as opposed to molecular fluorophores or quantum dots and their nontoxic features provide a versatile means for exploiting them in biological media.

Undoubtedly, biotemplated MNCs will play a key role in next-generation personalized nanomedicine, considering their enhanced treatment efficiency in terms of accurate diagnosis and targeted therapeutics. However, it should be noted that there are obstacles yet to be overcome needing clarifications. For example, controllable synthesis methods should be developed since up to now only empirical strategies have been applied, derived from the existing knowledge of synthesis methods of MNCs. The low quantum yield compared with that of organic dyes and quantum dots is another concern to be addressed, along with how synthesis conditions are associated with the activity of functional moiety and emission color. To this end, additional theoretical studies will unveil the interactions developing between MNCs and biosystems. Moreover, the utilization of low-cost metals, such as Cu, other than the noble ones should be exploited as well as protocols for large-scale production of MNCs should be examined.

By extension, future research is expected to achieve advances with the aid of those tiny MNCs and diseases or predisposition to diseases will be diagnosed earlier than it is possible at present.

Acknowledgments

Financial support through a PhD scholarship by the General Secretariat for Research and Technology (GSRT) – Hellenic Research Foundation for Research and Innovation (HFRI) to Malamatenia Koklioti (Grant 93) is acknowledged. This project has also received funding from the European Union's Horizon 2020 Research and Innovation Programme under the Marie Sklodowska-Curie grant agreement No. 642742. Partial financial support by the General Secretariat for Research and Technology, Greece, through project "Advanced Materials and Devices" (MIS: 5002409) is acknowledged.

References

1. Xie, J., Lee, S. and Chen, X. (2010). Nanoparticle-based theranostic agents, *Adv. Drug Deliv. Rev.*, **62**, pp. 1064–1079.
2. Mikami, Y., Dhakshinamoorthy, A., Alvaro, M. and Garcia, H. (2013). Catalytic activity of unsupported gold nanoparticles, *Catal. Sci. Technol.*, **3**, pp. 58–69.
3. Howes, P. D., Chandrawati, R. and Stevens, M. M. (2014). Colloidal nanoparticles as advanced biological sensors, *Science*, **346**, p. 1247390.
4. Doane, T. L. and Burda, C. (2012). The unique role of nanoparticles in nanomedicine: imaging, drug delivery and therapy, *Chem. Soc. Rev.*, **41**, pp. 2885–2911.
5. Schmid, G. (2008). The relevance of shape and size of Au_{55} clusters, *Chem. Soc. Rev.*, **37**, pp. 1909–1930.
6. Jin, R. (2010). Quantum sized, thiolate-protected gold nanoclusters, *Nanoscale*, **2**, pp. 343–362.

7. Wilcoxon, J. P. and Abrams, B. L. (2006). Synthesis, structure and properties of metal nanoclusters, *Chem. Soc. Rev.*, **35**, pp. 1162–1194.
8. Diez, I. and Ras, R. H. A. (2011). Fluorescent silver nanoclusters, *Nanoscale*, **3**, pp. 1963–1970.
9. Qian, H., Zhu, M., Wu, Z. and Jin, R. (2012). Quantum sized gold nanoclusters with atomic precision, *Acc. Chem. Res.*, **45**, pp. 1470–1479.
10. Lu, Y. and Chen, W. (2012). Sub-nanometre sized metal clusters: from synthetic challenges to the unique property discoveries, *Chem. Soc. Rev.*, **41**, pp. 3594–3623.
11. Shang, L., Dong, S. and Nienhaus, G. U. (2011). Ultra-small fluorescent metal nanoclusters: synthesis and biological applications, *Nano Today*, **6**, pp. 401–418.
12. Koklioti, M. A. and Tagmatarchis, N. (2016). Hybrids of metal nanoclusters and graphene-based materials: preparation, properties and applications, *ChemNanoMat*, **2**, pp. 1065–1072.
13. Qian, H., Zhu, M., Wu, Z. and Jin, R. (2012). Quantum sized gold nanoclusters with atomic precision, *Acc. Chem. Res.*, **45**, pp. 470–1479.
14. Li, J., Zhu, J.-J. and Xu, K. (2014). Fluorescent metal nanoclusters: from synthesis to applications, *Trends Anal. Chem.*, **58**, pp. 90–98.
15. Xie, J., Zheng, Y. and Ying, J. Y. (2009). Protein-directed synthesis of highly fluorescent gold nanoclusters, *J. Am. Chem. Soc.*, **131**, pp. 888–889.
16. Li, Z., Sun, Q., Zhu, Y., Tan, B., Xu, Z. P. and Dou, S. X. (2014). Ultra-small fluorescent inorganic nanoparticles for bioimaging, *J. Mater. Chem. B*, **2**, pp. 2793–2818.
17. Li, M.-B., Tian, S.-K., Wu, Z. and Jin, R. (2016). Peeling the core–shell Au_{25} nanocluster by reverse ligand-exchange, *Chem. Mater.*, **28**, pp. 1022–1025.
18. Yeh, H.-C., Sharma, J., Han, J. J., Martinez, J. S. and Werner, J. H. (2010). A DNA–silver nanocluster probe that fluoresces upon hybridization, *Nano Lett.*, **10**, pp. 3106–3110.
19. Yeh, H.-C., Sharma, J., Shih, I.-M., Vu, D. M., Martinez, J. S. and Werner, J. H. (2012). A fluorescence light-up Ag nanocluster probe that discriminates single-nucleotide variants by emission color, *J. Am. Chem. Soc.*, **134**, pp. 11550–11558.
20. Chen, Y.-A., Obliosca, J. M., Liu, Y.-L., Liu, C., Gwozdz, M. L. and Yeh, H.-C. (2015). Nanocluster beacons enable detection of a single N^6-methyladenine, *J. Am. Chem. Soc.*, **137**, pp. 10476–10479.

21. Wion, D. and Casadesus, J. (2006). N^6-methyl-adenine: an epigenetic signal for DNA-protein interactions, *Nat. Rev. Microbiol.*, **4**, pp. 183–192.

22. Teng, Y., Jia, X., Zhang, S., Zhu, J. and Wang, E. (2016). A nanocluster beacon based on the template transformation of DNA-templated silver nanoclusters, *Chem. Commun.*, **52**, pp. 1721–1724.

23. Petty, J. T., Giri, B., Miller, I. C., Nicholson, D. A., Sergev, O. O., Banks, T. M. and Story, S. P. (2013). Silver clusters as both chromophoric reporters and DNA ligands, *Anal. Chem.*, **85**, pp. 2183–2190.

24. Petty, J. T., Sergev, O. O., Kantor, A. G., Rankine, I. J., Ganguly, M., David, F. D., Wheeler, S. K. and Wheeler, J. F. (2015). Ten-atom silver cluster signaling and tempering DNA hybridization, *Anal. Chem.*, **87**, pp. 5302–5309.

25. Sharma, J., Yeh, H.-C., Yoo, H., Werner, J. H. and Martinez, J. S. (2011). Silver nanocluster aptamers: in situ generation of intrinsically fluorescent recognition ligands for protein detection, *Chem. Commun.*, **47**, pp. 2294–2296.

26. Yin, J., He, X., Wang, K., Qing, Z., Wu, X., Shi, H. and Yang, X. (2012). One-step engineering of silver nanoclusters-aptamer assemblies as luminescent labels to target tumor cells, *Nanoscale*, **4**, pp. 110–112.

27. Xiao, Y., Wu, Z., Wong, K.-Y. and Liu, Z. (2014). Hairpin DNA probes based on target-induced in situ generation of luminescent silver nanoclusters, *Chem. Commun.*, **50**, pp. 4849–4852.

28. Li, J., Zhong, X., Zhang, H., Le, X. C. and Zhu, J.-J. (2012). Binding-induced fluorescence turn-on assay using aptamer-functionalized silver nanocluster DNA probes, *Anal. Chem.*, **84**, pp. 5170–5174.

29. Yin, J., He, X., Wang, K., Xu, F., Shangguan, J., He, D. and Shi, H. (2013). Label-free and turn-on aptamer strategy for cancer cells detection based on a DNA–silver nanocluster fluorescence upon recognition-induced hybridization, *Anal. Chem.*, **85**, pp. 12011–12019.

30. Xu, S., Lu, X., Yao, C., Huang, F., Jiang, H., Hua, W., Na, N., Liu, H. and Ouyang, J. (2014). A visual sensor array for pattern recognition analysis of proteins using novel blue-emitting fluorescent gold nanoclusters, *Anal. Chem.*, **86**, pp. 11634–11639.

31. Fernandez-Iglesias, N. and Bettmer, J. (2014). Synthesis, purification and mass spectrometric characterisation of a fluorescent Au_9@BSA nanocluster and its enzymatic digestion by trypsin, *Nanoscale*, **6**, pp. 716–721.

32. Wen, Q., Gu, Y., Tang, L.-J., Yu, R.-Q. and Jiang, J.-H. (2013). Peptide-templated gold nanocluster beacon as a sensitive, label-free sensor for protein post-translational modification enzymes, *Anal. Chem.*, **85**, pp. 11681–11685.

33. Yang, J., Xia, N., Wang, X., Liu, X., Xu, A., Wu, Z. and Luo, Z. (2015). One-pot one-cluster synthesis of fluorescent and bio-compatible Ag_{14} nanoclusters for cancer cell imaging, *Nanoscale*, **7**, pp. 18464–18470.

34. Tao, Y., Lin, Y., Ren, J. and Qu, X. (2013). A dual fluorometric and colorimetric sensor for dopamine based on BSA-stabilized Au nanoclusters, *Biosens. Bioelectron.*, **42**, pp. 41–46.

35. Chan, P.-H., Ghosh, B., Lai, H.-Z., Peng, H.-L., Mong, K. K. T. and Chen, Y.-C. (2013). Photoluminescent gold nanoclusters as sensing probes for uropathogenic Escherichia coli, *PLoS One*, **8**, pp. e58064.

36. Jiang, H., Xu, G., Sun, Y., Zheng, W., Zhu, X., Wang, B., Zhang, X. and Wang, G. (2015). A "turn-on" silver nanocluster based fluorescent sensor for folate receptor detection and cancer cell imaging under visual analysis, *Chem. Commun.*, **51**, pp. 11810–11813.

37. Wang, Y., Chen, J.-T. and Yan, X.-P. (2013). Fabrication of transferrin functionalized gold nanoclusters/graphene oxide nanocomposite for turn-on near-infrared fluorescent bioimaging of cancer cells and small animals, *Anal. Chem.*, **85**, pp. 2529–2535.

38. Liu, X., Wang, F., Aizen, R., Yehezkeli, O. and Willner, I. (2013). Graphene oxide/nucleic-acid-stabilized silver nanoclusters: functional hybrid materials for optical aptamer sensing and multiplexed analysis of pathogenic DNAs, *J. Am. Chem. Soc.*, **135**, pp. 11832–11839.

39. Khandelia, R., Bhandari, S., Pan, U. N., Ghosh, S. S. and Chattopadhyay, A. (2015). Gold nanocluster embedded albumin nanoparticles for two-photon imaging of cancer cells accompanying drug delivery, *Small*, **11**, pp. 4075–4081.

40. Li, L., Zhang, L., Wang, T., Wu, X., Ren, H., Wang, C. and Su, Z. (2015). Facile and scalable synthesis of novel spherical Au nanocluster assemblies@polyacrylic acid/calcium phosphate nanoparticles for dual-modal imaging-guided cancer chemotherapy, *Small*, **11**, pp. 3162–3173.

41. Yahia-Ammar, A., Sierra, D., Mérola, F., Hildebrandt, N. and Le Guével, X. (2016). Self-assembled gold nanoclusters for bright fluorescence imaging and enhanced drug delivery, *ACS Nano*, **10**, pp. 2591–2599.

42. Zhang, X., Wu, F.-G., Liu, P., Wang, H.-Y., Gu, N. and Chen, Z. (2015). Synthesis of ultrastable and multifunctional gold nanoclusters

with enhanced fluorescence and potential anticancer drug delivery application, *J. Colloid Interface Sci.*, **455**, pp. 6–15.

43. Chen, T., Xu, S., Zhao, T., Zhu, L., Wei, D., Li, Y., Zhang, H. and Zhao, C. (2012). Gold nanocluster-conjugated amphiphilic block copolymer for tumor-targeted drug delivery, *ACS Appl. Mater. Interfaces*, **4**, pp. 5766–5774.

44. Wang, Y., Chen, J. and Irudayaraj, J. (2011). Nuclear targeting dynamics of gold nanoclusters for enhanced therapy of $HER2^+$ breast cancer, *ACS Nano*, **5**, pp. 9718–9725.

45. Zhou, F., Feng, B., Yu, H., Wang, D., Wang, T., Liu, J., Meng, Q., Wang, S., Zhang, P., Zhang, Z. and Li, Y. (2016). Cisplatin prodrug-conjugated gold nanocluster for fluorescence imaging and targeted therapy of the breast cancer, *Theranostics*, **6**, pp. 679–687.

46. Sarparast, M., Noori, A., Ilkhani, H., Bathaie, S. Z., El-Kady, M. F., Wang, L. J., Pham, H., Marsh, K. L., Kaner, R. B. and Mousavi, M. F. (2016). Cadmium nanoclusters in a protein matrix: synthesis, characterization, and application in targeted drug delivery and cellular imaging, *Nano Res.*, **9**, pp. 3229–3246.

47. Ghosh, R., Goswami, U., Ghosh, S. S., Paul, A. and Chattopadhyay, A. (2015). Synergistic anticancer activity of fluorescent copper nanoclusters and cisplatin delivered through a hydrogel nanocarrier, *ACS Appl. Mater. Interfaces*, **7**, pp. 209–222.

Chapter 8

Coupling Computational and Experimental Techniques for the Design, Characterization, and Performance of Self-Assembled Dendrimers for Heparin and DNA Binding

Domenico Marson, Erik Laurini, Maurizio Fermeglia, and Sabrina Pricl
Molecular Simulation Engineering (MOSE) Laboratory, Department of Engineering and Architecture (DIA), University of Trieste, Piazzale Europa 1 Trieste, 34127, Italy
sabrina.pricl@dia.units.it

8.1 Introduction

Managing anticoagulation in patients undergoing surgical procedures is a major challenge in medical practice. In fact, interrupting anticoagulation during an operation transiently increases the risk of thromboembolism. At the same time, surgery

Drug Delivery Nanosystems: From Bioinspiration and Biomimetics to Clinical Applications
Edited by Costas Demetzos, Stergios Pispas, and Natassa Pippa

ISBN 978-981-4774-92-5 (Hardcover), 978-0-429-49054-5 (eBook)
www.panstanford.com

and invasive procedures have associated bleeding risks that increase upon administration of anticoagulant agents for thromboembolism prevention. If the patient is subjected to bleeding during surgery, the anticoagulant treatment may need to be discontinued for a longer period, ultimately resulting in a longer period of increased thromboembolic risk. Therefore, the proper balance between reducing thromboembolism risk and preventing excessive bleeding must be *personalized* for each patient.

Heparin, the most charge-dense naturally occurring polyanion known in biological systems, is a linear polysaccharide consisting predominantly of one to four linked uronic acid and glucosamine subunits (Fig. 8.1).

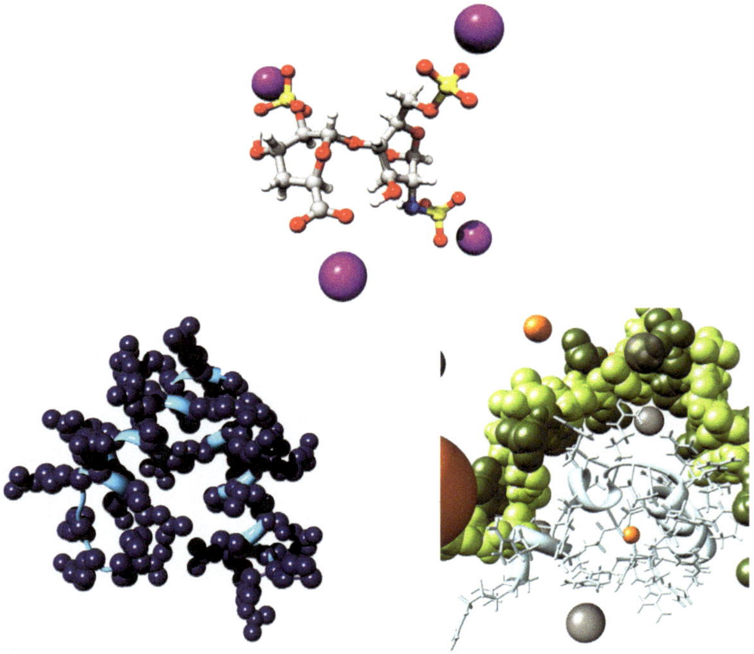

Figure 8.1 (Top) Molecular model of the predominant average repeat unit of heparin shown as colored sticks and balls (C, gray; O, red; N, blue; S, yellow; H, white). Na+ and Cl– counterions are portrayed as purple and green spheres, respectively. (Bottom, left) Molecular model of protamine structure (blue) and (bottom, right) of protamine bound to the major disaccharide repeat unit of heparin (alternating light- and dark-green units represent the two different saccharides).

Since 1935, heparin has been widely used as an anticoagulant in human surgery. The role of this sulfated polysaccharide is based on its interference with blood clotting cascade via interaction with naturally occurring thrombin inhibitors such as antithrombin III (ATIII). This heparin–ATIII interaction, mediated by the protease factor Xa, ultimately results in the inhibition of thrombin, the main protein involved in blood clotting [1].

To ensure the optimal level of heparin as an anticoagulant during medical operations, the quantification of this polyanion in blood is of paramount importance. In current practice, this is typically achieved via activated clotting time assays [2]. These measurements, however, suffer from several drawbacks, including (i) difficulty in determining the exact value of heparin levels, (ii) the amount of time required to complete the assays, and (iii) the impossibility of these tests to be carried out on a patient in a simple manner in situ. Moreover, once a surgical procedure in which heparin was used is concluded, there is an immediate need to neutralize its anticoagulant effect and allow blood clotting and recovery to begin. At the time being, the only Food and Drug Administration (FDA)-approved heparin antidote is protamine sulfate, a small, arginine-rich protein of shellfish origin. Protamine acts as a heparin neutralizer by forming a supermolecular complex (Fig. 8.1) driven by electrostatic interactions between the cationic arginine groups and the anionic heparin [3]. However, the binding is not selective for active or inactive heparin sequences. Furthermore, and most importantly, protamine can cause significant adverse effects, with major complications arising in 2.6% of cardiac surgeries, while up to 10% of patients treated with this protein experience different sorts of problems [4].

Given the clinical importance of heparin sensing and binding outlined above, the possibility of finding an effective and safer protamine replacement is one of the current hot topics in the field. It has to be noted here that establishing strong and selective binding in biological fluids, such as serum, plasma, or even whole blood, is a very complex challenge, as these media are highly competitive. Potential heparin-binding agents must therefore be carefully designed in order to operate effectively—furthermore, any protamine substitute must be endowed with the appropriate pharmacokinetic profile.

Gene therapy is a promising new technique for treating many serious incurable diseases, such as cancer and genetic disorders [5].

The main problem limiting the application of this strategy in vivo is the difficulty of transporting large, fragile, and negatively charged molecules, like DNA, into the nucleus of the cell without degradation [6]. The key to the success of gene therapy is to create safe and efficient gene delivery vehicles. Ideally, the vehicle must be able to remain in the bloodstream for a long time and avoid uptake by the mononuclear phagocyte system in order to ensure its arrival at the desired targets. Moreover, this carrier must also be able to transport the DNA efficiently into the cell cytoplasm, avoiding lysosomal degradation. Although viral vehicles are the most commonly used carriers for delivering DNA and have long been used for their high efficiency, their ability to elicit dangerous immunological responses make them problematic in clinical settings. Consequently, nonviral carriers are currently being designed and developed until alternative techniques for encapsulating nucleic acids can be found. Within the latter group, self-assembling multivalent (SAMul) amphiphilic dendrons are emerging as promising nanovectors by virtue of their well-defined structure, intriguing features of multivalency, and high cargo payload confined within a nanosized volume [7]. Multivalency is an effective and widely employed way of achieving high-affinity interactions between nanoscale surfaces. However, covalent multivalent systems often involve complex multistep syntheses and may persist in vivo long after they have had their desired effect. One approach to making multivalent systems that are synthetically simpler and more responsive is to design low-molecular-weight drug-like amphiphilic molecules, which spontaneously self-assemble into a nanoscale ligand array (Fig. 8.2).

In the last years, our laboratory, in collaboration with different international research groups, has designed and produced a plethora of amphiphilic molecules bearing dendritic portions as polar heads and different hydrocarbon chains as hydrophobic moieties, able to self-assemble into nanosized supramolecular structures of various sizes and shapes for drug and gene delivery [8–13]. In particular, in the most recent times, our attention has been focused on the problem of designing and synthesizing SAMul units with a unique capability of selectively binding different biological polyanions, such as DNA and heparin [14–20]. During this exciting scientific experience, we identified several critical design parameters that endow each SAMul-derived nanostructure with specific characteristics. Among these parameters, three deserve special attention: (i) the nature and charge of the cationic SAMul amphiphile end group [21], (ii) the capacity of generating highly ordered hierarchical nanoscale structures in solution per se and upon binding a specific polyanion [22], and (iii) the effect of the environmental conditions in which these SAMul nanomicelles operate their polyanion intramolecular recognition and complexation [23].

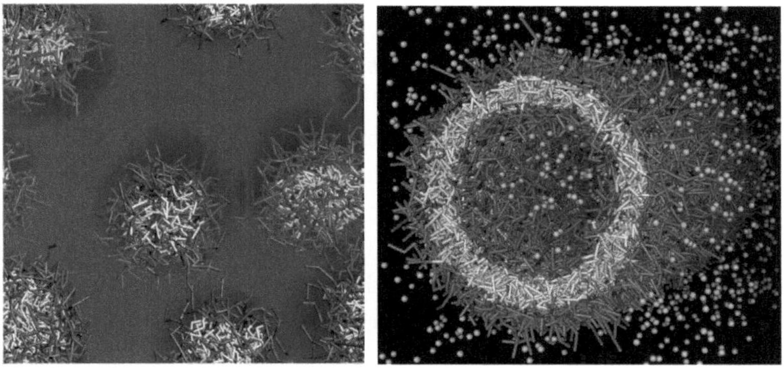

Figure 8.2 Computer models of spherical (left) and cylindrical (right) micelles generated from different SAMul molecules. Adapted from Refs. [8] and [9] with permission of The Royal Society of Chemistry.

This chapter is dedicated to these three main aspects and to their study and characterization via a combined approach of experimental and computational techniques.

8.2 SAMul Ligand Displays and Their Selective Preference for Heparin and DNA Binding

The capacity of any given positively charged ligand to discriminate between different biological polyanions is a formidable task, given the similarity of the primary mechanism by which they can be bound, that is, electrostatic interactions. So far, most studies focused on a specific anion with a defined application in mind, for example, nucleic acid binding for gene delivery [24] and heparin binding for coagulation control [1]. Considering these two specific anions, DNA is negatively charged by virtue of the phosphate residues populating the double helix, while the polysaccharide backbone of heparin is decorated with anionic sulfates and carboxylates. Clearly, there are some inherent differences between these polyanions, but surprisingly, there has been relatively little interest in probing binding selectivity. Understanding the factors leading to preferential polyanion binding by a given positive charge–bearing ligand will therefore enable the development of systems able to intervene much more precisely in processes of biomedical relevance and better optimized for specific clinical applications.

In recent years, the concept of SAMul ligand nanovectors, in which multiple ligands noncovalently assemble to generate a nanoscale display that interacts with a binding partner, has gained a special momentum in the field of drug/biologics clinical applications [7]. SAMul is a tunable strategy because it only requires the synthesis of small molecules—it is therefore easy to introduce structural variation and explore structure-activity relationships.

From this perspective, by adopting a combination of experimental and computational approaches, we recently demonstrated [20] how modifying the ligands in SAMul displays has an impact on their binding selectivity toward the two above-mentioned nanoscale biological polyanions—heparin and DNA. Probing subtle differences in such nanoscale binding interfaces was a significant challenge, and as such, several experimental binding assays, namely competition assays and isothermal titration calorimetry (ITC), were employed to confirm differences in affinity and provide thermodynamic insights. Furthermore, given the dynamic nature and hierarchical binding processes involved in SAMul systems, we resorted to multiscale modeling to propose reasons for the origins of polyanion selectivity differences.

Specifically, we synthesized and tested three different amphiphilic molecules with different ligands (DAPMA = *N*,*N*-di-(3-aminopropyl)-*N*-methylamine, SPD = spermidine, and SPM = spermine), as shown in Fig. 8.3.

A multiscale molecular simulation [25] in 150 mM aqueous NaCl predicted the formation of spherical micelles for all SAMul compounds (see Fig. 8.4); yet, the simulation indicated that the compounds formed micelles with different packing densities. Specifically, the estimated aggregation number N_{agg} (i.e., the average number of SAMul molecules within the corresponding micelle) decreased in the order C_{16}-DAPMA (16) > C_{16}-SPD (13) > C_{16}-SPM (10). These results suggest that the hydrophobic C_{16} chain is less effective in packing together the more highly charged SPM ligands (3+) within a nanomicelle. As a result of the decrease in N_{agg} for C_{16}-SPM, the calculated micellar electrostatic potential ψ also decreases in the same order (172.4, 153.3, and 144.6 mV), leading to simulated values of the zeta potentials ζ of 50.2, 45.1, and 41.8 mV for C_{16}-DAPMA, C_{16}-SPD, and C_{16}-SPM, respectively. Interestingly, these values are in agreement with the corresponding experimental data (51.9, 44, and 40.5 mV, respectively) as determined by dynamic light scattering (DLS).

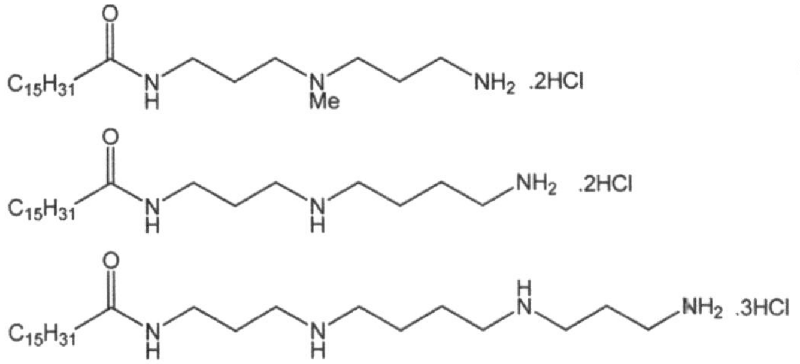

Figure 8.3 Structure of the three SAMul molecules, C_{16}-DAPMA, C_{16}-SPD, and C_{16}-SPM, with nominal ligand charges of +1, +2, +2, and +3, respectively, at physiological pH (7.4). Adapted from Ref. [21] with permission of The Royal Society of Chemistry.

The ability of SAMul nanostructures to bind the two polyanions of choice—DNA and heparin—was then tested experimentally via an ethidium bromide (EthBr) displacement assay (DNA) and a Mallard Blue (MalB) competition assay (heparin) [26]. These simple approaches allowed us to determine CE_{50} values (i.e., the cation/anion charge excess at which 50% of the dye is displaced in each case) and the corresponding EC_{50} values (i.e., the effective concentration of the binder at the same point. From these tests, we found that the C_{16}-SPM ligand (charge 3+) was the optimal DNA binder (CE_{50} = 4.3 and EC_{50} = 5.7 μM), whereas C_{16}-SPD and C_{16}-DAPMA were less effective in binding the nucleic acid (CE_{50} = 6 and 5 and EC_{50} = 11.9 and 10.1 μM, respectively). In contrast, C_{16}-SPD was found to be the most efficient heparin binder (CE_{50} = 0.34), significantly outperforming the other two SAMul micelles (for which CE_{50} = 0.49 [C_{16}-SPM] and 0.69 [C_{16}- DAPMA], respectively).

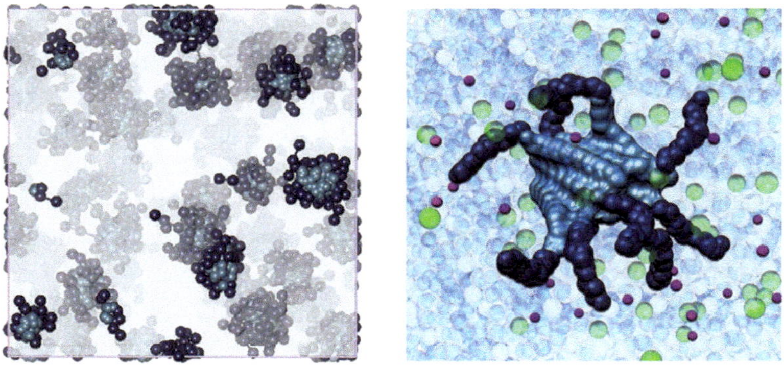

Figure 8.4 Mesoscopic (left) and atomistic (right) simulations of C_{16}-SPM self-assembling into micelles. The C_{16} hydrophobic portion is shown as steel-blue spheres, whereas the SPM residues are portrayed as navy-blue spheres. In the left panel, water, ions, and counterions are shown as a light-gray field; in the right panel, water molecules are depicted as transparent light-blue spheres; some Na+ and Cl– ions are shown as purple and green spheres, respectively. Reproduced from Ref. [21] with permission of The Royal Society of Chemistry.

To find a rationale for this apparent polyanion selectivity by the different SAMul micelles, we used ITC experiments. ITC data in terms of apparent binding affinity between the SAMul micelles and each polyanion (ΔG_{bind}) were in agreement with the trends obtained from EthBr/MalB assays. Indeed, C_{16}-SPM was the most effective DNA binder (ΔG_{bind} = –7.3 kJ/mol) and C_{16}-SPD (ΔG_{bind} = –4.9 kJ/mol) was the most effective heparin binder. Furthermore, as in the dye displacement assays, for DNA binding C_{16}-DAPMA > C_{16}-SPD, whereas for heparin binding C_{16}-SPD > C_{16}-DAPMA.

Further understanding of the polyanion selectivity by the SAMul nanostructures was derived again from atomistic simulations. Accordingly, the C_{16}-SPM micelles effectively engaged 9 out of 10 SPM residues in binding DNA (Fig. 8.5, top panel), resulting in a calculated, charge-normalized per-effective-residue free energy of binding ΔG^* of –14.32 kJ/mol. Conversely, C_{16}-SPD and C_{16}-DAPMA micelles only used 7 and 8 (out of 13 and 16) residues, to effectively bind DNA. This resulted in lower per-effective-residue interactions

(ΔG^* = –9.76 and –10.80 kJ/mol, respectively) with respect to C_{16}-SPM. The simulated ΔG^* values therefore yielded the same trend as experimental CE_{50} values and ITC data: C_{16}-SPM > C_{16}-DAPMA > C_{16}-SPD.

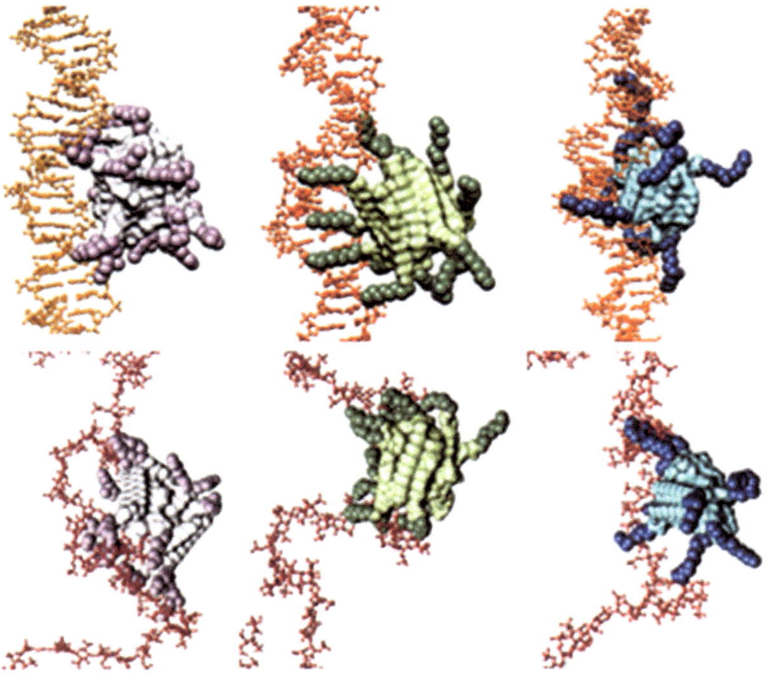

Figure 8.5 Equilibrated atomistic molecular dynamics simulation snapshots of SAMul micelles binding DNA (upper panel, orange) and heparin (lower panel, firebrick). In both panels, from left to right: C_{16}-DAPMA (light gray, C_{16}; and plum, DAPMA), C_{16}-SPD (lime green, C_{16}; and forest green, SPD), and C_{16}-SPM (steel blue, C_{16}; and navy blue, SPM). Hydrogen atoms, water molecules, ions, and counterions are not shown to maintain clarity. Reproduced from Ref. [21] with permission of The Royal Society of Chemistry.

For heparin binding (Fig. 8.5, bottom), the micelles formed by C_{16}-SPD employed 12 out of 13 available ligands in productive binding, resulting in a ΔG^* value of –14.98 kJ/mol. However, C_{16}-DAPMA and C_{16}-SPM nanostructures only exploited 9/16 and 6/10 ligands, yielding ΔG^* values of –8.65 and –11.97 kJ/mol, respectively. Once again, the predicted ΔG^* values were thus in agreement with the trend of experimental data: C_{16}-SPD > C_{16}-SPM > C_{16}-DAPMA.

To better appreciate the reasons the two negatively charged biological macromolecules show different selectivity toward the SAMul nanostructures, we decomposed the overall ΔG^* values into their enthalpic (ΔH^*) and entropic ($T\Delta S^*$) components. Let's first consider the case of DNA binding from the perspective of each effective SAMul cationic charge (see Fig. 8.6A). In the case of micelles formed by C_{16}-SPM (3+), Fig. 8.6A clearly shows that the entropic cost associated with ligand organization upon polyanion binding is largely compensated for by the favorable enthalpic gain. This is in agreement with ITC data, according to which for C_{16}-SPM $\Delta H = -6.6$ kJ/mol and $T\Delta S = 0.7$ kJ/mol. The other two less charged ligands (both 2+) gain less in enthalpy; accordingly, they bind DNA less well—in full agreement with the experimental ITC data ($\Delta H = -1.4$ and -3.9 kJ/mol for C_{16}-DAPMA and C_{16}-SPD, respectively). The shorter, slightly more rigid ligand (C_{16}-DAPMA) pays less entropic penalty than C_{16}-SPD on binding, slightly favoring its DNA binding over C_{16}-SPD. Once again, this is in agreement with ITC data ($T\Delta S = 2.9$ and 0.4 kJ/mol for C_{16}-DAPMA and C_{16}-SPD, respectively).

Applying the same analysis, but from the standpoint of each anionic DNA charge involved at the binding interface (Fig. 8.6B), ΔG^*, ΔH^*, and $T\Delta S^*$ are practically independent of the ligand nature, that is, from the perspective of DNA, all interactions are seen as equally good. In other words, the selectivity of the SAMul micelles for the nucleic acid can be ascribed only to ligand optimization. To summarize the concept, we suggest that, in this respect, DNA is a *shape-persistent polyanion*, which simply binds to and organizes the SAMul display with which it is presented.

For heparin binding, starting again from the perspective of the effective charge of the SAMul (Fig. 8.6C), the C_{16}-SPD ligand experiences the largest enthalpic gain when its interaction with the polysaccharide is reorganized and optimized with respect to its other two counterparts—C_{16}-DAPMA and C_{16}-SPM—in line with the ITC data ($\Delta H = -4.9$, -1.9, and 2.6 kJ/mol for C_{16}-SPD, C_{16}-DAPMA, and C_{16}-SPM, respectively). Notwithstanding the fact that the entropic penalty for C_{16}-SPD/heparin is not the best of the series, the most favorable being that estimated for C_{16}-SPM ($T\Delta S = 0$, 0.3, and 2.3 kJ/mol for C_{16}-SPD, C_{16}-DAPMA, and C_{16}-SPM, respectively), the overall binding remains enthalpy driven in nature, confirming that

C_{16}-SPD has the best heparin-binding properties. When SAMul/heparin binding is considered from the perspective of each heparin sugar (Fig. 8.6D), a different behavior can also be observed, depending on the ligand nature. Each heparin residue offsets the entropic cost of binding SPD with a greater enthalpic gain of its own. This is in stark contrast to DNA, where each anion behaves identically, irrespective of the ligand. As such, the more effective binding of C_{16}-SPD induces more effective binding from each residue of the heparin chain via an enthalpy/entropy optimization, mediated through polyanion structural adaptation—that is, heparin can be defined as an adaptive polyanion that not only binds to the SAMul display but also, importantly, is able to adapt itself in response.

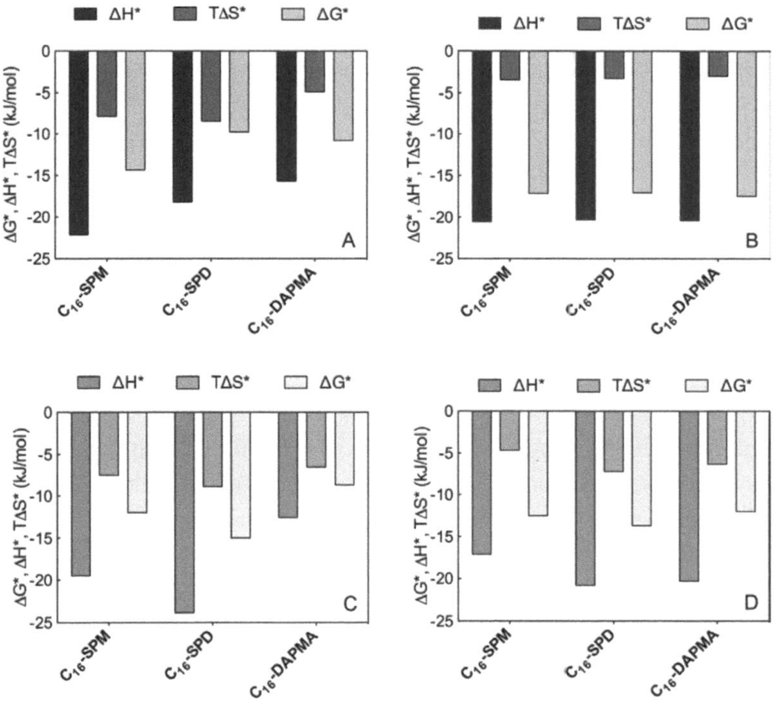

Figure 8.6 Charge-normalized per-effective-residue free energy of binding (ΔG^*), and enthalpic (ΔH^*) and entropic ($T\Delta S^*$) components for (A) each SAMul micelle ligand-type complexed with DNA, (B) DNA bases complexed with each of the SAMul micelles, (C) each SAMul micelle ligand-type complexed with heparin, and (D) heparin sugars complexed with each of the SAMul micelles. Reproduced from Ref. [21] with permission of The Royal Society of Chemistry.

In conclusion, this work demonstrated that the ligand choice in SAMul displays can have an influence on apparent binding selectivity. As such, electrostatic ion-ion binding depends on structural details, not only charge density, as confirmed by the complementary experimental methods of competition binding assays, ITC, and molecular modeling.

8.3 Highly Ordered Hierarchical Nanoscale Structures in SAMul Cationic Micelles/Heparin Systems

The previous section has revealed that a simple SAMul system based on the amphiphilic molecule C_{16}-DAPMA is an excellent heparin binder. Bearing in mind the clinical interest in heparin binding for the reversal of anticoagulation therapy following surgical intervention, we wanted to characterize this SAMul heparin binder in greater structural detail [22]. To this purpose, we also considered the homologous compound C_{14}-DAPMA, for which heparin-binding performance was only slightly inferior to its longer chain counterpart, that is, CE_{50} = 0.88 and EC_{50} = 48 μM. We began our study using transmission electron microscopy (TEM). TEM images were obtained for both SAMuls before and after binding to heparin.

As can be seen from Fig. 8.7, compound C_{16}-DAPMA formed spherical nanostructures upon self-assembly (analogous results were obtained for C_{14}-DAPMA). Remarkably, on binding to heparin, both systems formed highly organized semicrystalline nanostructured arrays. These TEM observations clearly suggest that the self-assembled micelles formed by C_{14}-DAPMA and C_{16}-DAPMA have excellent stability and appear to remain intact without disruption or reorganization, even in the presence of heparin, with which they can form very strong electrostatic interactions. The diameters of the micelles observed by TEM prior to and upon assembly with heparin are in good agreement with the micellar diameters observed by DLS, that is, 5.8 and 6.2 nm for C_{14}- and C_{16}-DAPMA, respectively.

It should be noted that TEM imaging was performed on dried samples. Given the fact that the drying process might induce some morphological change in the systems, we deemed it very important to ascertain whether the highly ordered hierarchical nanoscale aggregates revealed by TEM for C_{14}-DAPMA and C_{16}-DAPMA were preserved in solution. To this purpose, first mesoscopic dissipative particle dynamics (DPD) simulations [27, 28] were carried out to predict the self-assembly and spatial organization of these two amphiphiles in solution in the presence of heparin (Fig. 8.8).

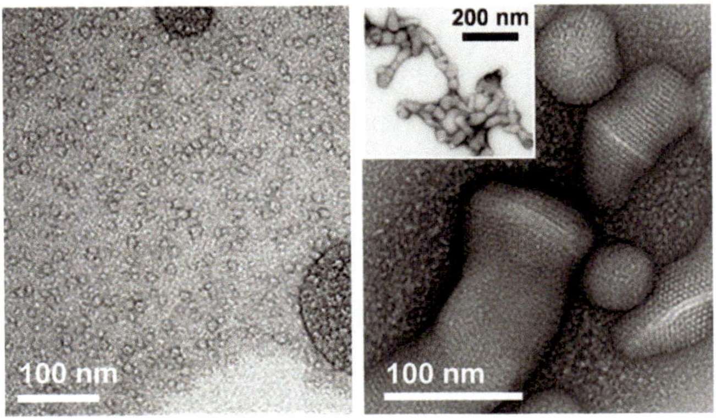

Figure 8.7 TEM images of C_{16}-DAPMA (left) and C_{16}-DAPMA with heparin (right); the inset shows the full image indicating the overall nanoscale aggregate made up of smaller nanocrystalline subunits. Adapted from Ref. [22] with permission of The Royal Society of Chemistry.

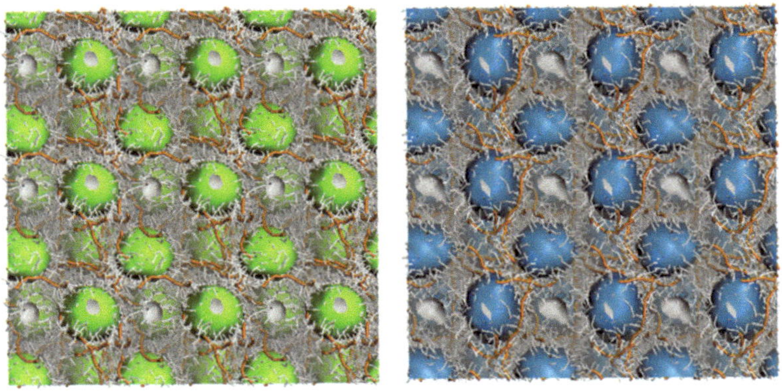

Figure 8.8 DPD snapshots of C_{14}-DAPMA (left) and C_{16}-DAPMA (right) self-assembly in the presence of heparin (2:1 binder:heparin ratio). The hydrophobic micellar core is highlighted as green and blue isosurfaces, respectively. Hydrophilic moieties of each aggregate are shown as white sticks, while heparin molecules are visualized as orange rods. A continuous light-gray field portrays the aqueous medium. Reproduced from Ref. [22] with permission of The Royal Society of Chemistry.

In agreement with TEM, DPD simulations showed that both types of amphiphiles self-assemble into highly ordered spherical nanostructures that remain intact in the presence of heparin. In both cases, the nanomicelles assume a face-centered cubic (fcc) organization (Fig. 8.8). The predicted lattice constants, *a*, are 8.1 nm and 8.6 nm for C_{14}-DAPMA and C_{16}-DAPMA micelles, respectively. The corresponding center-to-center distance ($a\sqrt{2}$) is 5.7 nm for C_{14}-DAPMA and 6.1 nm for C_{16}-DAPMA, in good agreement with the micelle diameters from DLS reported above.

Next, the nanostructures of the aqueous binder–heparin complexes were investigated by small-angle X-ray scattering (SAXS). The 2D diffraction patterns (Fig. 8.9, inset) show, for both binder-heparin supermolecular structures, a distinct feature of polycrystalline samples with isotropic orientation of multiple crystals [29], namely a Debye ring with a diffuse symmetric halo that does not present intensity differences. For the C_{14}-DAPMA-heparin complex, the positions of the diffraction peaks were located at q = 0.129 and 0.259 1/Å, assuming an fcc structure, in terms of crystal plane reflections with Miller indices corresponds to (*hkl*) = (111) and (222).

For the assembly of C_{16}-DAPMA and heparin, SAXS measurements (Fig. 8.9) showed diffraction peaks at q = 0.122, 0.138, and 0.246 1/Å, corresponding to crystal plane reflections with Miller indices (*hkl*) = (111), (200), and (222), again assuming an fcc structure. The quadratic Miller indices were next plotted against the measured $q(hkl)$ values for both SAMul-heparin complexes (Figs. 8.9b and 8.9c), and the lattice constant *a* was estimated by linear regression. For cubic phases $a = 2\pi\sqrt{h^2 + k^2 + l^2/q(hkl)}$; accordingly, *a* was found to be equal to 8.5 and 8.9 nm for C_{14}-DAPMA and C_{16}-DAPMA, respectively, in agreement with the corresponding values obtained from simulations. The center-to-center distance $a\sqrt{2}$ of the micelles was thus calculated as 6 nm for C_{14}-DAPMA and 6.3 nm for C_{16}-DAPMA, again in line with mesoscale predictions (see above).

As the last step, data from simulations and SAXS of SAMul/heparin systems were compared with the corresponding TEM images, as illustrated in Fig. 8.10.

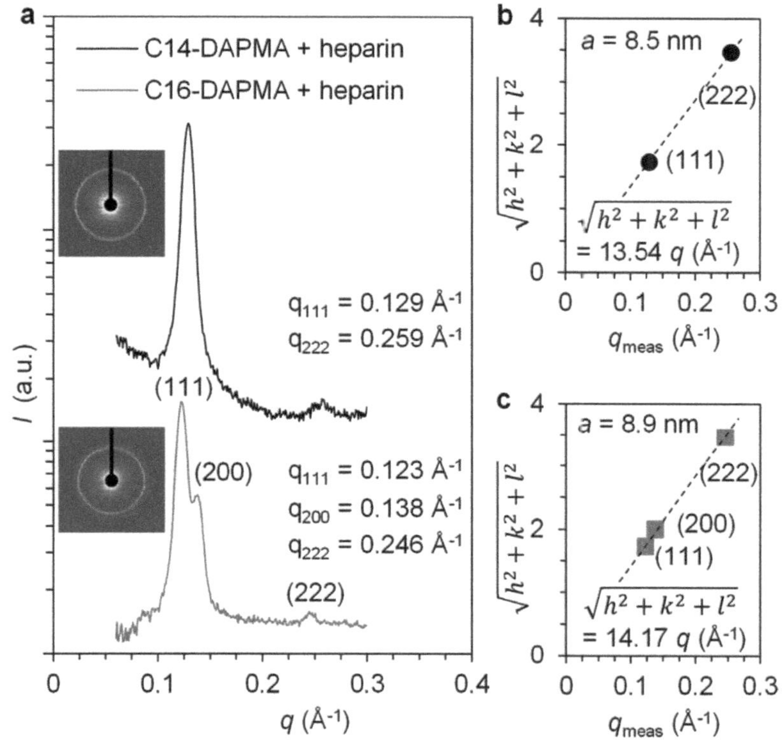

Figure 8.9 SAXS characterization of C_{14}-DAPMA and C_{16}-DAPMA in the presence of heparin. (a) Integrated SAXS curves measured from self-assembled C_{14}-DAPMA and C_{16}-DAPMA in the presence of heparin. Inset: 2D scattering pattern of C_{14}-DAPMA and C_{16}-DAPMA with heparin. Quadratic Miller indices of assigned reflections for the fcc structure versus measured q-vector positions for indexed peaks, related with (b) heparin-binding C_{14}-DAPMA and (c) heparin-binding C_{16}-DAPMA. Reproduced from Ref. [22] with permission of The Royal Society of Chemistry.

Specifically, the top-left panel in Fig. 8.10 shows the crystal projection viewed along the [110] zone axis. The analysis of the linear profile over the crystal projection gives an average period (ap) of 4.5 nm, corresponding to an fcc lattice constant a of 7.8 nm for C_{14}-DAPMA and of 8 nm for C_{16}-DAPMA, respectively. These values are in excellent agreement with the corresponding values obtained by DPD and SAXS—the slight reduction in the unit cell size being ascribable to the drying effect on the TEM grid. Fast Fourier transform calculations (Fig. 8.10 inset) from the crystalline area and filtering the inverse Fourier transform from selected Fourier components gave an image that represents the unit cell of the crystal viewed along the [110] zone axis (Fig. 8.10, bottom left panel). This was confirmed (Fig. 8.10, middle panel) by overlaying the image and a model of the unit cell shown in the right panel of Fig. 8.10. The center-to-center distances of 5.5 nm and 5.6 nm, calculated for C_{14}-DAPMA and C_{16}-DAPMA, respectively, were again in very good agreement with the micelle diameters measured by DLS and the corresponding center-to-center distances estimated from DPD and SAXS. In aggregate, these combined experimental/simulation studies demonstrate remarkably high stability of these SAMul micelles, even when forming strong electrostatic interactions with heparin, and provide structural insights into nanoscale hierarchical electrostatic assemblies.

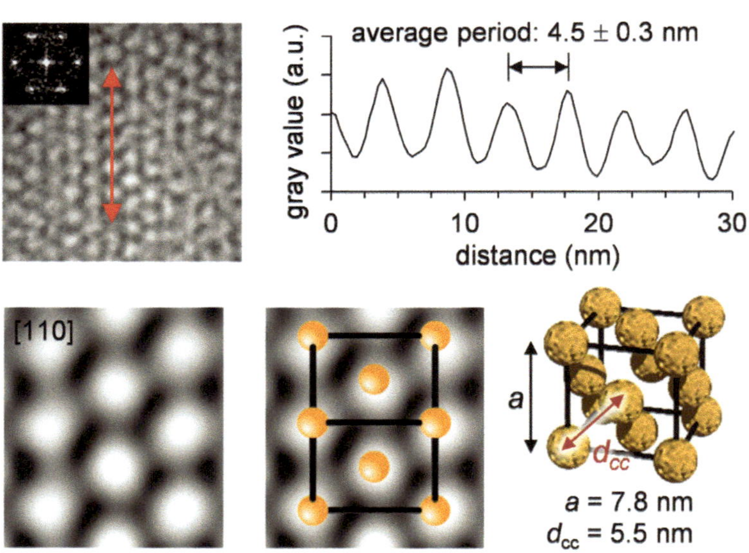

Figure 8.10 A crystalline area for C_{14}-DAPMA (top left, inset: fast Fourier transform) and a line profile analysis (right) along the red line. (Bottom) Filtered inverse Fourier transform from selected Fourier components for C_{14}-DAPMA (left), overlay of the image and the fcc unit cell (middle), and model of the fcc unit cell with key dimensions (right). Micelles shown in yellow; diameter reduced for clarity. Reproduced from Ref. [22] with permission of The Royal Society of Chemistry.

8.4 Effect of Buffer at Nanoscale Molecular Recognition Interfaces

When one is dealing with biomolecular recognition, competitive aqueous mediums are selected to mimic biological environments, as complex formation between any ligand and any target receptor must withstand high electrolyte concentrations and the presence of different physiological buffers. While the outcomes of the former have been the subject of a plethora of studies, the impact of the buffer is a field substantially less explored. Accordingly, in the last stage of this saga we have endeavored to analyze the effect of three different buffers, namely 2-amino-2-(hydroxymethyl)propane-1,3-diol-HCl (Tris-HCl), 2-[4-(2-hydroxyethyl)piperazin-1-yl]ethanesulfonic acid (HEPES), and phosphate-buffered saline (PBS), on the heparin binding of self-assembled multivalent C_{16}-DAPMA cationic micelles [23].

As the first step, MalB-based competition assays [26] were adopted to rapidly test the relative heparin binding of C_{16}-DAPMA micelles in each buffer. The results are listed in Table 8.1.

Table 8.1 CE_{50} and EC_{50} values obtained for C_{16}-DAPMA using a MalB competition assay (10 mM buffer, 150 mM NaCl, pH 7)

Sample	CE_{50}	EC_{50} (μM)
Tris	0.64 ± 0.02	34 ± 1
HEPES	1.02 ± 0.02	55 ± 1
PBS	2.24 ± 0.0334	121 ± 18

MalB = 25 μM and heparin = 27 μM (on the basis of a typical disaccharide repeat unit with an assumed –4 charge)
Source: Reproduced from Ref. [23] with permission of The Royal Society of Chemistry.

As can be seen from Table 8.1, C_{16}-DAPMA is a strong heparin binder in Tris-HCl, as low loadings (34 μM) are required to displace 50% of the MalB dye. On the other hand, polyanion binding by the SAMul micelles is less efficient in HEPES (55 μM) and decidedly less so in PBS (121 μM). We then proceeded by performing an ITC experiment (Fig. 8.11) to directly assess the binding between C_{16}-DAPMA and heparin. The numerical results of the ITC analysis are reported in Table 8.2.

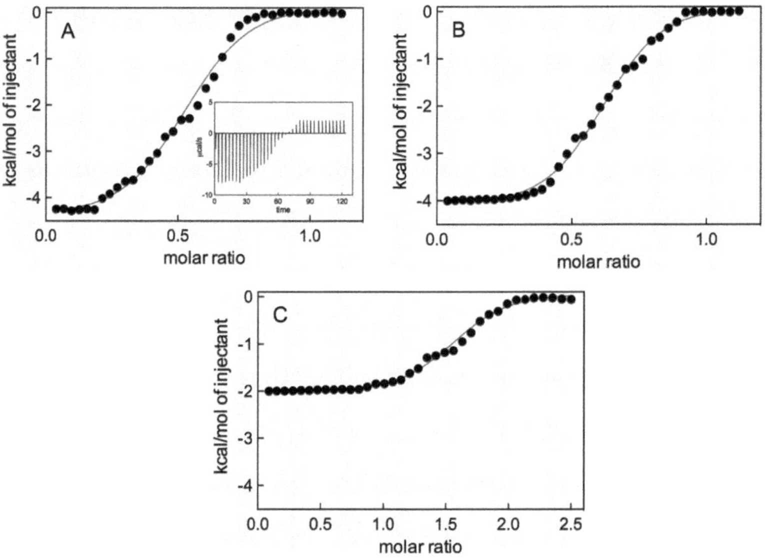

Figure 8.11 Representative integrated ITC profiles for the titration of heparin with SAMul micelles in (A) Tris-HCl (10 mM) + NaCl 150 mM, (B) HEPES (10 mM) + NaCl 150 mM, and (C) PBS at T = 25°C. The solid red lines are data fitting with a one-set-of-sites model. The inserts in panel A show the corresponding ITC raw data. All experiments were run in triplicate. Reproduced from Ref. [23] with permission of The Royal Society of Chemistry.

Table 8.2 Thermodynamic parameters obtained by ITC for C_{16}-DAPMA SAMul micelles titrated into heparin in different buffers (10 mM). ΔHobs, -$T\Delta S$ and ΔG are in kcal/mol, EOT is the end of titration point and K_d is the effective dissociation constant.

Buffer	NaCl (mM)	EOT	ΔH_{obs}	$-T\Delta S$	ΔG	K_d (μM)
Tris	150	0.8 ± 0.1	-4.31 ± 0.03	-3.77 ± 0.06	-8.08 ± 0.05	1.2 ± 0.1
HEPES	150	0.9 ± 0.1	-3.91 ± 0.08	-3.54 ± 0.11	-7.45 ± 0.06	3.5 ± 0.4
PBS	140	2.1 ± 0.1	-2.18 ± 0.06	-4.13 ± 0.06	-6.31 ± 0.07	24 ± 3

Source: Adapted from [23] with permission of the Royal Society of Chemistry.

In terms of the so-called thermodynamic signature, heparin binding was negative (i.e., favorable), as could be expected for a multivalent electrostatic process. On the other hand, the change in entropy was always positive (i.e., favorable), being mainly associated with the release of ions, counterions, and water molecules from the binding interface to the bulk solvent. Accordingly, the values of the free energy of binding of the C_{16}-DAPMA micelles to heparin in all three buffers considered are always negative (i.e., favorable, Table 8.2), leading to spontaneous supermolecular association. However, ITC data unequivocally demonstrate that the affinity of the SAMul micelles for heparin is highly dependent on the buffer adopted, Tris-HCl being the most effective medium (ΔG = −8.08 kcal/mol), followed by HEPES (ΔG = −7.45 kcal/mol) and the substantially less effective PBS (ΔG = −6.31 kcal/mol). Looking into the binding thermodynamics in more detail, the most favorable enthalpic contribution is experienced in TRIS-HCl (ΔH_{obs} = −4.31 kcal/mol), while in the other two buffers the binding process is sensibly less exothermic (ΔH_{obs} = −3.91 and −2.18 kcal/mol in HEPES and PBS, respectively). This detrimental effect is likely due to the progressively increasing competition of buffer molecules for the SAMul micelle negative surface in passing from Tris-HCl to PBS. Contextually, the release of ions/counterions and water molecules from the micelle-/polyanion-binding interface, which results in an overall system entropy increase, is favored in (nearly) the reverse order (i.e., PBS > HEPES > Tris-HCl, for which $-T\Delta S$ = −4.13, −3.54, and −3.77 kcal/mol, respectively). Yet, in the case of PBS, the large, favorable entropic contribution is not enough to compensate for the small, enthalpic term, ultimately resulting in the smallest affinity value between the two binding partners.

In summary, the fundamental general take-home message of this investigation of the buffer effect on self-assembled nanostructures on polyanion binding is that, when dealing with electrostatic supermolecular binding events, great care must be taken to select the relevant buffer, as final results are strongly dependent on the underlying choice. Specifically, it would be highly advisable to conduct binding experiments in a noninteractive buffer, such as Tris-HCl in a background electrolyte. Since, however, any real biological medium contains many other anionic species (e.g., phosphates), the specific effects of these anions on electrostatic (and other) binding processes must be carefully considered when developing recognition systems for in vivo testing.

8.5 Conclusions

The series of examples of coupled experimental/modeling investigations in the field of self-assembled multivalent nanovectors for biological polyanion binding illustrated and discussed in this chapter, taken from our own experience in the field, emphasize both the fundamental role and the potentiality played by this approach in the pre- and postdevelopment of nanodevices for DNA and heparin binding and the hurdles that this field has to face before it can be translated into the clinical setting. Despite its rapid growth and extraordinary potential, the branch of nanomedicine is still in its infancy, is highly interdisciplinary, and aims at solving problems of extraordinary and unprecedented complexity. In such a scenario, multiscale molecular modeling coupled with targeted experiments could contribute to the success of nanomedicine and make the difference between several years of unfruitful research and the development of new, revolutionary therapeutic strategies readily available to the human society.

Acknowledgments

The authors wish to acknowledge the invaluable, long-lasting collaboration with Prof. David Smith (University of York, UK) and his group. Also, the generous financial support from the Italian Association for Cancer Research (AIRC, Grant IG 17413 to SP) is gratefully acknowledged.

References

1. Bromfield, S. M., Wilde, E. and Smith, D. K. (2013). Heparin sensing and binding: taking supramolecular chemistry towards clinical applications, *Chem. Soc. Rev.*, **42**, pp. 9184–9195.
2. Hirsh, J., Warkentin, T. E., Shaughnessy, S. G., Anand, S. S., Halperin, J. L., Raschke, R., Granger, C., Ohman, E. M. and Dalen, J. E. (2001). Heparin and low-molecular-weight heparin: mechanisms of action, pharmacokinetics, dosing, monitoring, efficacy, and safety, *Chest*, **119**, pp. 64S–94S.

3. Vandiver, J. W. and Vondracek, T. G. (2012). Antifactor Xa levels versus activated partial thromboplastin time for monitoring unfractionated heparin *Pharmacotherapy*, **32**, pp. 546–558.

4. Chu, Y. Q., Cai, L. J., Jiang, D. C., Jia, D., Yan, S. Y. and Wang, Y. Q. (2010). Allergic shock and death associated with protamine administration in a diabetic patient, *Clin. Ther.*, **32**, pp. 1729–1732.

5. Naldini, L. (2015). Gene therapy returns to center stage, *Nature*, **526**, pp. 351–360.

6. Moss, J. A. (2014). Gene therapy review, *Radiol. Technol.*, **86**, pp. 155–180.

7. Barnard, A. and Smith, D. K. (2012). Self-Assembled multivalency: dynamic ligand arrays for high-affinity binding, *Angew. Chem. Int. Ed. Engl.*, **51**, pp. 6572–6581.

8. Barnard, A., Posocco, P., Fermeglia, M., Tschiche, A., Calderon, M., Pricl, S. and Smith, D. K. (2014). Double-degradable responsive self-assembled multivalent arrays – temporary nanoscale recognition between dendrons and DNA, *Org. Biomol. Chem.*, **12**, pp. 446–455.

9. Welsh, D. J., Posocco, P., Pricl, S. and Smith, D. K. (2013). Self-assembled multivalent RGD-peptide arrays--morphological control and integrin binding, *Org. Biomol. Chem.*, **11**, pp. 3177–3186.

10. Hinman, S. S., Ruiz, C. J., Cao, Y., Ma, M. C., Tang, J., Laurini, E., Posocco, P., Giorgio, S., Pricl, S., Peng, L. and Cheng, Q. (2017). Mix and match: coassembly of amphiphilic dendrimers and phospholipids creates robust, modular, and controllable interfaces, *ACS Appl. Mater. Interfaces*, **9**, pp. 1029–1035.

11. Chen, C., Posocco, P., Liu, X., Cheng, Q., Laurini, E., Zhou, J., Liu, C., Wang, Y., Tang, J., Dal Col, V., Yu, T., Giorgio, S., Fermeglia, M., Qu, F., Liang, Z., Rossi, J. J., Liu, M., Rocchi, P., Pricl, S. and Peng, L. (2016). Mastering dendrimer self-assembly for efficient siRNA delivery: from conceptual design to in vivo efficient gene silencing, *Small*, **12**, pp. 3667–3676.

12. Wei, T., Chen, C., Liu, J., Liu, C., Posocco, P., Liu, X., Cheng, Q., Huo, S., Liang, Z., Fermeglia, M., Pricl, S., Liang, X. J., Rocchi, P. and Peng, L. (2015). Anticancer drug nanomicelles formed by self-assembling amphiphilic dendrimer to combat cancer drug resistance, *Proc. Natl. Acad. Sci. U.S.A.*, **112**, pp. 2978–2983.

13. Liu, X., Zhou, J., Yu, T., Chen, C., Cheng, Q., Sengupta, K., Huang, Y., Li, H., Liu, C., Wang, Y., Posocco, P., Wang, M., Cui, Q., Giorgio, S., Fermeglia, M., Qu, F., Pricl, S., Shi, Y., Liang, Z., Rocchi, P., Rossi, J. J. and Peng, L. (2014). Adaptive amphiphilic dendrimer-based nanoassemblies as robust and

versatile siRNA delivery systems, *Angew. Chem. Int. Ed. Engl.*, **53**, pp. 11822–11827.

14. Rodrigo, A. C., Bromfield, S. M., Laurini, E., Posocco, P., Pricl, S. and Smith, D. K. (2017). Morphological control of self-assembled multivalent (SAMul) heparin binding in highly competitive media, *Chem. Commun.*, **53**, pp. 6335–6338.
15. Albanyan, B., Laurini, E., Posocco, P., Pricl, S. and Smith, D. K. (2017). Self-assembled multivalent (SAMul) polyanion binding-impact of hydrophobic modifications in the micellar core on DNA and heparin binding at the peripheral cationic ligands, *Chem. Eur. J.*, **23**, pp. 6391–6397.
16. Chan, C. W., Laurini, E., Posocco, P., Pricl, S. and Smith, D. K. (2016). Chiral recognition at self-assembled multivalent (SAMul) nanoscale interfaces - enantioselectivity in polyanion binding, *Chem. Commun.*, **52**, pp. 10540–10543.
17. Bromfield, S. M., Posocco, P., Chan, C. W., Calderon, M., Guimond, S. E., Turnbull, J. E., Pricl, S. and Smith, D. K. (2014). Nanoscale self-assembled multivalent (SAMul) heparin binders in highly competitive, biologically relevant, aqueous media, *Chem. Sci.*, **5**, pp. 1484–1492.
18. Barnard, A., Posocco, P., Pricl, S., Calderon, M., Haag, R., Hwang, M. E., Shum, V. W., Pack, D. W. and Smith, D. K. (2011). Degradable self-assembling dendrons for gene delivery: experimental and theoretical insights into the barriers to cellular uptake, *J. Am. Chem. Soc.*, **133**, pp. 20288–20300.
19. Jones, S. P., Gabrielson, N. P, Wong, C. H., Chow, H. F., Pack, D. W., Posocco, P., Fermeglia, M., Pricl, S. and Smith, D. K. (2011). Hydrophobically modified dendrons: developing structure-activity relationships for DNA binding and gene transfection, *Mol. Pharmaceutics*, **8**, pp. 416–429.
20. Posocco, P., Pricl, S., Jones, S. P., Barnard, A. and Smith, D. K. (2010). Less is more – multiscale modeling of self-assembling multivalency and its impact on DNA binding and gene delivery, *Chem. Sci.*, **1**, pp. 393–404.
21. Fechner, L. E., Albanyan, B., Vieir, V. M. P., Laurini, E., Posocco, P., Pricl, S. and Smith, D. K. (2016). Electrostatic binding of polyanions using self-assembled multivalent (SAMul) ligand displays – structure–activity effects on DNA/heparin binding, *Chem. Sci.*, **7**, pp. 4653–4659.
22. Vieira, V. M. P., Liljeström, V., Posocco, P., Laurini, E., Pricl, S., Kostiainen, M. P. and Smith, D. K. (2017). Emergence of highly-ordered hierarchical nanoscale aggregates on electrostatic binding of self-assembled

multivalent (SAMul) cationic micelles with polyanionic heparin, *J. Mater. Chem. B*, **5**, pp. 341–347.

23. Rodrigo, A. C., Laurini, E., Vieira, V. M. P., Pricl, S. and Smith, D. K. (2017). Effect of buffer at nanoscale molecular recognition interfaces – electrostatic binding of biological polyanions, *Chem. Commun.*, **53**, pp. 11580–11583.
24. Srinivas, R., Samanta, S. and Chaudhuri, A. (2009). Cationic amphiphiles: promising carriers of genetic materials in gene therapy, *Chem. Soc. Rev.*, **38**, pp. 3326–3338.
25. Posocco, P., Laurini, E., Dal Col, V., Marson, D., Karatasos, K., Fermeglia, M. and Pricl, S. (2012). Tell me something I do not know. Multiscale molecular modeling of dendrimer/dendron organization and self-assembly in gene therapy, *Curr. Med. Chem.*, **19**, pp. 5062–5087.
26. Bromfield, S. M., Barnard, A., Posocco, P., Fermeglia, M., Pricl, S. and Smith, D. K. (2013). Mallard blue: a high-affinity selective heparin sensor that operates in highly competitive media, *J. Am. Chem. Soc.*, **135**, pp. 2911–2914.
27. Hoogerbrugge, P. J. and Koelman, J. M. V. A. (1992). Simulating microscopic hydrodynamic phenomena with dissipative particle dynamics, *Europhys. Lett.*, **19**, pp. 155–160.
28. Groot, R. D. and Warren, P. B. (1997). Dissipative particle dynamics: bridging the gap between atomistic and mesoscopic simulation, *J. Chem. Phys.*, **107**, pp. 4423–4435.
29. Terentjev, E. M. and Weitz, D. A. (2015). *The Oxford Handbook of Soft Condensed Matter*, Oxford University Press, UK, pp. 297–331.

Chapter 9

Synthetic and Therapeutic Development of Spherical Nucleic Acids

Stanislav Rangelov and Ivaylo Dimitrov
Institute of Polymers, Bulgarian Academy of Sciences, Akad. G. Bonchev 103-A, Sofia 1113, Bulgaria
rangelov@polymer.bas.bg; dimitrov@polymer.bas.bg

Spherical nucleic acids (SNAs) represent a rapidly emerging class of nanoparticle-based therapeutics. They are composed of highly oriented and densely grafted oligonucleotides on the surface of a nanoparticle that can be inorganic, hollow, or organic. The spherical architecture of the oligonucleotide shell imparts unique advantages over traditional nucleic acid delivery methods, including cellular uptake with no need of transfection agents, resistance to nuclease degradation, and ability to overcome different biological barriers. In this chapter, the preparation methods and biomedical applications of SNAs are discussed. Special attention is paid to the very recently developed SNAs with organic (polymeric or liposomal) cores.

Drug Delivery Nanosystems: From Bioinspiration and Biomimetics to Clinical Applications
Edited by Costas Demetzos, Stergios Pispas, and Natassa Pippa

ISBN 978-981-4774-92-5 (Hardcover), 978-0-429-49054-5 (eBook)
www.panstanford.com

9.1 Introduction

Spherical nucleic acid (SNA) hybrid nanostructures of spherical morphology with densely functionalized and highly oriented oligonucleotides covalently attached to the surface of originally inorganic nanoparticles (NPs) were firstly introduced by Mirkin et al. [1] in 1996. SNAs have emerged as a new class of nanostructures exhibiting a wide variety of novel properties. The 3D arrangement of the oligonucleotides (Fig. 9.1) has been considered responsible for the unique properties that are substantially different from those of their linear counterparts.

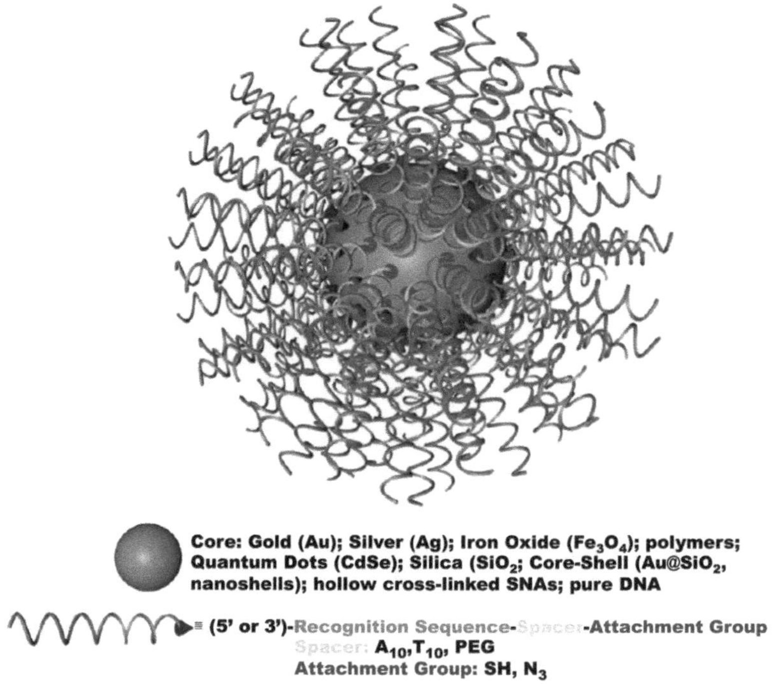

Figure 9.1 Structure of a spherical nucleic acid. Reprinted with permission from Ref. [2]. Copyright (2012) American Chemical Society.

An SNA typically consists of an inorganic core that is densely functionalized with oligonucleotides containing three segments: a recognition sequence, a spacer segment, and a chemical attachment group (Fig. 9.1). The oligonucleotides form the shell of these nanostructures. They are typically short (10–50 bases in length) and can be single-stranded (ss) and double-stranded DNA [3], small interfering RNA (siRNA) [4], micro-RNA (miRNA) [5], and modified nucleic acids. The attachment group is used to link the oligonucleotides to the NP surface and is selected depending on the chemistry of the latter. Thus, for gold (Au) NPs typical attachment groups are propyl or hexylthiol groups. SNAs from silver (Ag) NPs are typically prepared from oligonucleotides with multiple cyclic disulfide anchoring groups [6], whereas copper-catalyzed alkyne-azide "click" chemistry is used to prepare SNAs from superparamagnetic iron oxide NPs [7]. The spacer segment pushes the recognition sequence away from the NP surface, which gives more free volume of the former to interact with incoming strands [8]. Common spacers are composed of short (up to 10) sequences of DNA bases such as adenine and thymine or synthetic oligo(ethylene glycol) moieties [9]. The recognition sequence can be tailored for each investigation or technological use. It can be composed of any unit that can be incorporated via phosphoramidite chemistry. Additionally, other functional groups, such as dye molecules, quenchers, modified bases, and drugs, can be attached along any segment of the oligonucleotide [2].

The oligonucleotides are radially oriented and adopt an extended (brush-like) conformation, thus forming a dense monolayer shell on the NP surface. The thickness of the shell is governed by both the length of the oligonucleotides and their surface density, which, in turn, is dependent on the particle size and shape. On the surface, the geometric configuration confers a natural deflection angle between strands (Fig. 9.2A). Due to the higher curvature of smaller particles, the angle is greater on them, which results in a reduction in the coulombic repulsion at the termini of the strands and, hence, higher densities in the overall structure. Hill et al. reported that 10 nm Au NPs can typically support around 2×10^{13} oligonucleotides/cm^2, while the surface coverage on a macroscopic planar Au NP is considerably lower (approx. -5.8×10^{12} oligonucleotides/cm^2) [8].

The composition of the spacer segment has been shown to play a significant role since the oligonucleotide bases interact with the NP surface to varying degrees [10]: for example, the affinity of adenine to the gold surface is larger than that of thymine. Accordingly, for 15 nm Au NPs, the density of the oligonucleotides is higher when a spacer based on thymine is used (38 pmol/cm^2) rather than one based on adenine (19 pmol/cm^2). Higher densities (56 pmol/cm^2) have been reported if polyethylene glycol, which minimally interacts with the gold surface, is used as a spacer [9]. The same authors have reported facilitation of kinetics of immobilization, orientation, and packing of the oligonucleotides on the surface of the particles by sonication or, alternatively, upon increasing the temperature [9]. The density of the oligonucleotides can also be controlled in part by salt concentration (Fig. 9.2B). Increasing the salt concentration allows for a greater number of strands per particle, since the NaCl added screens the negatively charged phosphate-sugar backbones [8].

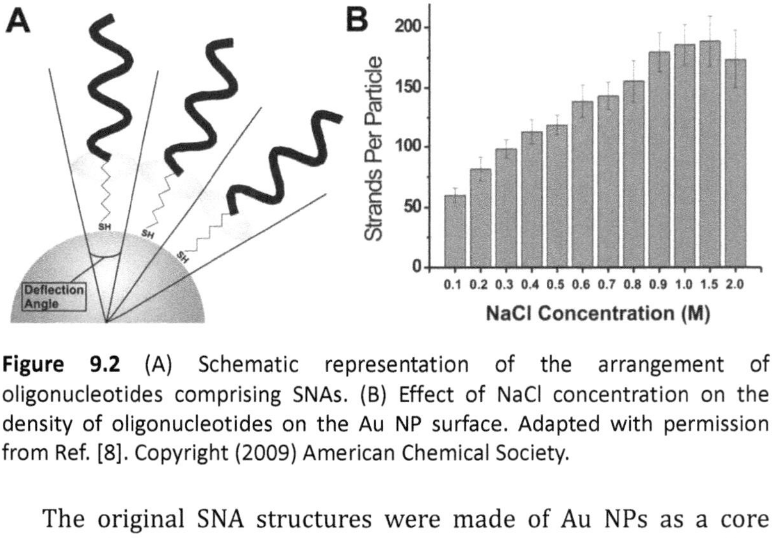

Figure 9.2 (A) Schematic representation of the arrangement of oligonucleotides comprising SNAs. (B) Effect of NaCl concentration on the density of oligonucleotides on the Au NP surface. Adapted with permission from Ref. [8]. Copyright (2009) American Chemical Society.

The original SNA structures were made of Au NPs as a core material [1]. Au NPs were chosen as initial candidates because they are easily synthesized over a range of particle sizes. To date these are the most common type of SNAs used in biomedical applications. However, SNAs have been prepared in a variety of different forms and with a variety of inorganic core compositions, including gold, silver, silica, iron oxide, and semiconductor quantum dots (QDs) [2, 5–7, 11–16]. Initially, it has been considered that the NP core typically plays little role in determining the chemical and biological properties of the corresponding SNAs and that most of the properties stem from the dense layer of oriented oligonucleotides. Subsequent studies have shown that the inorganic NPs serve two purposes [2]: (i) they provide novel physical and chemical properties (e.g., plasmonic, catalytic, scattering, and quenching) and (ii) they act as a scaffold for assembling and orienting the oligonucleotides into a dense arrangement that gives rise to many of their functional properties. Very recent studies report on preparation of metal-free SNAs. These are architectures with organic (polymeric, small molecule, drug conjugate, liposomal) cores, as well as hollow SNA structures that are held together by cross-linked oligonucleotides or silica shells [13, 17].

SNAs exhibit a variety of novel properties that are substantially different from those of their linear counterparts. Largely, the emergent properties, unique for SNAs, stem from the density and orientation of the oligonucleotides on the outer region of the nanostructures. Examples, demonstrating the markedly different properties, are given in Table 9.1. SNAs behave unlike any other forms of nucleic acids in binding experiments, exhibiting higher binding constants [18]. Other intriguing and unique properties are the rapid cellular uptake of high quantities of SNAs without the need for cationic (and typically cytotoxic) transfection agents [19] and the enhanced resistance to many forms of enzymatically enhanced cleavage. The former is believed to occur by scavenger-mediated endocytosis; the scavenger receptors are found on the surface of the cells and are known to widely recognize and take up macromolecules having a negative charge density [19]. It is noteworthy that, unlike their linear counterparts, SNAs do not elicit an immune response when taken up into cells [21]. For the latter, Seferos et al. proposed that the steric congestion and high salt concentration associated with the densely packed oligonucleotides in this architecture inhibit enzyme activity [20].

SNAs have been utilized in a number of important biomedical applications. Many extracellular solution-phase and surface-based diagnostic assays for detecting biomarkers for cancers and other diseases have been developed. SNAs are also leading to intracellular diagnostics and imaging tools and platforms. Due to their rapid and efficient cellular uptake, they are especially attractive as gene regulation materials and for the development of various therapeutic schemes.

Table 9.1 Comparison of properties of SNAs and linear nucleic acids

Property	SNAs	Linear nucleic acids
Melting transition	Cooperative and narrow (2°C ≈ 8°C)	Broad (~20°C)
Cellular uptake	Transfection agents not required	Transfection agents required
Immune response	Minimal [22]	Elevated interferon-β levels [22]
Stability	Nuclease resistance [20]	Subject to degradation by nucleases
Properties from inorganic core	Plasmonic, catalytic [17], magnetic [7], and luminescent [11]	n/a
Binding strength	$K_{eq} = 1.8 \times 10^{14}$	$K_{eq} = 1.8 \times 10^{12}$

Source: Reprinted with permission from Ref. [2]. Copyright (2012) American Chemical Society.

9.2 Spherical Nucleic Acids with Inorganic Nanoparticle Cores

SNAs with gold particle cores are most commonly used due to metal inertness and its ability to quench fluorescent molecules in a distance-dependent manner [23]. Citrate-capped Au NPs are usually prepared applying the Frens method, in which sodium citrate is used to reduce chloroauric acid ($HAuCl_4$) [24]. Thus, highly uniform Au NPs with sizes ranging from 5 to 150 nm in diameter are formed. The particles serve as templates for the subsequent attachment of nucleic acids and thus play an important role in determining the overall size of the final nanostructure. The core size should be properly chosen according to the specific application of the SNA. The most commonly used SNAs for diagnostic applications have 10–15 nm gold cores with various attachments [23]. Moreover, evaluating the toxicity of functionalized Au NPs with diameters ranging from 0.8 to 15 nm it was found that particles 1.4 nm in diameter were toxic, whereas particles 15 nm in diameter were nontoxic, even at up to hundredfold higher concentrations [25].

The so-called nanoflares, SNA-Au NPs conjugates, functionalized with oligonucleotide hybrid sequences that are designed to be complementary to genes of interest are used for gene detection and diagnostic purposes [26]. The conjugated strands are referred to as the recognition or antisense strands. A short internal complementary strand containing a terminal fluorophore is hybridized onto the antisense strand. Once the fluorophore is bound in close proximity to the gold particle, the fluorescence of the fluorophore is quenched. However, in the presence of a messenger RNA (mRNA) target complementary to the antisense sequence, the target forms a longer, more stable duplex and displaces the shorter flare strand. Displacement of the fluorophore from the NP surface results in a "turn-on" of a fluorescence signal proportional to the concentration of the target transcripts (Fig. 9.3).

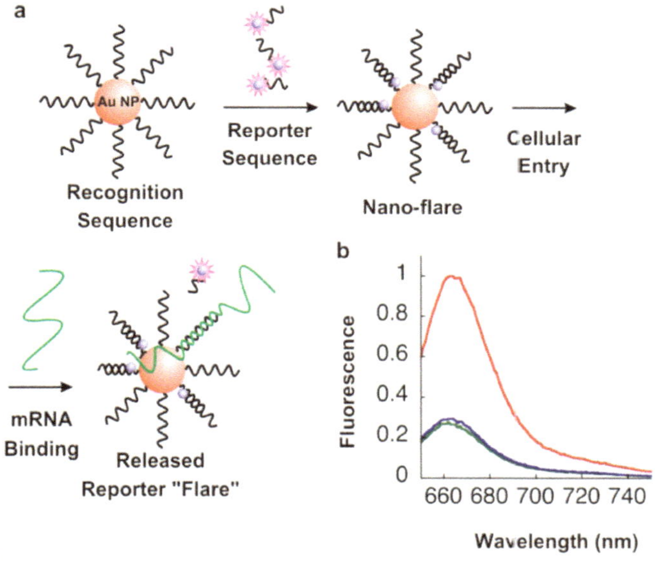

c

Recognition Sequence: 5'-CTT GAG AAA GGG CTG CCA AAA AA-SH-3'
Reporter Sequence: 3'-CCC GAC GGT T-Cy5-5'

Target Region: 3'-GAA CTC TTT CCC GAC GGT-5'

Figure 9.3 (a) Schematic representation of sequence-specific recognition of target RNA using nanoflares. (b) Fluorescence response of nanoflares alone (green) and nanoflares in the presence of the target (red) compared to the noncomplementary sequence (blue). (c) Oligonucleotide sequences. Reprinted with permission from Ref. [26]. Copyright (2007) American Chemical Society.

The nanoflare concept is further developed to yield a sticky flare, allowing quantification and real-time tracking of RNA in live cells [27]. With a simple design modification the flare sequence is made longer and complementary to the target RNA transcript. In contrast to the nanoflare where the fluorophore-labeled oligonucleotide reporter is floating freely in the cytoplasm, the flares from the sticky flare bind transcripts and act as fluorescent labels for intracellular tracking.

Song et al. report on multimodal, cell-permeable, Gd^{III}-enriched polyvalent DNA–Au NP conjugates for cellular magnetic resonance imaging (MRI) [28]. They represent a new class of contrast agents with the capability of highly efficient cell penetration and accumulation, providing sufficient contrast enhancement for imaging small cell populations with micromolar Gd^{III} incubation concentrations. The conjugates are prepared by reacting stabilized Au NPs (~13 nm in diameter) with thiol-labeled 24-mer deoxythymine (dT) oligonucleotides, each of them modified with five azide-containing conjugation sites. Alkyne functionalized Gd^{III} complexes are covalently attached through the highly efficient click chemistry. When modified with a fluorophore (such as Cy3 dye), the conjugates can be used as multimodal imaging agents and fluorescence microscopy shows that the particles localize in the perinuclear region inside cells (Fig. 9.4).

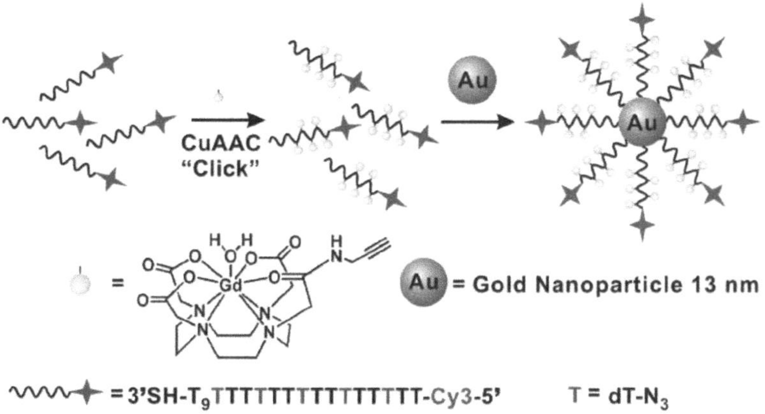

Figure 9.4 Synthetic route to Cy3-DNA-Gd^{III} Au NP conjugates. Reproduced from Ref. [28] with permission from John Wiley and Sons.

More recently, following similar synthetic scheme, a conjugate modified with terminal haloalkane moieties was prepared and used for targeted delivery to the HaloTag reporter protein and for detection of protein expression by MRI [29].

The ability to tune the oligonucleotide sequence of SNAs is an extremely powerful tool for the design of SNA-based cancer therapeutics. Actually, the oligonucleotide sequence can be synthesized in such manner to target any mRNA of interest. Thus, SNAs could be theoretically used for the treatment of any genetic disease. In vitro evaluations of various gold-core SNAs have shown gene knockdown of model targets, such as enhanced green fluorescent protein (eGFP) [3] and luciferase [4]. Moreover, they seem to be promising nanoscale gene regulation platforms toward targets involved in tissue engineering and cancer cell growth and proliferation [30, 31]. To evaluate SNAs for potential treatment of glioblastoma multiforme (GBM), a neurologically debilitating disease considered to be one of the deadliest brain tumors, Jensen et al. [31] designed an SNA conjugate consisting of a 13 nm Au NP core conjugated to thiolated siRNA duplexes targeting the GBM oncogene Bcl2L12. The latter is an effector caspase and p53 inhibitor overexpressed in most GBM tumors [32] It was found that in the absence of any auxiliary transfection strategies or chemical modifications, SNAs efficiently entered primary and transformed glial cells in vitro. In the following in vivo evaluations, the SNAs penetrated the blood-brain barrier and blood-tumor barrier to disseminate throughout xenogeneic glioma explants. Overall, SNAs targeting the oncoprotein were effective in knocking down endogenous Bcl2L12 mRNA and protein levels and sensitized glioma cells toward therapy-induced apoptosis by enhancing effector caspase and p53 activity. Furthermore, systemically delivered SNAs reduced Bcl2L12 expression in intracerebral GBM, increased intratumoral apoptosis, and reduced tumor burden and progression in xenografted mice without any side effects.

It has been demonstrated that microRNAs (miRNAs) are important regulators of GBM pathogenesis and therapeutic susceptibility [33]. Recently, Kouri et al. [34] identified miR-182 as a potential miRNA candidate that regulates Bcl2L12 expression. miR-182 acts as a regulator of apoptosis, growth, and differentiation programs whose expression level is correlated with GBM patient survival. To evaluate miR-182-related tumor-suppressive functions as a therapeutic agent in vitro and in vivo, the authors synthesized gold-core SNAs functionalized with mature miR-182 sequences (182-SNAs). It was demonstrated that 182-SNAs effectively decrease Bcl2L12 protein levels, enhance apoptotic responses to chemotherapy, drastically reduce tumor burden, and extend survival of GBM-xenografted mice. Moreover, the lack of detectable side effects or toxicity makes 182-SNAs a promising novel platform for delivering therapeutic miRNAs in GBM.

In another scientific report Wang et al. [35] demonstrated the development of an anti-miR99b gold-core SNA-NP conjugate (SNA-$NC^{anti\text{-}miR99b}$). It was designed for targeting of milk fat globule–EGF 8 (MFG-E8), which maintains intestinal homeostasis by enhancing enterocyte migration and attenuating inflammation (Fig. 9.5). Usually the sepsis is associated with downregulation of intestinal MFG-E8 and impairment of enterocyte migration. Administration of SNAs rescued intestinal MFG-E8 expression and restored enterocyte migration in lipopolysaccharide (LPS)-induced septic mice, most likely via a miR-99b-dependent mechanism.

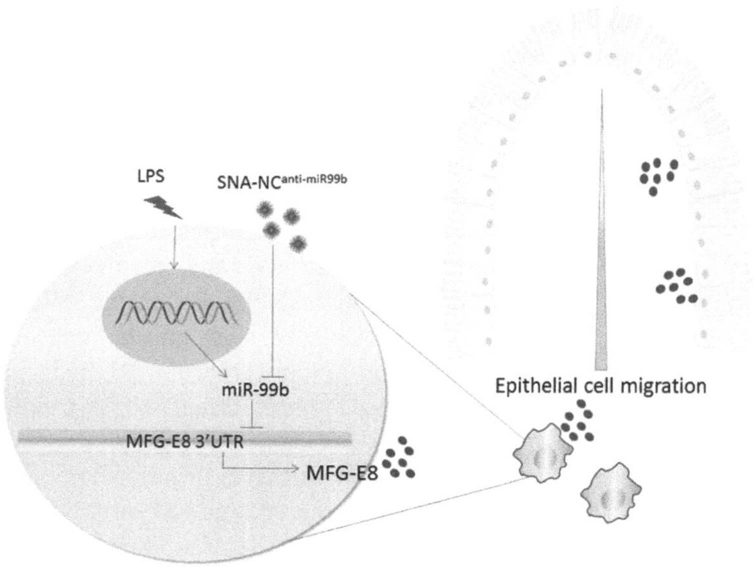

Figure 9.5 A schematic model of the effect of targeting MFG-E8 gene expression in macrophages on intestinal epithelial homeostasis. Reproduced with permission from Ref. [35]. Copyright © 2016, Nature Publishing Group.

The versatility of solid-phase DNA synthesis allows the addition of specific chemical functional groups onto oligonucleotides. These functional groups can be further used to attach various drugs, other small molecules, or markers of interest to oligonucleotides. Conjugation of such modified oligonucleotides with Au NPs enables the formation of SNAs with more than one function. Thus, Dhar et al. [36] synthesized oligonucleotide-bearing terminal alkylamine functionality. Carboxylic acid–modified Pt(IV) prodrug was attached to the oligonucleotide via amide linkage applying the carbodiimide coupling method (Fig. 9.6). In vitro evaluations of functional SNAs performed on cancer cell lines of various origins showed significant cytotoxicity, whereas the parent prodrug did not show any significant killing under the same conditions.

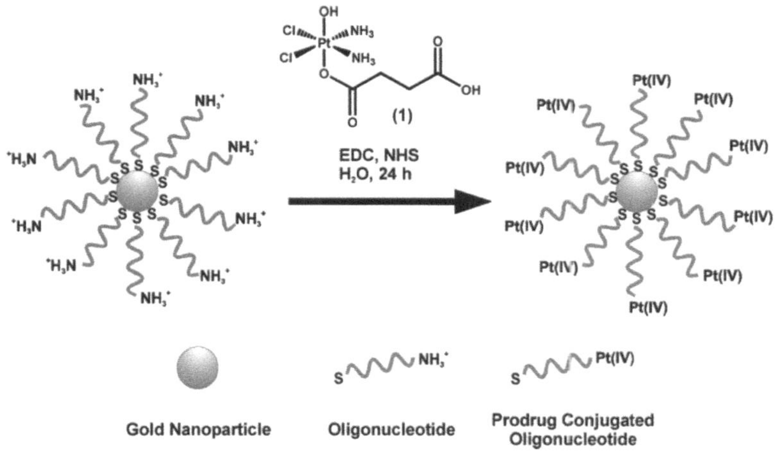

Figure 9.6 Scheme for the synthesis of Pt(IV)-terminated SNAs. Reprinted with permission from Ref. [36]. Copyright (2009) American Chemical Society.

Applying the same synthetic route, gold-core SNAs, modified with another anticancer drug, paclitaxel (PTX), were successfully prepared [37]. The oligonucleotide linkers were additionally labeled with a fluorophore, affording the visualization of SNA-conjugates within cells. The incorporation of PTX into the SNAs increases more than fiftyfold the drug solubility in aqueous media. The internalized PTX-modified conjugates revealed increased activity compared with the free drug toward different cancer cell lines, including a PTX-resistant cell line.

Besides drugs and other small molecules, larger structures, such as antibodies, could be attached to the SNAs and evaluated for potential therapeutic applications. Thus, to enhance SNA association with target cells, Zhang et al. conjugated a monoclonal antibody (mAb) to antisense gold-core DNA-SNAs, creating cellular targeting antisense DNA-SNAs [38]. Initially, the authors utilized click chemistry to conjugate a human epithelial growth factor receptor 2 (HER2) to fluorophore-labeled sense DNA sequence, specifically linking an azide-functionalized HER2 mAb to DNA with a 3′ alkyne group (Fig. 9.7). Once the mAb-DNA conjugates were isolated and purified, they were hybridized to the complementary antisense sequences comprising the surface of a gold-core SNA. In vitro evaluations performed on SKOV-3 ovarian cancer cells revealed that hybridization-based tethering of the HER2 mAb to SNAs imparts cell selectivity to these particles, allowing faster cell uptake and more efficient gene knockdown than the native SNA structures of the same sequence. Moreover, the antibody-modified conjugates exhibit many of the same attributes as exhibited by the nontargeted SNA structures. The imparted cellular targeting capabilities of the SNA constructs will allow for the systemic targeting of genetically based diseases, including many forms of cancer. More important, the proposed general hybridization approach for SNA functionalization can be extended to a wide variety of antibodies and other targeting moieties.

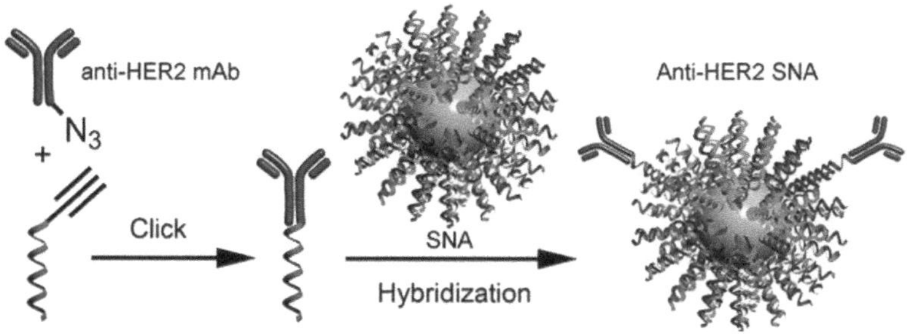

Figure 9.7 Synthetic route to anti-HER2 SNA preparation. Adapted with permission from Ref. [38]. Copyright (2012) American Chemical Society.

Despite the fact that most of currently developed SNA conjugates are based on Au NPs, there are examples of other inorganic cores used for the construction of SNAs. For example, Lee et al. have developed a method for synthesizing stable DNA-functionalized Ag NPs that exhibit distance-dependent optical and highly cooperative binding properties [6]. The method exploits the strong affinity of multiple cyclic disulfide-anchoring moieties for the Ag NP surface. Oligonucleotides of desired sequences were synthesized, modified with terminal cyclic disulfide groups, and successfully attached to Ag NPs (~30 nm in diameter). Upon combination of Ag NPs functionalized with complementary sequences, a reversible assembly to DNA-linked NP networks occurs.

In another work, Ag NPs were conjugated with thiol-terminated oligonucleotides and methoxy polyethylene glycol [15]. The antibacterial properties of the silver-core SNAs were evaluated. The obtained results are optimistic, particularly against the challenging drug-resistant gram-negative infections.

QD SNAs were first synthesized in 1999 by covalently attaching oligonucleotides directly to the QD core [11]. Initially, CdSe QDs were stabilized with trioctylphosphine oxide and trioctylphosphine followed by surface modification with 3-mercaptopropionic acid. After the surface carboxylic group deprotonation with 4-(dimethylamino)pyridine, QDs were readily dispersed in water and were able to immobilize thiol-terminated oligonucleotides. Later, a method for noncovalent immobilization of ssDNA on the surface of aliphatic ligand–protected CdSe/ZnS QDs by reacting them with amphiphilic polymers functionalized with DNA was reported [12]. Briefly, oleylamine-protected CdSe/ZnS core/shell QDs were modified with an amphiphilic polymer containing both hydrophobic alkyl chains (which intercalated with the hydrophobic capping ligands on the NP) and hydrophilic polyethylene glycol–bearing clickable end group. The particles were then functionalized with DNA applying click chemistry to produce a dense DNA shell. Fluorophore-labeled oligonucleotide QD SNAs were used to follow the intracellular events that occur following their cellular uptake [39].

Cutler et al. developed a strategy for the immobilization of oligonucleotides on the surface of superparamagnetic iron oxide NPs SPIONPs applying click chemistry [7]. Azide surface modification was achieved through the reaction of aminated SPIONPs with succinimidyl 4-azidobutyrate. Oligonucleotides modified with terminal alkyne groups were densely attached onto the particle surface via a highly efficient aqueous copper(I)-catalyzed azide-alkyne cycloaddition. The SPIONPs densely functionalized with DNA are able to cross HeLa (cervical cancer) cell membranes with no need to use any transfection agents. Moreover, the NP core properties predetermine potential applications such as MRI and magnetic hyperthermia therapy strategies.

A new class of core-free SNA conjugates consisting of a biocompatible porous silica shell has been developed [13]. Silica-coated Au NPs were used as templates, which can be easily functionalized with nucleic acids, applying a wide variety of coupling strategies and relatively simple and readily available coupling molecules. The silica shell acts as a cross-linked scaffold to assemble the nucleic acids into a densely packed and highly oriented form. The shell's porous architecture enables the chemical dissolution of the gold core. The resulting hollow silica SNAs maintain the unique properties of the SNA–Au NP conjugates. They do not show any cytotoxicity and have been used to effectively silence the eGFP gene in mouse endothelial cells through an antisense approach.

9.3 Spherical Nucleic Acids with Organic Cores

The organic cores introduce great versatility in the chemistry, structure, and properties of the SNAs. Of particular importance are the concerns about the long-term toxicity and metabolitic fate of the SNAs with metallic cores, which have inspired the use of organic templates. A variety of nucleic acid conjugates with organic molecules, proteins, drugs, and polymers have been reported in the literature, but none of them have been developed and optimized with regard to general SNA features and intracellular biological activity [40]. Only a few recent studies describe structures with organic cores that exhibit the hallmark properties of conventional SNAs to which specificities of the properties of the organic core material are added.

Hong et al. report on the assembly of two complementary small molecule–DNA hybrids into well-defined, narrowly dispersed spherical NPs [41]. The hybrids are composed of a tetraphenylmethane core and 18-base DNA that are linked together through $(CH_2)_4$-triazole spacers. Their sizes can be easily tuned by controlling the concentration, assembly time, and NaCl content. However, the particles continued to aggregate over time at room temperature through hybridization events between unhybridized strands on the surfaces of the neighboring particles. This was minimized by capping one of these two types of unhybridized strands with complementary ssDNA strands, thus transforming the initial particles into SNAs. The authors demonstrated also that the initial particles could be stabilized with two different sets of functionalized capping strands and that the whole platform would bear two different functional groups. The resulting particles exhibited features typical for SNAs, such as efficient cellular uptake and enhanced resistance to a DNase I enzyme.

A drug-cored SNA, which exploits the opposing hydrophilicity of nucleic acids and the anticancer drug PTX, is reported elsewhere [42]. PTX was attached to a norbornenyl group and prepolymerized (degree of polymerization of 10) by ring-opening metathesis polymerization and terminated with an azide-containing end-cap, allowing for clicking of a single DNA strand functionalized with a dibenzocyclooctyne group. The hydrophobic drug component allows for the conjugate to self-assemble in an aqueous solution into a small (about 15 nm) dense, spherical form, which enables rapid endocytosis (Fig. 9.8). The linker contained a disulfide bond, which was cleaved under the reducing environment of the cell, thus allowing free drug to be released upon cellular uptake (Fig. 9.8). For the novel structures, the authors found cell internalization to be ca. 100 times faster than free DNA, increased nuclease stability, and cytotoxicity nearly identical to that of the free drug. It is noteworthy that the nucleic acid component acted as both a therapeutic payload for intracellular gene regulation and a delivery vehicle for the drug component.

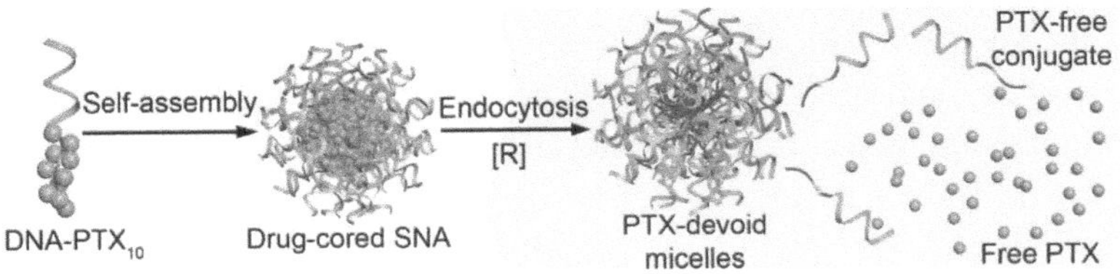

Figure 9.8 Schematic representation of the formation of DNA-paclitaxel$_{10}$ structures and their intended actions. Adapted with permission from Ref. [42]. Copyright (2016) American Chemical Society.

Similarly, Banga et al. have employed ring-opening metathesis polymerization to prepare short (up to 45 kDa) amphiphilic block copolymers consisting of a doxorubicin-conjugated block and a hydrophilic carboxy-terminated poly(ethylene oxide) block [43]. NPs with an average hydrodynamic diameter (D_h) of 63 ± 7 nm were obtained applying the solvent exchange method. The surface modification of the resulting NPs with 3′-amino-terminated oligonucleotides was achieved using EDC/NHS coupling (N-(3-dimethylaminopropyl)-*N*′-ethylcarbodiimide hydrochloride, hydroxysulfosuccinimide). The modification resulted in an increase in the size (D_h = 88 ± 7 nm) and a shift of the ζ potential to a higher negative value, whereas the spherical morphology was retained. The authors calculated an average of 1200 oligonucleotide strands per particle, corresponding to the surface density of ~7 pmol/cm^2. The dense oligonucleotide shell greatly increased the colloidal stability of the polymeric SNAs in biological media under physiological conditions and enhanced the cellular uptake.

In another approach Zhang et al. [40] describe SNAs based on brush-block copolymer micelles (Fig. 9.9). The copolymer was synthesized by grafting multiple DNA strands onto the terminal segments of a diblock copolymer based on polycaprolactone. In particular, polycaprolactone (M_w = 14 kDa) was used as a macroinitiator for polymerization of α-chloro-ε-caprolactone followed by conversion of the pendant chlorides into azides. The grafting of the azide-functionalized diblock copolymer was achieved by treating it with an excess of cyclooctyne-terminated DNA strands, resulting in the formation of a brush-block copolymer with an average of 10 DNA strands on each polymer chain (Fig. 9.9b). The self-assembly in water resulted in the formation of well-defined, spherical structures with an average D_h of 44 nm and a strongly negative (−48.5 mV) ζ potential. The number of DNA strands and surface density (302 and 22 pmol/cm^2, respectively) were comparable with those of Au NP–based SNAs of a similar size. Structures from a linear copolymer were prepared as well. They exhibited comparable hydrodynamic dimensions, less negative ζ potential (−27.9 mV), and a lower number of both strands and surface density (190 and 15.6 pmol/cm^2, respectively) compared to the structures prepared from the brush-block copolymer. The as-synthesized micellar SNAs did not have measurable cellular toxicity, even with an incubation time of up to four days. The biodegradability was evaluated in buffers of varied pH to mimic different intracellular environments. The agarose gel electrophoresis indicated degradation of the structures, which was faster at lower pH. Both structures exhibited the ability to enter cells without the assistance of cationic transfection agents, but the uptake of the SNAs based on the brush-block copolymer was more efficient, presumably due to the higher surface density of their DNA. Furthermore, the DNA strands were designed as an antisence sequence against eGFP mRNA. The results indicated that the micellar structures could effectively bind the cytosolic mRNA and alter the expression of its associated protein. Again, the constructs of the brush-block copolymer were more effective than those of the linear one.

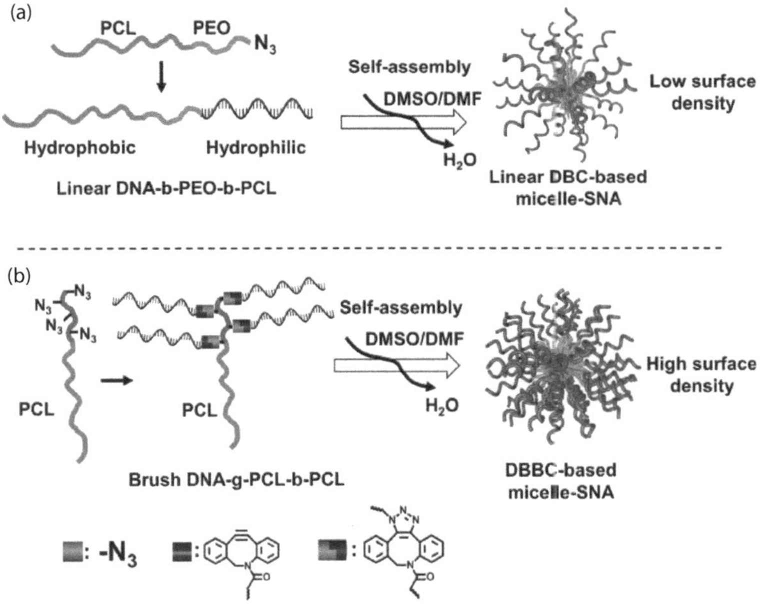

Figure 9.9 Synthesis of (a) the linear DNA-*b*-PEO-*b*–PCL block copolymer and the corresponding formation of low-surface-density micelle SNAs; (b) the brush DNA-*g*-PCL-*b*-PCL block copolymer and the formation of high-suface-density micelle SNAs. Reproduced from Ref. [40] with permission from John Wiley and Sons.

A novel class of metal-free SNAs held together via noncovalent bonds is described elsewhere [44, 45]. These are based on

30 nm liposomal cores that are stabilized with a dense shell of oligonucleotides, intercalated via a hydrophobic residue in the phospholipid bilayer of the liposomes (Fig. 9.10). The liposomes were prepared from 1,2-dioleyl-*sn*-glycero-3-phosphocholine in 4-(2-hydroxyethyl)-1-piperazine-1-ethanesulfonic acid (HEPES) buffer saline by sonication followed by extrusion through a polycarbonate membrane with a 30 nm pore size. The liposomal SNAs were synthesized by incubating the liposomal suspension with a nucleic acid derivative bearing a hydrophobic tocopherol moiety (Fig. 9.10) for 12 h at room temperature. The significant drop in the ζ potential from −1 to −23 mV and the increase in hydrodynamic diameter from ca. 30 to 46 nm indicated successful surface modification. The authors calculated an average of 70 DNA strands per particle, which was sufficient to exhibit the typical properties of SNAs [44]. The liposomal SNAs displayed enhanced stability resulting from the repulsive forces between the negatively charged nucleic acid strands and the ability to cooperatively bind complementary nucleic acids and to enter cells without the need for ancillary transfection agents. The potential to affect both cellular transfection and gene regulation was demonstrated as well [44].

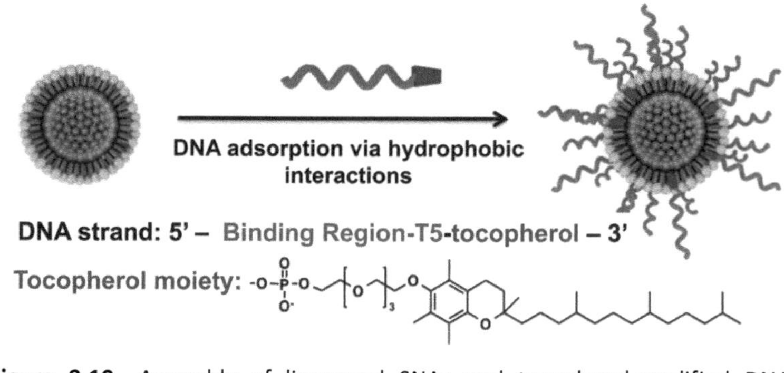

Figure 9.10 Assembly of liposomal SNAs and tocopherol-modified DNA. Reprinted with permission from Ref. [44]. Copyright (2014) American Chemical Society https://pubs.acs.org/doi/abs/10.1021/ja504845f. Further permissions related to the material excerpted should be directed to the American Chemical Society.

In a subsequent paper [45], the delivery of antisence oligonucleotides to the nucleus utilizing liposomal SNAs has been explored. Targeted knockdown of the nuclear-retained metastasis–

associated lung adenocarcinoma transcript 1 (Malat1, a key oncogenic long noncoding RNA involved in metastasis of several cancers) upon treatment with liposomal SNAs as well as the consequent upregulation of tumor suppressor mRNA associated with Malat1 were shown. Obviously, this form of liposomal SNA was able to escape, in full or in part, the endosome to an extent that it could effectively reach and bind the target in the nucleus. Of key importance was the dynamic character of the noncovalently assembled liposomal SNAs, allowing for uptake of the intact SNA and slow release of the antisence oligonucleotides comprising the latter in order to interact with nucleic acids in the nucleus.

Surface modification of Pluronic F127 micelles has been readily achieved by intercalation of a lipid-mimetic tail attached covalently to DNA [46]. The nucleic acid strands contained a block of five amine-functionalized bases, which was used for cross-linking with bis(succinimidyl)penta(ethylene glycol) after intercalation in the initial micelles (Fig. 9.11). An average surface coverage of about 150 DNA strands per particle resulting in doubling of the size to ~26 nm and a shift to a more negative ζ potential was calculated. With their extended stability and enhanced intracellular activity, the cross-linked micellar SNAs showed a strong potential for therapeutic development.

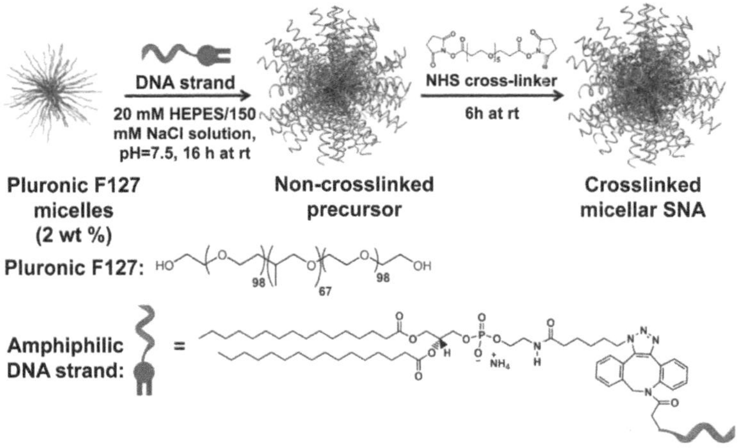

Figure 9.11 Assembly of cross-linked micellar SNAs from Pluronic F127 templates and amphiphilic DNA. Reprinted with permission from Ref. [46]. Copyright (2017) American Chemical Society.

9.4 Conclusions

A novel 3D nucleic acid architecture, referred to as the SNA, is described in this chapter. An SNA is typically a small (sub-100 nm) 3D structure composed of a gold core to which a shell of functionalized oligonucleotides is attached. These structures are characterized with a set of properties distinct from those of the linear forms of nucleic acids with the same sequence. They exhibit increased colloidal stability, superior cellular uptake via scavenger receptor-mediated endocytosis, and enhanced stability against nuclease degradation compared to the linear counterparts. The capability of SNAs to interact with biological materials in unique ways, resulting from the arrangement of oligonucleotides into highly oriented, densely packed structures, provides venues for them to be used in molecular diagnostics, gene regulation, and medicine. Besides gold, the core compositions may include silver, iron oxide, silica, and QDs, which contribute to diversification of the properties of SNAs while preserving those that stem from the specific arrangement and density of oligonucleotides on the core surface. Very recently SNAs with organic cores have been described and are beginning to be explored. Considering the versatility of these materials, their inherent biocompatibility and tolerability to biological matter, the possibilities to impart various functions, and their biodegradability, one may anticipate a strong potential for therapeutic and diagnostic development of SNAs with organic (polymer and liposomal) cores.

References

1. Mirkin, C. A., Letsinger, R. L., Mucic, R. C. and Storhoff, J. J. (1996). A DNA-based method for rationally assembling nanoparticles into macroscopic materials, *Nature*, **382**, pp. 607–609.
2. Cutler, J. I., Auyeung, E. and Mirkin, C. A. (2012). Spherical nucleic acids, *J. Am. Chem. Soc.*, **134**, pp. 1376–1391.
3. Rosi, N. L., Giljohann, D. A., Thaxton, C. S., Lytton-Jean, A. K., Han, M. S. and Mirkin, C. A. (2006). Oligonucleotide-modified gold nanoparticles for intracellular gene regulation, *Science*, **312**, pp. 1027–1030.
4. Giljohann, D. A., Seferos, D. S., Pridogich, A. E., Patel, P. C. and Mirkin, C. A. (2009). Gene regulation with polyvalent siRNA-nanoparticle conjugates, *J. Am. Chem. Soc.*, **131**, pp. 2072–2073.

5. Hao, L., Patel, P. C., Alhasan, A. H., Giljohann, D. A. and Mirkin, C. A. (2011). Nucleic acid–gold nanoparticle conjugates as mimics of microRNA, *Small*, **7**, pp. 3158–3162.
6. Lee, J. S., Lytton-Jean, A. K. R., Hurst, S. J. and Mirkin, C. A. (2007). Silver nanoparticle-oligonucleotide conjugates based on DNA with triple cyclic disulfide moieties, *Nano Lett.*, **7**, pp. 2112–2115.
7. Cutler, J. L., Zheng, D., Xu, X. Y., Giljohann, D. A. and Mirkin, C. A. (2010). Polyvalent oligonucleotide iron oxide nanoparticle "click" conjugates, *Nano Lett.*, **10**, pp. 1477–1480.
8. Hill, H. D., Millstone, J. E., Banholzer, M. J. and Mirkin, C. A. (2009). The role radius of curvature plays in thiolated oligonucleotide loading on gold, *ACS Nano*, **3**, pp. 418–424.
9. Hurst, S. J., Lytton-Jean, A. K. R. and Mirkin, C. A. (2006). Maximizing DNA loading on a range of gold nanoprticle sizes, *Anal. Chem.*, **78**, pp. 8313–8318.
10. Storhoff, J. J., Elghanian, R., Mirkin, C. A. and Letsinger, R. I. (2002). Sequence-dependent stability of DNA-modified gold nanoparticles, *Langmuir*, **18**, pp. 6666–6670.
11. Mitchell, G. P., Mirkin, C. A. and Letsinger, R. L. (1999). Programmed assembly of DNA functionalized quantum dots, *J. Am. Chem. Soc.*, **121**, pp. 8122–8123.
12. Zhang, C., Macfarlane, R. J., Young, K. L., Choi, C. H. J., Hao, L., Auyeung, E., Liu, G., Zhou, X. and Mirkin, C. A. (2013). A general approach to DNA-programmable atom equivalents, *Nat. Mater.*, **12**, pp. 741–746.
13. Young, K. L., Scott, A. W., Hao, L., Mirkin, S. E., Liu, G. and Mirkin, C. A. (2012). Hollow spherical nucleic acids for intracellular gene regulation based upon biocompatible silica shells, *Nano Lett.*, **12**, pp. 3867–3871.
14. Xue, C., Chen, X., Hurst, S. J. and Mirkin, C. A. (2007). Self-assembled monolayer mediated silica coating of silver triangular nanoprisms, *Adv. Mater.*, **19**, pp. 4071–4072.
15. Rische, C. H., Goel, A., Radovic-Moreno, A. F. and Gryaznov, S. M. (2016). Antibacterial silver core spherical nucleic acids, *Mater. Today Commun.*, **9**, pp. 30–40.
16. Yao, D., Song, T., Sun, X., Xiao, S., Huang, F. and Liang, H. (2015). Integrating DNA-strand-displacement circuitry with self-assembly of spherical nucleic acids, *J. Am. Chem. Soc.*, **137**, pp. 14107–14113.
17. Cutler, J. I., Zhang, K., Zheng, D., Auyeung, E., Prigodich, A. E. and Mirkin, C. A. (2011). Polyvalent nucleic acid nanostructures, *J. Am. Chem. Soc.*, **133**, pp. 9254–9257.

18. Lytton-Jean, A. K. R. and Mirkin, C. A. (2005). A thermodynamic investigation into the binding properties of DNA functionalized gold nanoparticle probes and molecular fluorophore probes, *J. Am. Chem. Soc.*, **127**, pp. 12754–12755.
19. Patel, P. C., Giljohann, D. A., Daniel, W. L., Zheng, D., Prigodich, A. E. and Mirkin, C. A. (2010). Scavenger receptors mediate cellular uptake of polyvalent oligonucleotide-functionalized gold nanoparticles, *Bioconjugate Chem.*, **21**, pp. 2250–2256.
20. Seferos, D. S., Prigodich, A. E., Giljohann, D. A., Patel, P. C. and Mirkin, C. A. (2009). Polyvalent DNA nanoparticle conjugates stabilize nucleic acids, *Nano Lett.*, **9**, pp. 308–311.
21. Prigodich, A. E., Seferos, D. S., Massich, M. D., Giljohann, D. A., Lane, B. C. and Mirkin, C. A. (2009). Nano-flares for mRNA regulation and detection, *ACS Nano*, **3**, pp. 2147–2152.
22. Massich, M. D., Giljohann, D. A., Seferos, D. S., Ludlow, L. E., Horvath, C. and Mirkin, C. A. (2009). Regulating immune response using polyvalent nucleic acid-gold nanoparticle conjugates, *Mol. Pharmaceutics*, **6**, pp. 1934–1940.
23. Giljohann, D. A., Seferos, D. S., Daniel, W. L., Massich, M. D., Patel, P. C. and Mirkin, C. A. (2010). Goldnanoparticles for biology and medicine, *Angew. Chem. Int. Ed.*, **49**, pp. 3280–3294.
24. Frens, G. (1973). Controlled nucleation for regulation of particle-size in monodisperse gold suspensions, *Nat. Phys. Sci.*, **241**, pp. 20–22.
25. Pan, Y., Neuss, S., Leifert, A., Fischler, M., Wen, F., Simon, U., Schmid, G., Brandau, W. and Jahnen-Dechent, W. (2007). Size-dependent cytotoxicity of gold nanoparticles, *Small*, **3**, pp. 1941–1949.
26. Seferos, D. S., Giljohann, D. A., Hill, H. D, Prigodich, A. E. and Mirkin, C. A. (2007). Nano-flares: probes for transfection and mRNA detection in living cells, *J. Am. Chem. Soc.*, **129**, pp. 15477–15479.
27. Briley, W. E., Bondy, M. H., Randeria, P. S., Dupper, T. J. and Mirkin, C. A. (2015). Quantification and real-time tracking of RNA in live cells using Sticky-flares, *Proc. Natl. Acad. Sci. U.S.A.*, **112**, pp. 9491–9492.
28. Song, Y., Xu, X., MacRenaris, K. W., Zhang, X.-Q., Mirkin, C. A. and Meade, T. J. (2009). Multimodal gadolinium-enriched DNA–gold nanoparticle conjugates for cellular imaging, *Angew. Chem. Int. Ed.*, **48**, pp. 9143–9147.
29. Vistain, L. F., Rotz, M. W., Rathore, R., Preslar, A. T. and Meade, T. J. (2016). Targeted delivery of gold nanoparticle contrast agents for reporting gene detection by magnetic resonance imaging, *Chem. Commun.*, **52**, pp. 160–163.

30. Rink, J. S., McMahon, K. M., Zhang, X., Chen, X., Mirkin, C. A., Thaxton, C. S. and Kaufman, D. B. (2013). Knockdown of intra-islet IKKβ by spherical nucleic acid conjugates prevents cytokine-induced injury and enhances graft survival, *Transplantation*, **96**, pp. 877–884.

31. Jensen, S. A., Day, E. S., Ko, C. H., Hurley, L. A., Luciano, J. P., Kouri, F. M., Merkel, T. J., Luthi, A. J., Patel, P. C., Cutler, J. I., Daniel, W. L., Scott, A. W., Rotz, M. W., Meade, T. J., Giljohann, D. A., Mirkin, C. A. and Stegh, A. H. (2013). Spherical nucleic acid nanoparticle conjugates as an RNAi-based therapy for glioblastoma, *Sci. Transl. Med.*, **5**, pp. 209ra152.

32. Stegh, A. H. and DePinho, R. A. (2011). Beyond effector caspase inhibition Bcl2L12 neutralizes p53 signaling in glioblastoma, *Cell Cycle*, **10**, pp. 33–38.

33. Huse, J. T. and Holland, E. C. (2009). Yin and yang: cancer-implicated miRNAs that have it both ways, *Cell Cycle*, **8**, pp. 3611–3612.

34. Kouri, F. M., Hurley, L. A., Day, E. S., Hua, Y., Merkel, T. J., Queisser, M. A., Peng, C.-Y., Ritner, C., Hao, L., Daniel, W. L., Zhang, H., Sznajder, J. I., Chin, L., Giljohann, D. A., Kessler, J. A., Peter, M. E., Mirkin, C. A. and Stegh, A. H. (2015). miR-182 integrates apoptosis, growth and differentiation programs in glioblastoma, *Genes Dev.*, **29**, pp. 732–745.

35. Wang, X., Hao, L., Bu, H.-F., Scott, A. W., Tian, K., Liu, F., De Plaen, I. G., Liu, Y., Mirkin, C. A. and Tan, X.-D. (2016). Spherical nucleic acid targeting microRNA-99b enhances intestinal MFG-E8 gene expression and restores enterocyte migration in lipopolysaccharide-induced septic mice, *Sci. Rep.*, **6**, p. 31687.

36. Dhar, S., Daniel, W. L., Giljohann, D. A., Mirkin, C. A. and Lippard, S. J. (2009). Polyvalent oligonucleotide gold nanoparticle conjugates as delivery vehicles for platinum(IV) warheads, *J. Am. Chem. Soc.*, **131**, pp. 14652–14653.

37. Zhang, X.-Q., Xu, X., Lam, R., Giljohann, D., Ho, D. and Mirkin, C. A. (2011). Strategy for increasing drug solubility and efficacy through covalent attachment to polyvalent DNA–nanoparticle conjugates, *ACS Nano*, **5**, pp. 6962–6970.

38. Zhang, K., Hao, L., Hurst, S. J. and Mirkin, C. A. (2012). Antibody-linked spherical nucleic acids for cellular targeting, *J. Am. Chem. Soc.*, **134**, pp. 16488–16491.

39. Wu, X. A., Choi, C. H. J., Zhang, C., Hao, L. and Mirkin, C. A. (2014). Intracellular fate of spherical nucleic acid nanoparticle conjugates, *J. Am. Chem. Soc.*, **136**, pp. 7726–7733.

40. Zhang, Ch., Hao, L., Calabrese, C. M., Zhou, Y., Choi, Ch. H. J., Xing, H. and Mirkin, C. A. (2015). Biodegradable DNA-brush block copolymer

spherical nucleic acids enable transfection agent-free intracellular gene regulation, *Small*, **11**, pp. 5360–5368.

41. Hong, B. J., Eryazici, I., Bleher, R., Thaner, R. V., Mirkin, C. A. and Nguyen, S. T. (2015). Directed assembly of nuclei acid-based polymeric nanoparticles from molecular tetravalent cores, *J. Am. Chem. Soc.*, **137**, pp. 8184–8191.

42. Tan, X., Lu, X., Jia, F., Liu, X., Sun, Y., Logan, J. K. and Zhang, K. (2016). Blurring the role of oligonucleotides: spherical nucleic acids as a drug delivery vehicle, *J. Am. Chem. Soc.*, **138**, pp. 10834–10837.

43. Banga, R. J., Krovi, S. A., Narayan, S. P., Sprangers, A. J., Liu, G., Mirkin, C. A. and Nguyen, S. T. (2017). Drug-loaded polymeric spherical nucleic acids: enhancing colloidal stability and cellular uptake of polymeric nanoparticles through DNA surface functionalization, *Biomacromolecules*, **18**, pp. 483–489.

44. Banga, R. S., Chernyak, N., Narayan, S. P., Nguyen, S. T. and Mirkin, C. A. (2014). Liposomal spherical nucleic acids, *J. Am. Chem. Soc.*, **136**, pp. 9866–9869.

45. Sprangers, A. J., Hao, L., Banga, R. J. and Mirkin, C. A. (2017). Liposomal spherical nucleic acids for regulating long noncoding RNAs in the nucleus, *Small*, **13**, p. 1602753.

46. Banga, R. J., Meckes, B., Narayan, S. P., Sprangers, A. J., Nguyen, S. T. and Mirkin, C. A. (2017). Cross-linked micellar spherical mucleic acids from thermoresponsive templates, *J. Am. Chem. Soc.*, **139**, pp. 4278–4281.

Chapter 10

Radiolabeled Nanoparticles as Diagnostic and Therapeutic Agents of Cancer

Charalampos Tsoukalas,[a] Maria-Argyro Karageorgou,[a,b] and Penelope Bouziotis[a]
[a]*Radiochemical Studies Laboratory, Institute of Nuclear and Radiological Sciences & Technology, Energy & Safety, National Center for Scientific Research "Demokritos," Patriarchou Grigoriou and 27 Neapoleos Street 15341 Aghia Paraskevi, Athens, Greece*
[b]*Department of Solid State Physics, National and Kapodistrian University of Athens, University Campus, Zografou, Athens 15784, Greece*
bouzioti@rrp.demokritos.gr

In recent years, the field of nanotechnology has emerged as an approach with the potential to produce novel diagnostics and therapeutics. Nanomedicine is rapidly expanding and has proven to be a promising approach for producing efficient methods for the diagnosis and treatment of a multitude of diseases. Nanooncology is the application of nanobiotechnology in cancer and it is the most important chapter of nanomedicine. Various applications in the

Drug Delivery Nanosystems: From Bioinspiration and Biomimetics to Clinical Applications
Edited by Costas Demetzos, Stergios Pispas, and Natassa Pippa

ISBN 978-981-4774-92-5 (Hardcover), 978-0-429-49054-5 (eBook)
www.panstanford.com

diagnosis and therapy of cancer are discussed in this chapter. The aim of this unit is to show how nanotechnology is applied in the study of cancer and to discuss the various applications of nanotechnology in the diagnosis and treatment of this disease.

10.1 Introduction

According to the most recent World Health Organization report, the number of new cancer cases in 2012 stood at 14 million and is expected to reach the staggering number of 22 million cases by the year 2030 [1]. Despite advances in treatment, diagnosis, and prevention options, cancer deaths over the same period are predicted to rise from 8.2 million a year to 13 million. These statistics indicate that there is a pressing need to develop novel treatments and approaches that will enhance the survival rates.

Even though much work has been dedicated to optimizing cancer treatment, the strategy still remains the same: surgery, chemotherapy, and/or radiation. We have witnessed great advances in treatment protocols with chemotherapy, but efficient drug delivery to the tumor site still has many obstacles to overcome, among which are high systemic toxicity and poor pharmacokinetics. Furthermore, many cancers are characterized by low survival rates, which can be attributed to late diagnosis.

In recent years, nanoscale materials (nanoparticles [NPs]) have been developed for a wide range of purposes related to drug delivery, cancer treatment, and diagnosis. These materials present numerous opportunities to improve the current state of cancer diagnosis and treatment available to patients. A material is considered an NP when at least one dimension is on the order of 10–100 nm. A number of parameters must be taken into account when designing novel NPs for application in oncology. The NP size will determine whether the NPs will be cleared via the kidneys or will be taken up by the reticuloendothelial system (RES). Hydrodynamic size is not the only parameter that determines the in vivo fate of an NP; the surface is also very important. After NPs are injected into the bloodstream, they are rapidly coated by plasma proteins in a process known as opsonization. The NPs are then recognized by plasma membrane receptors found on monocytes and macrophages and are thus taken up by the body's main defense system, the RES, also known as the mononuclear phagocyte system. The liver, spleen, and bone marrow are rich in macrophages, thus becoming the most accessible tissues to NPs.

The development of novel imaging tools with improved imaging characteristics would lead to an early identification of the disease and, consequently, to improved patient management. The development of targeted NPs that can deliver cytotoxic agents (drugs, radioisotopes, toxins) directly to cancer cells may provide better efficacy and have lower toxicity in the treatment of primary and advanced metastatic tumors. Finally, the development of multimodal imaging systems has led to a boom in dual-mode molecular imaging probes that are targeted for very specific clinical applications, such as the imaging of tumors.

The present chapter provides an overview of radiolabeled NPs as imaging and therapeutic agents, with examples from recent literature.

10.2 Radiolabeled Nanoparticles in Cancer Imaging

Molecular imaging of cancer is crucial to modern-day cancer management. The evaluation of new imaging agents will lead to the development of cancer imaging probes that are highly target specific and biocompatible, have high sensitivity, have a high signal-to-noise ratio, and have optimum pharmacokinetic and pharmacodynamic profiles.

Radioisotopes have been extensively used in the development of NP-based imaging agents. Radiolabeled NPs can circulate for longer periods of time than small-molecule single-photon emission computed tomography/positron emission tomography (SPECT/PET) tracers, thus carrying a larger radionuclide payload [2]. The radiolabeled NP must be designed in such a way so as to get stable radiolabeling and a high specific activity product [3]. The delivery of the radiolabeled NP to the disease site can be achieved via either passive targeting or active targeting.

The enhanced permeability and retention effect (EPR) is important for NP delivery to cancer tissue because nanostructures such as NPs extravasate from tumor tissue due to leaky vasculature and remain there because of dysfunctional lymphatic drainage [4, 5]. Although NPs can accumulate in tumors due to the EPR effect, they cannot be considered molecular imaging agents in the strict sense of the term.

Active targeting is achieved by functionalizing the NP surface with various targeting ligands, such as small molecules, antibodies, peptides, and aptamers, which recognize characteristic epitopes at the surface of the diseased cells, thus increasing specific cell uptake [6]. Tumor-specific, radiolabeled NPs can be prepared in four different ways: (i) by coating NPs with an already radiolabeled targeting vector directed against tumor antigens, (b) by coating NPs with a targeting vector and, consequently, labeling the targeting vector, (c) by radiolabeling the NP either directly or via an adequate chelator conjugated onto the NP surface already functionalized by a targeting molecule, and (d) by incorporating the radiolabel into the NP core, during synthesis of the NP, and then conjugating a targeting vector onto the NP surface.

10.2.1 Nanoparticles and SPECT Imaging

SPECT is based on noncoincident γ-rays generated by radioisotopes (Table 10.1). Consequently, the sensitivity of SPECT is about an order of magnitude lower than that of PET and its quantification is somewhat more difficult. Prototypic examples of radioisotopes used in SPECT are technetium-99m (^{99m}Tc), Indium-111 (^{111}In), and Iodine-125/131 ($^{123/125}$I). In contrast to PET, energies routinely used in SPECT are different, and energy-dependent imaging enables the assessment of different radiotracers and thus of different radiolabeled (nano)probes at the same time. The most straightforward approach consists in the direct radiolabeling of NPs through the addition of radioisotope during NP synthesis or the utilization of chelator-free methods [7–9].

The most common NP radiolabeling approach with radiometals utilizes a two-step procedure in which chelates are first conjugated to preformed NPs, which are then subsequently labeled by mixing with the radioisotope [10]. Alternatively, NPs can be labeled via covalent radioiodination. Commercially available reagents chloramine-T and Iodogen can be used to oxidize radioiodide into a mixed halogen species, which readily iodinates activated aromatic groups via electrophilic substitution [11, 12]. In the following paragraphs an overview of the recent literature on radiolabeled NPs for SPECT imaging can be found.

Table 10.1 SPECT radioisotopes for nanoparticle labeling

Radioisotope	Type of emission	Half-life	E_{max} (keV)	Radiolabeling methods
^{99m}Tc	g	6.1 h[a]	140	HMPAO/glutathiones, biphosphonate, HYNIC, DTPA, and direct labeling
^{111}In	Auger, γ	2.8 d[b]	245	Oxine/nitrilotriacetic acid, CHX-DTPA, DOTA, and DTPA
^{125}I	Auger, γ	60.1 d	36	Tyrosine electrophilic substitution, iodogen or chloramine-T catalyzed, Bolton–Hunter reagent, and direct labeling
^{131}I	β, γ	8 d	364(γ)	

[a]h = hours
[b]d = days

10.2.1.1 Nanoparticles radiolabeled with ^{99m}Tc

Radiolabeled NPs can be used to assess the in vivo behavior of novel drug delivery NP systems. Curcumin is a hydrophobic polyphenol with antioxidant, anticarcinogenic, and anti-bacterial properties. However, its low bioavailability due to its low solubility prevents its use as a therapeutic agent. A way to circumvent this problem is to use solid lipid NPs (slns) as a drug carrier system. Ayan et al. proceeded to synthesize and radiolabel curcumin-loaded slns (C-slns) with ^{99m}Tc in order to evaluate their in vivo biodistribution, and they found that C-slns could be used for liver-spleen imaging, with definitive advantages over the phytate colloid radiopharmaceutical commonly used in nuclear medicine. Furthermore, these C-slns could be used for the treatment of liver and spleen diseases due to their curcumin component [13].

Chloramphenicol (CHL) is an antibacterial drug that easily crosses the blood-brain barrier (BBB). However, its most serious side effect is bone marrow toxicity. Almost a decade ago, Halder et al. developed CHL-loaded, poly(lactic-*co*-glycolic acid) (PLGA)-based NPs coated with PS-80 surfactant, which reduces the uptake of the NPs by phagocytic cells of the RES [14]. Direct radiolabeling with ^{99m}Tc in the presence of $SnCl_2$ as the reducing agent showed that these NPs could be a promising drug delivery system, as they resulted in higher brain and reduced bone marrow uptake.

PLGA NPs have also been investigated in sentinel lymph node (SLN) imaging after their direct radiolabeling with ^{99m}Tc, as described above. Gamma (γ) scintigraphy and biodistribution studies showed localization in the SLN, albeit lower than the uptake observed for Nanocis, the radiopharmaceutical commercially available for SLN detection 15]. More recently, the same group proceeded to surface-modify these PLGA derivatives with diethylenetriamine pentaacetic acid (DTPA), a chelator suitable for ^{99m}Tc complexation [16]. This modification led to improved radiolabeling yields under milder reaction conditions and improved uptake in the SLN. Another SLN imaging agent was developed by Ocampo-García et al. by conjugating hydrazinonicotinamide-Gly-Gly-Cys-NH_2 (HYNIC-GGC) peptide (for labeling with ^{99m}Tc) and a mannose derivative (for specific binding to mannose receptors overexpressed in lymph node macrophages) onto gold NPs (Au NP–mannose) and consequently labeling this construct with ^{99m}Tc [17]. After subcutaneous injection of the radiotracer into the footpad of rats, it was shown that ^{99m}Tc-Au-NP-mannose remained within the first lymph node for 24 h, with negligible uptake in all other tissues and minimal accumulation in the kidney; therefore, it can be considered a potential SLN imaging agent.

Mesoporous silica NPs (MSNs) are nontoxic, biocompatible nanomaterials with a high surface area and a large pore volume that can be used in drug delivery applications. However, they can also be used as imaging agents, when appropriately modified for consequent radiolabeling. Barros et al. functionalized MSNs with DTPA for labeling with ^{99m}Tc. Biodistribution experiments in healthy mice showed the expected high uptake by liver and extremely high specificity for the lung. What needs to be kept in mind is that MSNs could carry a significant drug load and at the same time could be used for theranostic purposes [18].

Liposomes are nanoparticulate systems widely used for drug delivery. A liposome is composed of a self-assembling lipid bilayer surrounding an aqueous "core" that can encapsulate hydrophilic or hydrophobic drugs. These drugs remain in the aqueous interior and are released, after the adherence of the liposome to cell membranes, via endocytosis. When radiolabeled with diagnostic radioisotopes, liposomes are an excellent tool for studying the pharmacokinetics of liposome-based drug delivery systems. One such example has been provided by Fragogeorgi et al., who assessed the in vivo behavior of liposomes labeled with the $^{99m}Tc(I)(CO)_3$ moiety by a direct labeling strategy via a carboxyl group of the liposome surface or by surface functionalization of the liposome with a pyridyl-ethyl-cysteine compound, which acts as the chelating agent [19]. Passive tumor accumulation was shown for liposomes labeled by both techniques.

An example of direct labeling of an NP for targeted delivery was provided by Polyáka and his group [20]. Self-assembled, folate-targeted NPs were prepared by conjugating folic acid (FA) to poly-γ-glutamic acid, followed by the addition of a chitosan solution. These NPs were directly labeled with ^{99m}Tc after the addition of pertechnetate eluate, in the presence of $SnCl_2$ as the reducing agent. In vitro results in tumor cells overexpressing folate receptors demonstrated efficient binding and internalization of such NPs, while in vivo studies showed their considerably higher uptake in the tumorous kidney, when compared to the normal one, thus offering the possibility of such NPs serving as a tumor-specific SPECT imaging agent. Subsequent studies by the same group on a spontaneously occurring animal model with oral carcinoma showed relatively high tumor uptake in the folate-expressing tumor [21].

Dendrimers are nanostructures synthesized from branched monomer units, which can easily be functionalized with a wide variety of groups on their surface. Their monodisperse nature and structural/chemical uniformity make them excellent candidates for drug delivery applications. Zhang et al. functionalized polyamidoamine (PAMAM) dendrimers with FA and consequently radiolabeled them with ^{99m}Tc via 1B4M-DTPA, which acts as the chelating agent [22]. Biodistribution and micro-SPECT imaging studies showed definitive accumulation in nude mice bearing folate receptor–positive KB tumors. Because of the significant kidney uptake of the FA dendrimer derivative, the group next reported on the synthesis of a dendrimer-avidin conjugate, which could be easily radiolabeled with ^{99m}Tc and showed excellent in vitro/in vivo stability, rapid blood clearance, and very low kidney uptake [23].

Another tumor-specific nanosystem, this time targeting the gastrin-releasing peptide receptor (GRPr), was developed by Mendoza-Sánchez et al. Au NPs were surface functionalized with Lys$_3$-bombesin, a peptide with high affinity to the GRPr, and HYNIC-GGC for radiolabeling with ^{99m}Tc [24]. Biodistribution studies in PC-3 tumor-bearing nude mice showed maximum tumor uptake of the radionanotracer at 1 h postinjection (p.i.), which was confirmed by micro-SPECT/CT imaging. These promising results prompted the group to develop a kit formulation for facile labeling of Au NPs conjugated to either Lys$_3$-bombesin (targeting the GRPr), cyclo[-Arg-Gly-Asp-D-Phe-Lys-] (c[RGDfK(C)]) (targeting $\alpha_v\beta_3$ integrins overexpressed in tumor angiogenesis), or thiol-mannose (for SLN detection) [25]. The development of such kits will greatly facilitate the preparation of radiolabeled NPs for target-specific applications.

10.2.1.2 Nanoparticles radiolabeled with ^{111}In and $^{125/131}$I

Pluronics are polymer-based nanocarriers composed of poly(ethylene oxide) (PEO) and poly(propylene oxide) (PPO). Arranja et al. investigated the biodistribution of Pluronic unimers (PEO-PPO-PEO) and micelles radiolabeled with ^{111}In, which is suitable for imaging compounds with prolonged blood circulation, due to its half-life of 63.7 h. Radiolabeling was afforded via the DTPA chelator, and showed high efficiency for the copolymers PEO-PPO-PEO (>95%), in comparison to the micelles (~50%). SPECT imaging studies provided valuable information regarding liver and renal clearance of these molecules, which can be used in further development of Pluronic-based nanocarriers [26].

Targeted NPs could be a useful tool in the noninvasive detection of vulnerable plaques in atherosclerotic regions. One such example has been provided by Ogawa et al., who developed liposomes bearing phosphatidylserine, which is recognized by macrophages found in these plaques, as a liposome-based imaging probe for vulnerable atherosclerotic plaque imaging [27]. Radiolabeling was accomplished with ^{111}In by incubating nitrilotriacetic acid (NTA)-encapsulated liposomes with ^{111}In-oxine, which diffuses across the lipid bilayer into the liposome aqueous core, where it is transchelated to NTA. In vitro and in vivo SPECT/CT results showed that phosphatidylserine modification of the liposomes led to macrophage targeting with the radiolabeled liposomes.

Another example of molecular targeting with NPs radiolabeled with ^{111}In has been provided by Ng et al., who directly labeled Au NPs with ^{111}In, leading to stable radiolabeling without the need to functionalize the surface of the NP with metal chelators, thus sparing the NP surface for modifications with targeting moieties [28]. The NP was then functionalized with an arginine-glycine-aspartic acid (RGD) peptide and was assessed in low- and high-$\alpha_v\beta_3$ integrin–expressing tumors. Biodistribution and imaging studies demonstrated molecular targeting with the ^{111}In-radiolabeled Au NPs.

A micelle is a spherical NP consisting of a hydrophobic core and a hydrophilic shell. Micelles are formed by block copolymers consisting of two or more polymer chains with different hydrophobicity. Their main advantage is their ability to encapsulate lipophilic drugs, thus facilitating transport of poorly soluble drugs to the site of interest. A new and easy method of radiolabeling polystyrene (PS)-block-PEO (PS-*b*-PEO) micelles has been developed by Laan et al., which does not require the conjugation of a chelating agent onto the micelle surface that might lead to altered biological behavior of the micelles and compromised stability of the radiolabel [29]. In this study tropolone, a lipophilic ligand, is labeled with ^{111}In and is consequently entrapped in the core of the micelle, leading to stably labeled micelles. Ex vivo biodistribution studies in healthy mice showed high accumulation in the spleen and liver and blood circulation even at 24 h p.i.

Ignjatović et al. used ^{125}I to investigate the possibility of obtaining an organ-targeting carrier based on hydroxyapatite (HAp) NPs [30]. Three different HAp NPs were evaluated: HAp, HAp coated with chitosan (HAp/Ch), and HAp coated with a chitosan-poly-D,L-lactide-*co*-glycolide polymer blend (HAp/Ch-PLGA). HAp was radiolabeled with ^{125}I, the ^{125}I-HAp was consequently coated with chitosan of chitosan-PLGA, and all three NPs were assessed for in vitro stability in saline and human serum. ^{125}I-HAp particles were proven to be the least stable (~47% after eight days of incubation), while the ^{125}I-HAp/Ch-PLGA particles were the most stable (~83% at eight days of incubation). Different biodistribution patterns were observed for the three iodinated NPs, after their administration in normal Wistar rats. ^{125}I-HAp exhibited fast clearance from systemic circulation and mainly accumulated in the liver, while the presence of chitosan increased their concentration in blood and their circulation half-life. The very high accumulation of ^{125}I-HAp/Ch-PLGA in the lungs (~80%) indicates aggregation of the particles.

Although silver (Ag) NPs are finding more applications in medicine, little is known about their in vivo behavior. Chrastina and Schnitzer developed a method for tracking Ag NPs after their systemic administration, by radiolabeling them with ^{125}I via chemisorption onto the Ag surface [31]. After intravenous (IV) administration of ^{125}I-Ag NPs, high uptake was observed in the liver and spleen, which could lead to toxicity issues and should be taken into account before clinical application.

Shao et al. investigated the ^{125}I radiolabeling of gold nanorods (GdNRs) functionalized with the anticellular adhesion molecule 1 (ICAM-1) for targeted imaging of inflammation in rheumatoid arthritis [32]. Three groups of rats were used for in vivo animal studies: Group A consisted of normal rats injected with ^{125}I-ICAM-GdNRs, Group B had arthritic rats injected with nontargeted ^{125}I-GdNRs, and Group C had arthritic rats injected with the targeted agent ^{125}I-ICAM-GdNRs. The highest uptake in arthritic ankle joints was demonstrated for the ^{125}I-ICAM-GdNRs. As the ICAM-1 biomarker is also overexpressed in several cancers, including melanoma, lung, and breast, NPs functionalized with this biomarker could also be useful for molecular imaging of cancer. Furthermore, if radiolabeled with an appropriate radioisotope of iodine (e.g., ^{131}I), they could find application in radiotherapy.

10.2.2 Nanoparticles and PET Imaging

PET is an imaging technique in which positron-emitting radioisotopes are visualized and quantified. The emitted positrons annihilate nearby electrons, thereby generating two 511 keV photons, which are detected by detectors embedded in PET scanners. Because of its high sensitivity, unlimited penetration depth, quantifiable results, and the broad range of available radioisotopes (Table 10.2), PET is highly suitable for monitoring the pharmacokinetics, biodistribution, and target site accumulation of nanomedicine formulations.

Table 10.2 PET radioisotopes for nanoparticle labeling

Radioisotope	Type of emission	Half-life	E_{max} (keV)	Radiolabeling methods
^{11}C	Positron	20.36 min.	960	Methyl iodine substitution
^{18}F	Positron	109.8 min.	650	Cu-catalyzed click chemistry between 2-[^{18}F]-fluoroethyl azide and alkyne-NHS spacer; direct encapsulation
^{68}Ga	Positron	67.71 min.	1899, 770	NOTA, NODAGA, and direct labeling
^{64}Cu	Positron	12.7 h	650	DOTA, TETA, BAT, DO3A, biphosphonate, and direct labeling
^{89}Zr	Positron	78.4 h	900	DFO and direct labeling

PET radiolabeling approaches consist of two main strategies—utilizing direct covalent chemistries and utilizing coordination chemistry [33]. Radioisotopes amenable to organic chemistry, including carbon-11 (^{11}C) and halogens like fluorine-18 (^{18}F), bromium-76, and ^{124}I, are usually bound covalently, while radiometals (gallium-68, ^{68}Ga; copper-64, ^{64}Cu; and zirconium-89, ^{89}Zr) are typically bound via chelation. Recent advances have been made that incorporate radiometals directly into or onto the NP for ligand-free radiolabeling approaches [34–36].

10.2.2.1 Nanoparticles radiolabeled with ^{18}F

$MnFe_2O_4$ and Fe_3O_4 magnetic NPs (MNPs), which exhibit excellent colloidal stability in water, show high affinity to fluoride ions and bisphosphonate groups due to the presence of an aluminum hydroxide, or $Al(OH)_3$, coating layer [37]. These NPs were incubated with ^{18}F and ^{64}Cu-bis(dithiocarbamate) bisphosphonate (^{64}Cu-$(DTCBP)_2$) at room temperature for 5 min., providing radiolabeled conjugates at high radiolabeling yields (97% and 100%, respectively). The PET/magnetic resonance (MR) imaging studies performed in normal mice revealed that the ^{18}F-labeled NPs accumulated in the liver and spleen, despite their small hydrodynamic size (21 nm), while there was a slow detachment of fluoride ions from the NPs, which increased with time. On the contrary, the same NPs labeled with ^{64}Cu showed no sign of outflow of radiotracer from these organs.

HAp and $Al(OH)_3$ are two biocompatible, low-toxicity inorganic materials that can be labeled quickly and efficiently with [^{18}F]-fluoride, providing sufficiently stable radiotracers for in vivo imaging [38]. The radiolabeled NPs demonstrated different in vivo behavior, depending on the route of administration. Furthermore, their in vivo stability was monitored by PET imaging, as [^{18}F]-fluoride released from the NPs would show uptake in the joints of the skeleton. Further modification of these NPs could lead to the development of targeted contrast agents exhibiting lower in vivo aggregation and uptake in the RES organs.

For radiolabeling with ^{18}F, Au NPs were functionalized with the peptides Cys-Leu-Pro-Phe-Phe-Asp (CLPFFD) and cysteinyllysin (CK) to obtain the conjugate C(Au-NP)LPFFD-C(Au-NP)K, which could consequently be radiolabeled by covalent binding of *N*-succinimidyl-4-[^{18}F]-fluorobenzoate ([^{18}F]-SFB), in order to evaluate their in vivo behavior [39]. In vivo biodistribution in rats revealed high accumulation of the radiolabeled Au NPs in the bladder and urine and a lower uptake in the intestine, where the NPs were progressively accumulated in accordance with the biliary excretion of the conjugate. Furthermore, ex vivo biodistribution indicated that the Au NPs were also accumulated in the RES organs, a fact that could be attributed to their negative surface charge, which is known to enhance the phagocytosis process by the macrophages.

The rapid reaction between tetrazine and *trans*-cyclooctenes was cleverly used by Emmetiere et al. for the rapid delivery of radiolabeled liposomes to the diseased site [40]. In this approach, liposomes that contain ^{18}F-labeled dipalmitoyl and the bio-orthogonal moiety *trans*-cyclooctene-labeled DSPE-PEG2k-TCO, were reacted with tumor tissues displaying a bio-orthogonal tetrazine pHLIP-TZ. These tetrazine-labeled tumors showed increased uptake of these radiolabeled liposomes when compared to tumors without the tetrazine label.

10.2.2.2 Nanoparticles radiolabeled with ^{64}Cu

^{64}Cu-radiolabeled liposomes were evaluated as potential PET radiotracers for imaging bone marrow [41]. Different liposomal formulations were prepared, with diameters of 90 and 140 nm, and were doped with DOTA-Bn-DSPE (DOTA stands for 1,4,7,10-tetraazacyclododecane-1,4,7,10-tetraacetic acid; Bn stands for benzyl; and DSPE stands for 1,2-distearoylphosphatidylethanolamine) for radiolabeling with ^{64}Cu. PET imaging and biodistribution studies of the radiolabeled liposomes revealed high accumulation in the bone marrow (15.18 ± 3.69% injected dose per gram [ID/g]) for the 90 nm liposomes, compared to the 7.01 ± 0.92% ID/g for 140 nm liposomes, 24 h p.i., while in tumor-bearing animal models the accumulation of the 90 nm liposomes was found to be 0.89 ± 0.48%ID/g in tumor and 14.22 ± 8.07%ID/g in bone marrow. The results indicated that these ^{64}Cu-radiolabeled liposomes show promise as an adequate PET imaging agent for bone marrow imaging.

Another method for radiolabeling liposomes with ^{64}Cu was described by Lee et al., which involved synthesizing PEGylated liposomal therapeutics loaded with a gradient loadable chelator diacetyl 4,4'-bis(3-(N,N-diethylamino)propyl)thiosemicarbazone (4-DEAP-ATSC) for radiolabeling with ^{64}Cu in high yields (>94%) [42]. The radiolabeled liposome ^{64}Cu-MM-302 was assessed for its in vitro stability in human plasma and in vivo stability, after its injection into CD-1 immunocompetent mice, where it was found to be highly stable for up to 48 h in vitro (>99%) and for up to 24 h in vivo (>94%). PET/CT imaging studies performed in tumor-bearing mice justify the application of these radiolabeled liposomes as PET tracers for in vivo liposome tracking.

Frellsen et al. used a chelator-free process to radiolabel Au NPs with ^{64}Cu [43]. Specifically, the group synthesized Au NPs embedded with ^{64}Cu, where the absorbed ^{64}Cu ions are covered by a controllable layer of gold, embedding them deeper inside the NPs, resulting in a highly stable conjugate. The group studied the in vivo biodistribution of the ^{64}Cu–Au NPs with three different coatings—1-dodecanethiol and Tween 20, MeO-PEG_{5000}-SH, and sodium 10-mercaptodecanesulfonic acid and (10-mercaptodecyl)trimethylammonium bromide)—by PET imaging performed in tumor-bearing mice. The results showed that the polyethylene glycol (PEG)-coated Au NPs exhibited long circulation time and satisfactory tumor uptake (3.9% ID/g) compared to the Au NPs with other coatings used in the study.

The copper-free click chemistry approach was used to radiolabel glycol chitosan NPs (CNPs) with ^{64}Cu [44]. According to this method, the cyclooctyne derivative dibenzocyclooctyne (DBCO) conjugated to the DOTA chelating agent was initially radiolabeled with ^{64}Cu (DBCO-PEG$_4$-Lys-DOTA-^{64}Cu). This radiolabeled construct was consequently conjugated to the azide-functionalized CNPs, creating radiolabeled NPs (^{64}Cu-CNPs) at a high radiolabeling yield (>98%). A microPET study in tumor-bearing animal models showed a gradually increased tumor accumulation with prolonged blood circulation time of the ^{64}Cu-CNPs. These biodistribution results indicated that copper-free click chemistry has the potential to be used as an efficient preradiolabeling method for the evaluation of the in vivo pharmacokinetics of radiolabeled NPs.

Shaffer et al. demonstrated a radiolabeling procedure to radiolabel silica NPs with softer radioisotopes, like ^{64}Cu [45]. The group used silica NPs functionalized with thiols (soft electron donors) to achieve a thermodynamically stable bond with ^{64}Cu, expanding the use of radiolabeled silica NPs, with both hard and soft radiometal ions, in molecular imaging.

10.2.2.3 Nanoparticles radiolabeled with ^{68}Ga

Biocompatible glucose-coated Au NPs were labeled with ^{68}Ga to explore the BBB permeability with PET imaging [46]. Specifically, small-sized (2 nm) Au NPs were coated with glucose in order to obtain the appropriate stability and solubility and were further conjugated with the 1,4,7-triazacyclononane-1,4,7-triacetic acid (NOTA) chelator (for ^{68}Ga radiolabeling) and also with BBB-permeable neuropeptides (for targeted delivery to the brain). In vivo biodistribution studies showed that the targeted Au NPs exhibited a threefold higher brain accumulation (0.020 ± 0.0050% ID/g) compared to the nontargeted Au NPs (0.0073 ± 0.0024% ID/g).

In their study, Burke et al. reported the synthesis and radiolabeling of silica-coated iron oxide nanorods with various ratios of PEG and DOTA chelator to assess their potential application as PET/MR imaging agents [47]. The group observed that all the silica-coated iron oxide nanorods were successfully radiolabeled with ^{68}Ga, noting that even those synthesized with no chelator formed highly stable radiolabeled complexes. Further work from the same group demonstrated that these nanorods coated with PEG can also be directly radiolabeled within 15 min. of incubation with ^{68}Ga radionuclide, resulting in highly stable radiolabeled nanorods in vivo, suitable for PET/MR imaging of liver malignancies. The group indicated that the radiolabeling was achieved due to the interaction of ^{68}Ga radionuclide with the silica coating, proving not only that the use of a chelating agent is unnecessary but also that the attachment of ^{68}Ga is not solely a property of PEG [48].

Polyaka et al. synthesized and evaluated ^{68}Ga-labeled porous zirconia NPs (^{68}Ga-DOTA-Zr-NP), with the aim to assess their applicability as potential PET/CT imaging drug delivery nanoplatforms [49]. In brief, after the adsorption of the DOTA chelator on the surface of Zr NPs, the DOTA–Zr NPs (with hydrodynamic size 94 ± 19 nm) were incubated with ^{68}Ga, leading to high radiolabeling yields (90.5%–97.5%). The radiolabeled complex was also found to be very stable in vitro (80.2%–94.7%) in human blood serum. μPET/CT imaging results showed higher uptake of the NPs in the RES organs but also low uptake in the lungs, indicating the lack of aggregates, extended blood retention time, and slow kidney clearance. Consequently, the encouraging in vivo biodistribution results enhanced the possibility for further study of ^{68}Ga-labeled porous zirconia NPs for use as drug delivery systems.

Graphene oxide (GO) has attracted great attention for use in many biomedical applications due to its remarkable physicochemical properties along with the enhanced EPR in tumors. For this reason, Fazaeli et al. synthesized ^{68}Ga magnetite (Fe_3O_4)-GO nanocomposite (MGO) to be assessed as a potential drug delivery system [50]. Briefly, MGO was synthesized via a coprecipitation method and radiolabeled with ^{68}Ga. In vitro stability studies of ^{68}Ga-MGO performed in fresh human serum showed no detachment of the radioisotope from the complex, while in vivo biodistribution studies revealed that the grafting of Fe_3O_4 in GO reduces NP uptake from the RES organs. Along with the its high uptake by vital organs and fast clearance from kidneys and the liver, ^{68}Ga-MGO could serve as a promising agent for PET imaging.

10.2.2.4 Nanoparticles radiolabeled with other positron-emitting radioisotopes

^{89}Zr-labeled antibodies represent a powerful PET imaging agent for the in vivo evaluation of various radiolabeled complexes used for therapy. In their study, Karmani et al. assessed the biodistribution of cetuximab labeled with ^{89}Zr via a desferal moiety [51]. Furthermore, they conjugated the ^{89}Zr-cetuximab to small-sized Au NPs (with a radiolabeling yield >75%) using carbodiimide chemistry to further evaluate their behavior. In vivo biodistribution studies performed for both radiolabeled complexes showed that the ^{89}Zr-cetuximab-conjugated Au NPs accumulated in the tumor without any alteration up to 72 h p.i., indicating that the conjugation of cetuximab onto the Au NPs did not alter its tumor-targeting efficacy.

Boros et al. reported a robust and simple chelate-free, heat-induced metal ion–binding reaction to radiolabel iron oxide NPs, creating stable radiolabeled complexes [52]. Addition of ^{89}Zr to ferumoxytol (FH) NPs demonstrated binding of the metal ion to the surface of the magnetite core at high radiolabeling yields (93% ± 3%), in vitro stability in ligand change and plasma studies, and the ability to use the same radiochemical conditions to radiolabel FH with other radioisotopes (including $^{64}Cu^{2+}$, $^{89}Zr^{4+}$, and $^{111}In^{3+}$). PET/CT imaging and biodistribution of ^{89}Zr-FH NPs indicated that the radiolabeling did not alter the initial physicochemical properties of FH NPs.

MSNs were directly labeled with ^{89}Zr, leading to a product with high in vivo stability due to the presence of deprotonated silanol groups inside or on the surface of MSNs [53]. The direct radiolabeling process, along with the exhibited long-term stability of the ^{89}Zr-MSN, paves the way for the use of radiolabeled MSNs as a PET tracer for tracking drug delivery.

Li et al. described an efficient method for radiolabeling various liposomal NPs with ^{89}Zr, based on a ligand exchange reaction at room temperature, at high radiochemical yields [54]. In brief, as an alternative to the conjugation of ^{89}Zr onto the surface of liposomes reported elsewhere, ^{89}Zr is introduced into the liposomal cavity to achieve ligand exchange with encapsulated desferrioxamine (DFO). The group synthesized and evaluated three ^{89}Zr liposomal NPs that proved to be highly stable in phosphate-buffered saline (PBS) and rat serum for 48 h, while PET imaging and biodistribution studies gave evidence for their in vivo pharmacokinetics.

10.2.3 Radiolabeled Nanoparticles as Multimodality Imaging Agents

Techniques for imaging of cancer in multiple modalities using a single agent in a single session have been developed, and these techniques are categorized under what is known as "multimodality imaging." There has been a great deal of interest in combining imaging modalities to more accurately interpret disease and abnormalities in vivo. The combination of two or more imaging techniques can provide more precise information regarding a disease, such as its location, extent, metabolic activity, blood flow, and function of the target tissue, resulting in better characterization of disease processes.

One of the exciting features of NP platforms is their versatility. Researchers are actively investigating almost every permutation of the various imaging modalities in combination with NP carriers. The list of potential modalities includes computed tomography (CT), MR imaging, PET, SPECT, and optical imaging. NP radiolabeling opens a route toward novel diagnostic approaches utilizing simultaneous contrasts in multiple modalities. In this part of the chapter, we will elaborate on radiolabeled NPs that have shown promise in the development of multimodality imaging agents.

10.2.3.1 Dual-modality SPECT/MR imaging agents

To avoid the creation of degradation products of iron oxide NPs that increase free radical production, leading to cell death, Felber and Alberto coated the surface of each iron oxide NP with a gold shell, which in turn was coated with bifunctional ligands consisting of an anchor for the metal surface and chelators for the labeling of the constructs with the $[^{99m}Tc(CO)3]+$ moiety [55]. Alternatively, they first synthesized the ^{99m}Tc complexes, which were then attached to the gold surface. Both approaches resulted in satisfactory radiochemical yields and showed promise in the development of dual-modality SPECT/MR imaging agents.

PEG polymer conjugates capable of avoiding rapid sequestration of NPs by the RES were developed by Rosales and group. These conjugates contain a terminal 1,1-bisphosphonate group capable of binding to the surface of ultrasmall superparamagnetic iron oxide (USPIO) NPs [PEG(5)-BP-USPIO] [56]. Radiolabeling with ^{99m}Tc was afforded by adding ^{99m}Tc-DPA-ale (a bifunctional bisphosphonate that has previously been used for the radiolabeling of iron oxide NPs) to the PEG(5)-BP-USPIO (reference above). In vivo MR imaging studies showed that this nanostructure can be used as an effective MR imaging contrast agent with minor accumulation of USPIOs in the liver at low doses, while SPECT imaging allows tracking of the NPs in vivo.

In another study an ^{111}In-labeled antimesothelin antibody (mAbMB) was conjugated to a superparamagnetic iron oxide NP (SPION) for SPECT/MR imaging of mesothelin-expressing cancers. The ^{111}In-mAbMB was conjugated to the SPIONs after the carbodiimide coupling reaction, and the resulting conjugates possessed a hydrodynamic size of 76.6 nm. This ^{111}In-mAbMB-SPION had significantly ($p < 0.05$) higher tumor accumulation in mesothelin-expressing A431K5 tumors than in 431 control tumors, indicating the ability to bind specifically to mesothelin-expressing cells [57].

Ultrasmall iron oxide NPs functionalized with a novel RGD peptide (targeting integrin $\alpha_v\beta_3$ overexpressed in tumor cells and tumor endothelial cells in breast cancer [BC]) and consequently radiolabeled with ^{125}I were evaluated by Deng et al. [58]. Radiolabeling was accomplished by addition of chloramine-T to cyclic RGD (cRGD)-USPIO and consequent addition of Na^{125}I. The iodination reaction was stopped by the addition of sodium thiolsulfate. The radiolabeled nanoconstruct showed long blood circulation time, high tumor uptake, and moderate liver uptake, features that are desirable for an imaging agent. SPECT/MR imaging studies confirmed in vivo tumor targeting, thus indicating that ^{125}I-cRGD-USPIO shows promise as a dual-modality radiotracer for early tumor detection. Replacement of ^{125}I with other radioisotopes of iodine could lead to the development of PET radiotracers (^{123}I/^{124}I) or therapeutic agents (^{131}I).

10.2.3.2 Dual-modality PET/MR imaging agents

A direct method of radiolabeling SPIONs with arsenic isotopes (*As), on the basis of the high affinity of arsenic for magnetite surfaces was accomplished simply by mixing water-soluble SPIONS with *AsIII or

*AsV species. These SPIONs had been initially functionalized with oleic acid, which was then exchanged with polyacrylic acid (PAA), rendering them water soluble and highly stable in many biological solutions [59]. The maximum yield of radiolabeling was reached after a 24 h incubation (92.2%). Further coating of *As-SPIONs with a layer of PEG led to increased stability of the imaging tracer, which demonstrated high liver uptake and significantly decreased bladder uptake. PET imaging studies were in agreement with the ex vivo biodistribution results mentioned above.

^{11}C is a cyclotron-produced, positron-emitting radioisotope with a 20.4 min. half-life. It is produced as [^{11}C]-carbon dioxide ([^{11}C]-CO_2), which can be easily converted to precursor molecules such as [^{11}C]-methyl iodide ([^{11}C]-CH_3I), appropriate for radiolabeling particles functionalized with amine (–NH_2) and carboxylic acid (–COOH) groups, via N- and O-methylation reactions. Different NP systems were assessed in the study by Sharma et al., namely –COOH and –NH_2-functionalized IONPs, platinum NPs, and silicon dioxide NPs [60]. The lowest radiochemical yields were observed for the IONPs, which can be attributed to low surface coverage and a higher degree of agglomeration of these particles. However, it was shown that all particles containing either –COOH or –NH_2 groups could be labeled with ^{11}C and have sufficient radioactivity to perform PET imaging and biodistribution studies. Only the IONPs were used for dual-modality PET/MR imaging studies and showed excellent correlation of their biodistribution in both PET and MR images, with high liver uptake being observed within the first few minutes after injection.

AGuIX NPs are ultrasmall rigid NPs made of polysiloxane and surrounded by gadolinium chelates. With a hydrodynamic diameter of under 5 nm, they represent the first multifunctional silica-based NPs that are sufficiently small to escape hepatic clearance and enable animal imaging by four complementary techniques (MR imaging, SPECT after labeling by ^{111}In, fluorescence imaging, and CT). Thanks to their radiosensitizing properties, AGuIX NPs have proven to be an excellent tool for radiation therapy, and recent literature shows how MR imaging can be used to perform image-guided radiation therapy with these. However, a dual-modality PET/MR imaging agent that combines the advantages of both imaging modalities has more to offer than a single-modality, gadolinium MR imaging agent, and can be used as a companion diagnostic agent. Initial work from the group of Tillement has shown that AGuIX derivatives labeled with ^{68}Ga, via the DOTA chelator, are a promising imaging tool for simultaneous PET/MR imaging [61]. Ex vivo biodistribution studies on normal mice showed an extremely low residual activity in all untargeted tissues, especially in organs where NPs are classically sequestered, such as the liver and lung (<2% ID/g at 120 min. p.i.). Further work was performed on AGuIX NPs functionalized with another chelator for ^{68}Ga labeling, namely NODAGA, for more efficient labeling. Passive accumulation of ^{68}Ga-AGuIX@NODAGA in a U87MG tumor model was shown both by ex vivo biodistribution studies and in vivo PET and MR imaging studies. The integrity of these radiolabeled NPs in mice was evaluated, and it was shown that ^{68}Ga-AGuIX@NODAGA, when injected at a concentration that was appropriately tailored to the sensitivity of both PET and MR imaging modalities, remained unmetabolized in mice, thus providing a single-injection, dual-modality imaging agent adequate for both PET and MR imaging [62]. These same NPs, functionalized with a DFO chelator instead of NODAGA, have also been labeled with ^{89}Z for PET imaging applications [63].

Moon et al. developed a prostate-specific membrane antigen (PSMA)-targeting IONP for dual-modality PET/MR imaging of PSMA, a well-known biomarker of prostate cancer [64]. Amphiphiles containing DOTA (as the chelating agent for radiolabeling with ^{68}Ga) and glutamate-urea-lysine (GUL, a PSMA-targeting ligand) were used for encapsulation of IONPs (as the MR imaging contrast agent). An in vitro competitive binding study on PSMA-positive cells proved the specific binding of DOTA-IO-GUL to these cells. PSMA-positive and PSMA-negative tumors were established on the left and right flanks of mice for the in vivo imaging studies. The MR imaging study showed that DOTA-IO-GUL was taken up only by the PSMA-positive 22v1 tumor and not by the PSMA-negative PC-3 tumor. The PET images acquired after injection of the radiotracer in the same tumor model were consistent with the MR imaging results. The same group developed a dual-modality imaging agent targeting lymph nodes, on the basis of their previous studies, by encapsulation of IONPs in amphiphiles containing NOTA (a ^{68}Ga-chelating agent) and D-mannose (man, for lymph node targeting) [65]. ^{68}Ga labeling was straightforward and led to ^{68}Ga-NOTA-IO-man with a radiochemical purity >99% after purification, which was stable in serum up to 2 h. Both PET and MR imaging studies confirmed specificity of ^{68}Ga-NOTA-IO-man for the lymph nodes of rats. Encapsulation of IONPs in amphiphiles shows great promise in the area of dual imaging, as it can lead to the development of other target-specific imaging probes.

An alternative approach to dual-modality imaging of lymph nodes was presented by Thorek et al., who radiolabeled a clinically used iron oxide NP, namely FH, with the positron-emitter ^{89}Zr [66]. Minimal modification of the IONP surface with the DFO chelate for ^{89}Zr labeling led to ^{89}Zr-FH, with minimal effects on particle size and charge. Disease sites were detected with PET/MR imaging with high sensitivity and accuracy.

A biphosphonate agent appropriately modified to contain dithiocarbamate as a chelating group to bind ^{64}Cu—[^{64}Cu(dtcbp)$_2$— was synthesized and evaluated by de Rosales et al. [67]. Clinically available SPIONs (Endorem®/Feridex®) were radiolabeled with [^{64}Cu(dtcbp)$_2$] with high radiolabeling yields, while maintaining their colloidal stability. In vitro studies showed that ^{64}Cu(dtcbp)$_2$ remained bound quantitatively to the MNPs for at least 48 h. Transchelation toward excess ethylenediaminetetraacetic acid (EDTA) was also studied, showing that ^{64}Cu remains associated with Endorem for at least 24 h. MR imaging of an anesthetized C57BL/6 mouse, after injection of the radiocomplex in the footpads, showed significant decrease in signal and hence accumulation of Endorem in the popliteal lymph nodes, as compared to the preinjection images of the same mouse. PET-CT scanning results were in agreement with the MR imaging studies, revealing uptake in the popliteal lymph nodes and, to a lesser extent, in the iliac lymph nodes.

10.2.3.3 Other dual- or multimodality imaging agents

In vivo biodistribution of radiolabeled liposomes can provide valuable information on delivery of drugs encapsulated in liposomes. Nonetheless, it does report on drug release, drug uptake, and retention of the drug in the tumor. Lamichhane et al. have developed a single-agent, dual-modality SPECT/PET imaging agent based on a novel ^{18}F-labeled carboplatin drug derivative (([^{18}F]-FCP) encapsulated in an ^{111}In-labeled liposome ([^{18}F]-FCP-Lipo), which has the capacity to report on the delivery of the drug and the drug carrier [68]. PET and SPECT imaging at 1 h p.i. of [^{18}F]-FCP-

Lipo showed similar radiotracer accumulation in RES organs, which were consistent with the biodistribution data. This leads us to the conclusion that the ^{18}F radioactivity, which is attributed to [^{18}F]-FCP, is contained within the liposome.

Banerjee et al. attached a small-molecule PSMA-targeting ligand to a polylactic acid (PLA)/PEG copolymer in order to investigate its pharmacokinetics and biodistribution both with SPECT and fluorescence imaging [69]. ^{111}In labeling of PSMA-targeted (TNP) or untargeted (UNP) was achieved in a two-step, copper-assisted click chemistry reaction at 4°C, to ensure the stability of the PLA/PEG NPs. Ex vivo biodistribution studies of both TNP and UNP in mice bearing both PSMA-positive [(PSMA(+)PIP] and PSMA-negative [(PSMA(-)PC-3 flu] (control) tumors showed similar accumulation in all tissues at 96 h p.i. except in tumor and liver. The TNP showed a tumor uptake of 6.58% ID/g at 48 h, remaining practically stable up to 96 h p.i., while the UNP showed a tumor uptake of 8.17% ID/g but was significantly cleared at 96 h p.i. (2.37% ID/g). SPECT studies of the tumor-bearing mice were in agreement with the above results. Near-infrared fluorescence imaging confirmed the biodistribution and SCECT/CT findings, while microscopy studies demonstrated that accumulation of the UNP was less epithelium specific than that of the TNP and depended on a combination of EPR and phagocytosis by tumor-associated macrophages. The TNP were retained within the PSMA-positive tumor epithelial cells as well. The significance of such studies is that they can be utilized to predict the biodistribution and tumor accumulation of therapeutic NPs.

Polyamidoamine (PAMAM) was grafted onto silica NPs and conjugated to a fluorescent dye. The silica NPs were further functionalized with anti–human epithelial growth factor receptor 2 (HER2) antibodies, for targeted delivery to HER2-expressing tumors [70]. Radiolabeling with ^{99m}Tc provided a dual-modality imaging probe, which successfully targeted HER-expressing cells, as shown by in vitro and in vivo experiments. These functionalized silica NPs could prove to be an efficient platform for targeted delivery of antitumor agents of beta (β) emitters for therapy, with simultaneous imaging capabilities.

Li et al. entrapped Au NPs in dendrimers, the surfaces of which were modified with FA and which were then radiolabeled with ^{99m}Tc via the DTPA chelator on the dendrimer surface [71]. Thus, they integrated both SPECT (^{99m}Tc) and CT (Au NPs) imaging components onto a single NP system. In vitro and in vivo experiments showed that this multifunctional nanoprobe could be used for targeted SPECT/CT imaging of different types of tumors expressing the FA receptor.

MR imaging, PET, SPECT, and fluorescent imaging are biomedical imaging techniques suitable for noninvasively imaging stem cells (SCs) after transplantation. As a combination of imaging techniques could provide crucial information for in vivo tracking of SCs, Tang et al. developed a trimodal MR imaging/SPECT/fluorescent probe for quantitatively tracking mesenchymal stem cells (MSCs) [72]. Fluorescent silica-coated SPIONs were functionalized with *N*-succinimidyl-3-(tributyl stannyl)benzoate for radiolabeling with ^{125}I. Cell viability studies demonstrated that cell viability decreased with an increase in radiation dose. For intracerebral injection, in vivo SPECT/MR and ex vivo biodistribution studies showed that (^{125}I)-fSiO$_4$@SPIO-labeled MSCs were detected in the ischemic area (21.04% ± 7.2% and 35.14% ± 5.9% at 7 and 14 days after cell injection, while (^{125}I)-fSiO$_4$@SPIO were mainly found at the injection site. For IV injection, the (^{125}I)-fSiO$_4$@SPIO-labeled MSCs were trapped in the lung. Histological testing confirmed the above results.

10.3 Radiolabeled Nanoparticles as Cancer Therapeutic Agents

Over the past decade, there has been an increasing interest in the use of nanotechnology for cancer therapy. Targeted NPs that can deliver cytotoxic agents (drugs, radioisotopes, toxins) directly to cancer cells may provide better efficacy and lower toxicity for treating primary and advanced metastatic tumors. However, NP-based therapies are not limited to delivery of drug molecules. NPs are also being used to develop new cancer treatments such as photothermal and photodynamic therapies. Here we will focus on NPs radiolabeled with radioisotopes with β particle, alpha (α) particle, and Auger electron emissions, which are suitable for therapy.

The radioisotopes studied for targeted radiotherapy are listed in Table 10.3.

Table 10.3 Radioisotopes for nanoparticle radiotherapy

Radioisotope	Type of emission	Half-life	Nanoparticle platform
^{225}Ac	α, β	6.1 h[a]	Mineral lattice
^{111}In	Auger, γ	2.8 d[b]	Biotinylated streptavidin
^{177}Lu	β, γ	6.1 d	Liposomes; fullerene cages
^{125}I	Auger, γ	60.1 d	Biotinylated streptavidin
^{131}I	β, γ	8 d	Synthetic polymer
^{90}Y	b	64 d	Lipid–polymer hybrid
^{198}Au	b	2.7 d	Dendrimer
^{186}Re	β, γ	89 h	Liposome
^{188}Re	β, γ	17 h	IONPs
^{166}Ho	β, γ	27 h	Acetylacetone

[a]h = hours
[b]d = days

β emitters are the most widely used for therapy, having relatively long path lengths and low linear energy transfer (LET) (0.2 keV/μm). β particles kill cells by inflicting indirect damage on the DNA. They ionize water molecules in the cells, causing formation of free hydroxyl radicals, which interact with DNA and cause single strand breaks. α emitters produce high-energy particles (4–9 MeV) that travel very short distances (40–100 μm) and have high LET (100 keV/μm). The emission of α particles is highly cytotoxic because they cause double-stranded DNA breaks. Auger emitters have also been used for cancer radiotherapy. However, their use has been relatively restricted because of extreme toxicity. To date, the study of therapeutic radionanoparticles has involved a wide range of NP platforms combined with an even vaster array of radioisotopes.

10.3.1 Beta Decay Radionanoparticles

Radioisotopes decaying through β emission are perhaps the best studied agents for NP radiotherapy. With a path length of 1–10 mm, β particles traverse multiple cells while interacting, leading to a "cross fire" effect. Therefore, tagged NPs do not require cellular internalization to provide effective cell kill. The particle range may also allow for potential cell kill in areas of tumor lacking good vascular access. Khan et al. demonstrated the antitumor effect of dendrimer NPs carrying therapeutic loads of ^{198}Au. Researchers generated the radioactive composite nanodevice (CND) by simultaneous neutron activation and radiation polymerization of dendrimers tagged with ^{197}Au. Neutron capture formed ^{198}Au, which could then decay by β emission. In a melanoma model, tumors of mice injected with the ^{198}Au CND decreased in size by 45% compared to the untagged CND, with no observed toxicity [73]. Chanda et al. described a similar ^{198}Au NP with good therapeutic efficacy and low toxicity in a murine prostate cancer model [74]. Several other platforms have been developed for the delivery of internal β irradiation, like fullerene cage NPs tagged with lutetium-177 (^{177}Lu) for targeting Il-13 or incorporating ^{212}Pb, a β emitter with an α-emitting daughter radionuclide, ^{212}Bi [75, 76].

Reactive ionic radioisotopes such as Lu and Pb must be shielded from the microenvironment to prevent interaction. Fullerene cages are the most attractive NPs for this purpose because the ions are completely enclosed within the platform. Holmium-166 (^{166}Ho) is another appealing candidate radioisotope due to its concurrent γ and β decays as well as its high attenuation coefficient and paramagnetic properties. This combination suggests that it has wide-ranging potential as a true theranostic agent. With this in mind, Bult et al. successfully developed an acetylacetone NP labeled with ^{166}Ho [77]. Other radiolabels have been incorporated in liposomes. Glutathione-encapsulated liposomes have been radiolabeled with rhenium-186 (^{186}Re) and ^{188}Re for both diagnostic and therapeutic purposes using a rhenium-SNS/S complex [78]. More recent examples of work being done with NPs radiolabeled with β emitters are provided below.

Due to the strong antioxidant properties of epigallochatechin-gallate (ECGg), it was utilized as a reducing agent to prepare radioactive Au NPs from radioactive $H^{198}AuCl_4$ (radiochemical yield > 99%) [79]. ECGg also targets Laminin receptor (Lam67R) overexpressed on human prostate cancer cells. The ^{198}Au NP–ECGg nanoconstruct was evaluated for its in vivo targeting potential and therapeutic properties. In vitro experiments in PC-3 prostate cancer cells overexpressing Lam67R showed that a significant amount of ^{198}Au NP–ECGg was internalized into the cells, while blocking studies with native laminin demonstrated its binding specificity.

Intratumoral administration of ^{198}Au NP–ECGg in PC-3 tumor-bearing mice demonstrated an 80% reduction of tumor volumes after 28 days, in comparison to a control group of animals, which showed no tumor regression.

Radiolabeled Au NPs have been utilized for radiotherapy and plasmonic photothermal therapy (PTT) of cancer. Jiménez-Mancilla et al. developed a radiotherapy and thermal ablation system based on Au NPs radiolabeled with ^{99m}Tc and ^{177}Lu [80]. The multifunctional system was prepared by conjugating the (H-Arg-Lys-Lys-Arg-Arg-Gln-Arg-Arg-Arg-NH_2) (Tat)-bombesin peptide (GRPr targeting), ^{177}Lu-DOTA-GGC (radiotherapy), and ^{99m}Tc-HYNIC-TOC (γ imaging, Auger radiotherapy) to Au NPs (PTT). In vitro cell studies showed GRPr-positive cell accumulation in PC-3 cancer cells, due to active targeting of ^{99m}Tc/^{177}Lu-Au NPs-Tat-bombesi. Upon laser irradiation of PC-3 cells treated with Au NP-Tat-BN, cell viability was significantly reduced when compared to the viability of cells without NPs.

In another study by the same group, Au NPs were functionalized with cRGD for targeting the $\alpha_v\beta_3$ receptor and a DOTA chelate for radiolabeling with ^{177}Lu [81]. When compared to the nontargeted ^{177}Lu-Au NPs and the radiolabeled peptide ^{177}Lu-RGD, the ^{177}Lu-Au-NP-RGD showed the highest uptake and retention in tumors, consequently delivering a greater radiation absorbed dose to tumors. This nanoconstruct shows great potential as a theranostic agent, due to SPECT imaging properties of ^{177}Lu, targeted radiotherapy due to the RGD peptide and high β particle energy of ^{177}Lu, and PTT due to the Au NPs.

Au NPs radiolabeled with ^{177}Lu were utilized to study the stability of Au NPs conjugated to metal-chelated polymers (MCPs) via a single thiol (DOTA-PEG-ortho-pyridyl disulfide [OPSS]), a dithiol (DOTA-PEG-lipoic acid [LA]), or a multithiol end group (PEG-pGlu[DOTA]$_8$-LA$_4$) [82]. It was demonstrated that ^{177}Lu-PEG-pGlu(DOTA)$_8$-LA$_4$ was the most stable in plasma and less prone to aggregation, when compared to the other two radiolabeled species, and showed the lowest liver and highest spleen uptake after in vivo administration in mice. Therefore, this nanoconstruct exhibits the most promising properties for the preparation of ^{177}Lu-MCP-Au-NPs for radiation treatment of cancer. The same group studied gold nanoseeds modified with DOTA (for complexing ^{177}Lu) and panitumumab, an anti–epidermal growth factor receptor [EGFR] antibody targeting EGFRs overexpressed on BC cells (^{177}Lu-T-Au-NPs) [83]. Intratumoral injection of ^{177}Lu-T-Au-NPs was shown to be highly effective for inhibiting the growth of BC tumors in athymic mice.

Bovine serum albumin–poly-(ε-caprolactone) (BSA-PCL) is an amphiphilic, protein-based conjugate comprised of hydrophobic maleimide-functionalized PCL covalently linked to hydrophilic BSA. BSA-PCL NPs were functionalized with an anti-EGFR antibody and radiolabeled with ^{131}I in a direct radiolabeling protocol with chloramine-T (^{131}I-EGFR-BSA-PCL) [84]. Compared to the nontargeted ^{131}I-BSA-PCL, the targeted construct exhibited greater in vitro cytotoxicity, higher cellular uptake, and higher uptake in tumor tissues after in vivo administration in tumor-bearing mice.

Radovic et al. investigated the possible use of yttrium-90 (^{90}Y)-labeled magnetic microspheres in bimodal radionuclide and hyperthermia cancer therapy [85]. Magnetite NPs coated with citric acid were encapsulated with human serum albumin microspheres (HSAMMS) and then the resulting construct was labeled with ^{90}Y, a pure β emitter, in a chelator-free method, by directly adding $^{90}YCl_3$ to an HSAMMS suspension (radiolabeling yield ~67%). It was shown that ^{90}Y remained bound to HSAMMS for a time period sufficient for in vivo evaluation. Ex vivo biodistribution studies on Wistar rats showed dominant lung accumulation, which can be attributed to the size of these NPs. No toxic effects were observed in these studies, due to the small concentration of administered ^{90}Y-HSAMMS. Heating efficiency testing of HSAMMS showed that these particles could reach the temperature range required for thermally induced cell apoptosis by hyperthermia. Radiolabeled HSAMMS could potentially be used for combined radiotherapy/hyperthermia treatment.

10.3.2 Alpha Decay Radionanoparticles

Particles that decay through α emission may be attractive alternatives for targeting intravascular micrometastases due to high LET. These particles are limited by a penetration range of 40–100 μm, making them less well suited for bulky tumor deposits.

Within the context of in vivo α generator systems, and in order to retain the radioactive daughters of the parent radioisotope at the targeting site, lanthanide NPs doped with actinium-225 (^{225}Ac) and covered with a gold shell were investigated [86]. The lanthanide phosphate core of these NPs offers the radiation resistance required to encapsulate and contain atoms of the therapeutic mother radioisotope ^{225}Ac and its radioactive daughters, the gadolinium phosphate shell facilitates magnetic separation of the NPs, and the gold shell is exploited for NP functionalization with various targeting agents. These NPs were functionalized with 201b and antithrombomodulin antibody for targeted delivery to the lung epithelium [87]. Very high accumulation in the lungs was observed after in vitro autoradiography, ex vivo biodistribution, and in vivo SPECT/CT studies. Binding specificity was demonstrated after the administration of excess unlabeled antibody. Preinjection of clodronate liposomes resulted in the neutralization of macrophages associated with NP clearance, thus decreasing liver uptake and increasing lung uptake. The layered NP retained the daughter radioisotope ^{213}bismuth (Bi^{213}) in the lung up to ~90% at 24 h p.i. A therapy study was conducted on mice injected with EMT-6 cells, which form tumor colonies in lung tissue. The mice were separated into three groups: Group A was injected with PBS (control group), Group B was injected with unconjugated 201b antibody mixed with NP-201b conjugates, and Group C was injected with NP-201b conjugates. Seven days after tumor cell injection, Group C mice had the fewest tumor colonies per tumor section, thus demonstrating the tumoricidal properties of the targeted, radiolabeled NP construct.

Another α emitter used to radiolabel NPs is ^{213}Bi. It has recently been shown that the ^{213}Bi-labeled antibody, which targets cells overexpressing the HER2/neu antigen, was effective in treating HER2/neu-expressing micrometastases in a preclinical model. Lingappa et al. investigated the ^{213}Bi radiolabeling of a liposome functionalized with a DTPA moiety (for radiolabeling) and 7.16.4, a HER2/neu-targeting antibody (for targeted delivery of the radiolabeled construct to the diseased site) [88]. When compared to liposome-CHX-A''-DTPA-^{213}Bi, targeted liposome-CHX-A''-DTPA-^{213}Bi-7.16.4 was shown to exhibit a significant increase in median survival, similar to the results acquired with the radiolabeled antibody 213Bi-7.16.4. Cytotoxicity studies demonstrated that liposome-CHX-A''-DTPA-^{213}Bi-7.16.4 was more cytotoxic than the nontargeted liposomes but less effective than ^{213}Bi-7.16.4.

The radium(II) ion exhibits high affinity for HAp, a constituent of bone tissue. Both ^{222}/^{225}Ra isotopes target the bone and remain there, as does the α-emitting daughter of ^{225}Ra, ^{225}Ac. However, the decay daughters of ^{225}Ac migrate from bone to the kidneys. Lanthanum phosphate ($LaPO_4$) NPs were investigated as potential carriers of ^{223}Ra or ^{225}Ra/^{225}Ac parent radioisotopes, as well as their daughter isotopes. $LaPO_4$ were radiolabeled during their synthesis process, with an overall radiochemical yield of ~91% for ^{223}Ra and 94% and 95% for $LaPO_4$ containing ^{225}Ra/^{225}Ac. Further stabilization of the radioactive cores was afforded by deposition of one and two cold $LaPO_4$ shells onto the core (core +1 shell and core +2 shells NPs). The radiochemical yield of the +2 shells NPs was 80% for the ^{223}Ra-labeled NPs and 85% for the ^{225}Ra/^{225}Ac-radiolabeled NPs. In vitro release studies of the parent radioisotopes and their daughters from core +2 shells $LaPO_4$ demonstrated a reduced release of ^{223}Ra and its daughter ^{211}Pb (<0.1% over 27 days). Similar retention behavior was exhibited by the ^{225}Ra/^{225}Ac parents and their francium-225 and ^{213}Bi daughters, with a retention of >99.9% and ~80%, respectively. This is a great improvement when compared to the radiolabeling of NPs with such isotopes via chelators, which release the α emitters in vivo, thus limiting the dose that can be delivered to the diseased site [89].

10.3.3 Auger Decay Radionanoparticles

Due to their short range, Auger electrons rely on high selective cellular uptake and incorporation in cellular DNA to have a meaningful tumoricidal effect. To date, ^{111}In, ^{123}I, and ^{125}I have been studied as potential agents for this purpose [90–93].

In addition to γ emissions (for SPECT imaging), ^{111}In emits low-energy Auger electrons with a very short range but high LET, which can inflict lethal damage on DNA in cells, especially if these are released near the cell nucleus. Cai et al. surface-modified Au NPs with trastuzumab, an antibody targeting HER2-positive BC cells, and a DOTA derivative for ^{111}In chelation [94]. These modified NPs were surface-coated with PEG to stabilize the particles to aggregation and evade the RES organs. As the preliminary in vivo results showed low tumor uptake in MDA-MB-361 human BC xenografts and modest liver and high spleen uptake, the group proceeded to the intratumoral application of trastuzumab-Au-NP-^{111}In in athymic mice bearing MDA-MB 231 human BC xenografts and evaluated the Auger effect of ^{111}In on these tumors. Trastuzumab-Au-NP-^{111}In showed specific binding to SK-BR-3 and MDA-MB-361 cells, while internalization was more efficient for the targeted nanoconstruct than for Au NP–^{111}In. It also induced DNA double-strand breaks, thus reducing the surviving fraction of both SK-BR-3 and MDA-MB-361 cancer cells, as shown by clonogenic assays. Intratumoral injection in athymic mice bearing MDA-MB-361 xenografts halted tumor growth during the 70-day evaluation period, while no normal tissue toxicity was observed.

Song et al. showed an easy way to prepare ^{111}In-radiolabeled Au NPs targeting the EGFR, with a high radioactivity payload per NP [95]. The DTPA chelator was first coupled to EGF, which was then attached to Au NPs via Au-S bonds. Consequent addition of $^{111}InCl_3$ led to successful radiolabeling of the nanoconstruct (radiolabeling yield > 90%). Although nonlabeled EGF–Au NPs are toxic to MDA-MB-468, as shown by clonogenic assays, therapeutic efficacy was greatly enhanced through radiolabeling with this Auger-electron-emitting isotope.

10.4 Radiolabeled Nanoparticles as Theranostic Agents

Theranostics, the merging of diagnosis and therapy, is a new area of interest in nanotechnology. Engineering of an NP surface allows the surface area to bear therapeutic molecules, imaging agents, or targeting ligands. A single NP can be conjugated with a large number of targeting ligands, increasing the affinity of the NP to its biological target through a phenomenon known as multivalency. Subsequently, the NP can be linked to a large number of reporter molecules, thus increasing the signal-to-noise ratio in imaging applications. Finally, one or more types of anticancer drugs can be encapsulated in or conjugated to the NP. Thus, a theranostic NP represents a culmination of multiple strategies combined into a multifunctional NP, which would be able to carry a targeting moiety, an imaging agent, one or more drugs, a stimulus-sensitive part for controlled release of the drugs, and a polymer coating for biocompatibility of the NP [96–98]. This multifunctional NP would simultaneously target and image the diseased site, while treating the disease itself (Fig. 10.1). Some multimodal NPs have also been developed with a superparamagnetic core, which are used for MR imaging, and a gold shell, for PTT.

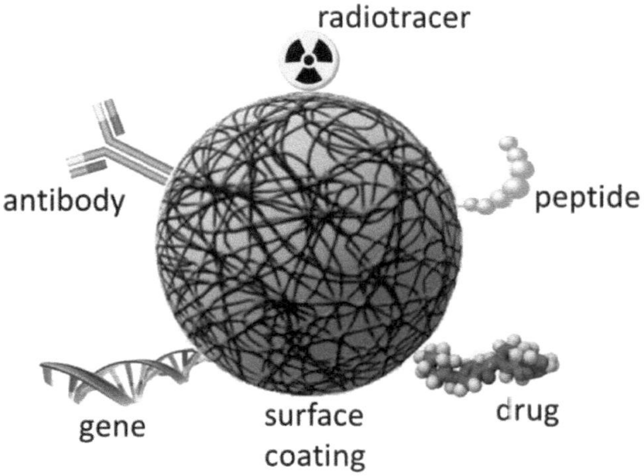

Figure 10.1 Surface-functionalized nanoparticles with theranostic properties. Republished with permission of Bentham Science Publishers Ltd., from Ref. [98b] 2013; permission conveyed through Copyright Clearance Center, Inc.

While there have been numerous studies on multifunctional NPs, they have yet to reach clinical translation. Thus, a lot of work still needs to be done, especially with regard to toxicity issues, before these new NP formulations are approved for human use.

A few examples of NP theranostic agents from recent literature are provided below.

^{166}Ho, a radioisotope with theranostic properties (SPECT imaging and therapy), was used to radiolabel dextran-coated SPIONS for the development of a potential theranostic agent [99]. Initially, the SPIONS were mixed and incubated with a DTPA chelator at room temperature for 1 h. Then, the DTPA-SPIONS were mixed gently with ^{166}Ho for 30 min. to create the radiolabeled conjugate. After purification of the radiolabeled conjugate to remove the unattached ^{166}Ho, its radiochemical purity was found to be 99%. The ^{166}Ho-SPIONs were found to be stable in human serum for at least 48 h, while in vivo biodistribution studies indicated high accumulation of

^{166}Ho-DTPA-SPIONS in the liver and spleen, revealing the efficacy of these NPs as RES theranostic agents.

Radovic et al. synthesized and compared the in vivo behavior of naked and PEG 600 diacid functionalized MNPs with the aim to assess their potential efficiency in therapeutic applications [100]. Both MNPs were radiolabeled with ^{90}Y, a β emitter suitable for radionuclide tumor therapy, in high yield (>97%) and evaluated for their in vitro stability in saline and human serum, indicating excellent results for ^{90}Y-PEG MNPs over a period of 72 h. Furthermore, in vivo biodistribution studies performed in healthy Wistar rats showed significant uptake in the liver for both MNPs but lower uptake in the lungs for the ^{90}Y-PEG MNPs compared to the naked MNPs. The difference in lung accumulation can be attributed to the presence of PEG, which prevents the in vivo agglomeration of MNPs. The results showed that ^{90}Y-PEG MNPs have great potential to be used as diagnostic and therapeutic agents, that is, for MR imaging–guided hyperthermia studies and radiotherapy of liver malignancies.

Cheng et al. developed an ^{131}I-labeled nanodelivery system for glioma SPECT imaging and radiotherapy [101]. In brief, PAMAM dendrimers were synthesized and loaded with 3-(4'-hydroxyphenyl) propionic acid-OSu (HPAO), an ^{131}I linker, while they were conjugated with Buthus martensii Karsch chlorotoxin (BmK CT) for specific delivery to the tumor. The ^{131}I-labeled dendrimers exhibited high radiochemical purity in vitro. Moreover, the ^{131}I-labeled dendrimers were assessed for their cytotoxicity on C6 glioma cells. A significant decrease in the viability of glioma cells exposed to the ^{131}I-labeled dendrimers was observed, compared to the nonradiolabeled dendrimers, which showed no inhibition effect on the cells. This result was attributed to the increased delivery of ^{131}I to the C6 glioma cells caused by the BmK CT. Thus, ^{131}I-labeled dendrimers conjugated with BmK CT could be used as a potential agent for SPECT imaging and radiotherapy of glioma.

^{68}Ga and ^{177}Lu-DOTA dendrimers conjugated with bombesin and folate, along with Au NPs within their cavity, were developed for use in theranostic applications [102]. The DOTA dendrimers were robustly labeled with ^{68}Ga and ^{177}Lu with a radiochemical purity of >95%. Fluorescence studies confirmed the potential of the Au NPs for optical imaging. Furthermore, studies performed in T47D BC tumor-bearing mice showed high specific cell uptake and retention in the tumors. These initial studies demonstrate that ^{177}Lu-DOTA dendrimers show potential as an optical imaging and targeted radiotherapeutic agent for BC.

Zolata et al. synthesized ^{111}In-labeled SPIONs to serve not only as SPECT/MR imaging agents but also as targeted drug delivery systems for tumor therapy [103]. The SPIONs were developed via thermal decomposition, surface-coated with 3-aminopropyltriethoxysilane-PEG to increase their blood retention time, conjugated with trastuzumab antibody (a targeting moiety) and doxorubicin (a chemotherapeutic agent) and radiolabeled with ^{111}In. The biodistribution results showed that these functionalized SPIONs were significantly accumulated in tumors due to the EPR tumor effect and HER2-specific uptake. Furthermore, their therapeutic efficacy was proved, as the mice injected with the functionalized SPIONs exhibited a decrease in their tumor volumes compared to the untreated ones.

Farrag et al. reported on the synthesis and radiolabeling of three types of Ag NPs with ^{125}I at high radiolabeling yields (>90%) [104]. The in vivo biodistribution results of the injected ^{125}I–Ag NPs in tumor-bearing mice showed higher uptake of the DOX-loaded ^{125}I–Ag NPs in the tumor 1 h p.i. compared to DOX-free ^{125}I–Ag NPs, along with high tumor/normal tissue and tumor/blood ratios, indicating that these radiolabeled Ag NPs can serve as promising agents for tumor imaging with high affinity and retention, promoting their theranostic effect.

SPIONs functionalized with targeting and detection elements along with drugs and radioisotopes have attracted significant attention due to their ability to combine PET/MR imaging and therapy of tumors. For this reason, Yang et al. synthesized multifunctional SPIONs with the aim to create a dual-modality PET/MR imaging and drug delivery agent for tumors that express integrin $\alpha_v\beta_3$ [105]. The PEG-coated SPIONs were conjugated with doxorubicin to achieve pH-controlled drug release and a cRGD peptide that served as a targeting moiety promoting the active targeting of the tumors. The SPIONs were also radiolabeled with ^{64}Cu via the NOTA macrocyclic chelator to perform in vivo PET imaging of their biodistribution and to evaluate their drug release efficacy at the tumor site. In vitro cytotoxicity studies revealed that ^{64}Cu-SPION-cRGD showed significant cytotoxicity to the tumor cells, indicating DOX release.

The in vivo PET imaging and biodistribution results showed higher tumor uptake for ^{64}Cu-SPION-cRGD compared to ^{64}Cu-SPIONs, while in vitro r2 MR imaging relaxivity measurements gave results comparable to a commercially available MR imaging contrast agent.

Wang et al. developed a tumor-targeting, dual-modality imaging agent by conjugating radiolabeled c(RGDyK) peptide to PEGylated Fe@Fe_3O_4 NPs (RGD-PEG MNPs) and then radiolabeling them with ^{125}I with the chloramine-T method [106]. High in vivo targeting of U87MG glioblastoma and low mononuclear phagocyte uptake were confirmed by SPECT/MR imaging. PTT conducted on mice injected with RGD-PEG MNPs showed satisfactory in vivo therapeutic efficacy.

Tsiapa et al. synthesized aminosilane-coated iron oxide NPs and evaluated both bare and peptide-decorated NPs after their radiolabeling with ^{99m}Tc [107]. Their results showed that the NPs functionalized with the $\alpha_v\beta_3$-targeting peptide RGD are a target-specific agent for molecular imaging of $\alpha_v\beta_3$ expression in tumor angiogenesis. Preliminary in vivo hyperthermia experiments demonstrated their potential as cancer therapeutic agents.

Manganese (as $MnCl_2$) has been used as a contrast agent for MR imaging; however, excessive intake could lead to cardiovascular toxicity. Thus, manganese-based NPs have been used as MR contrast agents to avoid the disadvantages of Mn^{2+}. In this scope, Gao et al. proceeded to disperse MnO_x NPs within the mesopores of MSNs and further labeled these with ^{99m}Tc for dual-modality imaging applications [108]. Doxorubicin loaded onto these NPs was shown to be efficiently released at lower pH values, such as those of the tumor environment. As these mesoporous NPs are excellent carriers of anticancer drugs, this construct could prove to be an ideal theranostic agent.

10.5 Conclusions

NPs have gained tremendous interest as tools for medical applications in recent years. Radioisotopes have grown to be an integral part of this field for purposes of both drug development and now diagnostic and therapeutic applications. The flexibility of NPs enables the utilization of radioisotopes in novel applications. Careful construction and evaluation of these NP probes using nuclear imaging methods provides considerable insight into their in vivo fate and their prospective utility in research and clinical application. Convergence of radiolabeling with the cornucopia of NPs for imaging and therapy has resulted in many particles capable of multimodal imaging. To move the field of multimodal imaging probes forward, there is a need for research that not only reports a new coating or combination of different components but also performs in-depth investigation on real diagnostic or therapeutic applications with potential for clinical translation. It is expected that improved NPs will be developed on the basis of the accumulated knowledge and technology in which radioisotopes promise to continue playing an important role. We hope that these multifunctional NPs for multimodal imaging and theragnosis can make great contributions to human health in the near future.

References

1. http://www.who.int/cancer/en/; Accessed August 2017.
2. Shokeen, M., Fettig, N. M. and Rossin, R. (2008). Synthesis, *in vitro* and *in vivo* evaluation of radiolabeled nanoparticles, *Q. J. Nucl. Med. Mol. Imaging*, **52**, pp. 267–277.
3. Liu, Y. and Welch, M. J. (2012). Nanoparticles labeled with positron emitting nuclides: advantages, methods and applications, *Bioconjugate Chem.*, **23**, pp. 671–682.
4. Maeda, H. (2010). Tumor-selective delivery of macromolecular drugs via the EPR effect: background and future prospects, *Bioconjugate Chem.*, **21**, pp. 797–802.
5. Brigger, I., Dubernet, C. and Couvreur, P. (2002). Nanoparticles in cancer therapy and diagnosis, *Adv. Drug Deliv. Rev.*, **54**, pp. 631–651.
6. Veiseh, O., Gunn, J. W. and Zhang, M. (2010). Design and fabrication of magnetic nanoparticles for targeted drug delivery and imaging, *Adv. Drug Deliv. Rev.*, **62**, pp. 284–304.
7. Madru, R., Kjellman, P., Olsson, F., Wingardh, K., Ingvar, C., Stahlberg, F., Olsrud, J., Lätt, J., Fredriksson, S., Knutsson, L. and Strand, S. E. (2012). ^{99m}Tc-labeled superparamagnetic iron oxide nanoparticles for multimodality SPECT/MRI of sentinel lymph nodes, *J. Nucl. Med.*, **53**, pp. 459–463.
8. Psimadas, D., Baldi, G., Ravagli, C., Bouziotis, P., Xanthopoulos, S., Franchini, M. C., Georgoulias, P. and Loudos, G. (2012). Preliminary

evaluation of a ^{99m}Tc labeled hybrid nanoparticle bearing a cobalt ferritecore: *in vivo* biodistribution, *J. Biomed. Nanotechnol.*, **8**, pp. 575–585.

9. Zeng, J., Jia, B., Qiao, R., Wang, C., Jing, L., Wang, F. and Gao, M. (2014). In situ ^{111}In-doping for achieving biocompatible and non-leachable ^{111}Inlabeled Fe_3O_4 nanoparticles, *Chem Commun. (Camb.)*, **50**, pp. 2170–2172.
10. Laverman, P., Dams, E. T., Oyen, W. J., Storm, G., Koenders, E. B., Prevost, R., van der Meer, J. W. M., Corstens F. H. M. and Boerman O. C. (1999). A novel method to label liposomes with ^{99m}Tc by the hydrazino nicotinyl derivative, *J. Nucl. Med.*, **40**, pp. 192–197.
11. Black, K. C., Akers, W. J., Sudlow, G., Xu, B., Laforest, R. and Achilefu, S. (2015). Dual-radiolabeled nanoparticle SPECT probes for bioimaging, *Nanoscale*, **7**, pp. 440–444.
12. Park, J. J., Lee, T. S., Kang, J. H., Song, R. and Cheon, G. J. (2011). Radioiodination and biodistribution of quantum dots using Bolton-Hunter reagent, *Appl. Radiat. Isot.*, **69**, pp. 56–162.
13. Ayan, A. K., Yenilmez, A. and Eroglu, H. (2017). Evaluation of radiolabeled curcumin-loaded solid lipid nanoparticles usage as an imaging agent in liver-spleen scintigraphy, *Mater. Sci. Eng. C*, **75**, pp. 663–670.
14. Halder, K. K., Mandal, B., Debnath, M. C., Bera, H., Ghosh, L. K. and Gupta, B. K. (2008). Chloramphenicol-incorporated poly lactide-co-glycolide (PLGA) nanoparticles: formulation, characterization, technetium-99m labeling and biodistribution studies, *J. Drug Target.*, **16**(4), pp. 311–320.
15. Subramanian, S., Dandekar, P., Jain, R., Pandey, U., Samuel, G., Hassan, P. A., Patravale, V. and Venkatesh, M. (2010). Technetium-^{99m}-labeled poly(dl-lactide-co-glycolide) nanoparticles as an alternative for sentinel lymph node imaging, *Cancer Biother. Radiopharm.*, **25**(6), pp. 637–644.
16. Subramanian, S., Pandey, U., Gugulothu, D., Patravale, V. and Samuel, G. (2013). Modification of PLGA nanoparticles for improved properties as a ^{99m}Tc-labeled agent in sentinel lymph node detection, *Cancer Biother. Radiopharm.*, **28**(8), pp. 598–606.
17. Ocampo-García, B. E., de M. Ramírez, F., Ferro-Flores, G., de León-Rodríguez, L. M., Santos-Cuevas, C. L., Morales-Avila, E., Arteaga de Murphy, C., Pedraza-López, M., Medinae, L. A. and Camacho-López, M. A. (2011). ^{99m}Tc-labelled gold nanoparticles capped with HYNIC-

peptide/mannose for sentinel lymph node detection, *Nucl. Med. Biol.*, **38**, pp. 1–11.

18. de Barros, A. L. B., de Oliveira Ferraz, K. S., Soares Dantas, T. C., Andrade, G. F., Nascimento Cardoso, V. and de Sousa, E. M. B. (2015). Synthesis, characterization, and biodistribution studies of ^{99m}Tc-labeled SBA-16 mesoporous silica nanoparticles, *Mater. Sci. Eng. C*, **56**, pp. 181–188.

19. Fragogeorgi, E. A., Savina, I. N., Tsotakos, T., Efthimiadou, E., Xanthopoulos, S., Palamaris, L., Psimadas, D., Bouziotis, P., Kordas, G., Mikhalovsky, S., Alavijeh, M. and Loudos, G. (2014). Comparative *in vitro* stability and scintigraphic imaging for trafficking and tumor targeting of a directly and a novel ^{99m}Tc (I)$(CO)_3$ labeled liposome, *Int. J. Pharm.*, **465**(1–2), pp. 333–346.

20. Polyáka, A., Hajdub, I., Bodnár, M., Trencsényi, G., Pöstényi, Z., Haász, V., Jánoki, G., Jánoki, G. A., Balogh, L. and Borbély, J. (2013). ^{99m}Tc-labelled nanosystem as tumour imaging agent for SPECT and SPECT/CT modalities, *Int. J. Pharm.*, **449**, pp. 10–17.

21. Polyák, A., Hajdu, I., Bodnár, M., Dabasi, G., Jóba, R. P., Borbély, J. and Balogh, L. (2014). Folate receptor targeted self-assembled chitosan-based nanoparticles for SPECT/CT imaging: demonstrating a preclinical proof of concept, *Int. J. Pharm.*, **474**, pp. 91–94.

22. Zhang, Y., Sun, Y., Xu, X., Zhu, H., Huang, L., Zhang, X , Qi, Y. and Shen Y. M. (2010). Radiosynthesis and micro-SPECT imaging of ^{99m}Tc-dendrimer poly(amido)-amine folic acid conjugate, *Bioorg. Med. Chem. Lett.*, **20**, pp. 927–931.

23. Xu, X., Zhang, Y., Wang, X., Guo, X., Zhang, X., Qi, Y. and Shen, Y. M. (2011). Radiosynthesis, biodistribution and micro-SPECT imaging study of dendrimer–avidin conjugate, *Bioorg. Med. Chem.*, **19**, pp. 1643–1648.

24. Mendoza-Sánchez, A. N., Ferro-Flores, G., Ocampo-García, B. E., Morales-Avila, E., de Marıa Ramírez, F., de León-Rodríguez, L. M., Santos-Cuevas, C. L., Medina, L. A., Rojas-Calderón, E. L. and Camacho-López, M. A. (2010). Lys_3-bombesin conjugated to ^{99m}Tc-labelled gold nanoparticles for *in vivo* gastrin releasing peptide-receptor imaging, *J. Biomed. Nanotechnol.*, **6**, pp. 375–384.

25. Ocampo-Garcıa, B., Ferro-Flores, G., Morales-Avila, E. and de Marıa Ramırez, F. (2011). Kit for preparation of multimeric receptor-specific ^{99m}Tc-radiopharmaceuticals based on gold nanoparticles, *Nucl. Med. Commun.*, **32**(11), pp. 1095–1104.

26. Arranja, A., Ivashchenko, O., Denkova, A. G., Morawska, K., van Vlierberghe, S., Dubruel, P., Waton, G., Beekman, F. J., Schosseler, F. and Mendes, E. (2016). SPECT/CT imaging of pluronic nanocarriers with

varying poly(ethylene oxide) block length and aggregation state, *Mol. Pharmaceutics*, **13**, pp. 1158–1165.

27. Ogawa, M., Umeda, I. O., Kosugi, M., Kawai, A., Hamaya, Y., Takashima, M., Yin, H., Kudoh, T., Seno, M. and Magata, Y. (2014). Development of ^{111}In-labeled liposomes for vulnerable atherosclerotic plaque imaging, *J. Nucl. Med.*, **55**, pp. 1–6.

28. Ng, Q. K. T., Olariu, C. I., Yaffee, M., Taelman, V. F., Marincek, N., Krause, T., Meier, L. and Walter, M. A. (2014). Indium-111 labeled gold nanoparticles for in-vivo molecular targeting, *Biomaterials*, **35**, pp. 7050–7057.

29. Laan, A. C., Santini, C., Jennings, L., de Jong, M., Bernsen, M. R. and Denkova, A. G. (2016). Radiolabeling polymeric micelles for *in vivo* evaluation: a novel, fast, and facile method, *EJNMMI Res.*, **6**, p. 12.

30. Ignjatović, N., Vranješ-Djurić, S., Mitić, Ž., Janković, D. and Uskoković, D. (2014). Investigating an organ-targeting platform based on hydroxyapatite nanoparticles using a novel in situ method of radioactive ^{125}Iodine labeling, *Mater. Sci. Eng. C*, **43**, pp. 439–446.

31. Chrastina, A. and Schnitzer, J. E. (2010). Iodine-125 radiolabeling of silver nanoparticles for *in vivo* SPECT imaging, *Int. J. Nanomed.*, **5**, pp. 653–659.

32. Shao, X., Zhang, H., Rajian, J. R., Chamberland, D. L., Sherman, P. S., Quesada, C. A., Koch, A. E., Kotov, N. A. and Wang, X. (2012). ^{125}I-labeled gold nanorods for targeted imaging of inflammation, *ACS Nano*, **5**(11), p. 2011.

33. Vallabhajosula, S. (2009). *Molecular Imaging: Radiopharmaceuticals for PET and SPECT*, Springer-Verlag Berlin Heidelberg.

34. Abou, D. S., Thorek, D. L., Ramos, N. N., Pinkse, M. W., Wolterbeek, H. T., Carlin, S. D., Beattie, B. J. and Lewis, J. S. (2013). Zr-labeled paramagnetic octreotide liposomes for PET-MR imaging of cancer, *Pharm. Res.*, **30**, pp. 878–888.

35. Shaffer, T. M., Wall, M. A., Harmsen, S., Longo, V. A., Drain, C. M., Kircher, M. F. and Grimm, J. (2015). Silica nanoparticles as substrates for chelator-free labeling of oxophilic radioisotopes, *Nano Lett.*, **15**, pp. 864–868.

36. Boros, E., Bowen, A. M., Josephson, L., Vasdev, N. and Holland, J. P. (2015). Chelate-free metal ion binding and heat-induced radiolabeling of iron oxide nanoparticles, *Chem. Sci.*, **6**, pp. 225–236.

37. Cui, X., Belo, S., Krüger, D., Yan, Y, de Rosales, R. T. M., Jauregui-Osoro, M., Ye, H., Su, S., Mathe, D., Kovács, N., Horváth, I., Semjeni, M., Sunassee, K.,

Szigeti, K., Green, M. A. and Blower, P. J. (2014). Aluminium hydroxide stabilised $MnFe_2O_4$ and Fe_3O_4 nanoparticles as dual-modality contrasts agent for MRI and PET imaging, *Biomaterials*, **35**, pp. 5840–5846.

38. Jauregui-Osoro, M., Williamson, P. A., Glaria, A., Sunassee, K., Charoenphun, P., Green, M. A., Mullen, G. E. D. and Blower, P. J. (2011). Biocompatible inorganic nanoparticles for [^{18}F]-fluoride binding with applications in PET imaging, *Dalton Trans.*, **40**, pp 6226–6237.

39. Guerrero, S., Herance, J. R., Rojas, S., Mena, J. F., Gispert, J. D., Acosta, G. A., Albericio, F. and Kogan, M. J. (2012). Synthesis and *in vivo* evaluation of the biodistribution of a ^{18}F-labeled conjugate gold-nanoparticle-peptide with potential biomedical application, *Bioconjugate Chem.*, **23**, pp. 399–408.

40. Emmetiere, F., Irwin, C., Viola-Villegas, N. T., Longo, V., Cheal, S. M., Zanzonico, P., Pillarsetty, N., Weber, W. A., Lewis, J. A. and Reiner, T. (2013). ^{18}F-labeled-bioorthogonal liposomes for *in vivo* targeting, *Bioconjugate Chem.*, **24**(11), pp. 1784–1789.

41. Lee, S., Gangangari, K., Kalidindi, T. M., Punzalan, B., Larson, S. M. and Pillarsetty, N. V. K. (2016). Copper-64 labeled liposomes for imaging bone marrow, *Nucl. Med. Biol.*, **43**, pp. 781–787.

42. Lee, H., Zheng, J., Gaddy, D., Orcutt, K. D., Leonard, S., Geretti, E., Hesterman, J., Harwell, C., Hoppin, J., Jaffray, D. A., Wickham, T., Hendriks, B. S. and Kirpotin, D. (2015). A gradient-loadable ^{64}Cu-chelator for quantifying tumor deposition kinetics of nanoliposomal therapeutics by positron emission tomography, *Nanomed. Nanotechnol. Biol. Med.*, **11**, pp. 155–165.

43. Frellsen, A. F., Hansen, A. E., Jølck, R. I., Kempen, P., Severin, G. W., Rasmussen, P. H., Kjær, A., Jensen, A. T. I. and Andresen, T. L. (2016). A mouse positron emission tomography study of the biodistribution of gold nanoparticles with different surface coatings using embedded copper-64, *ACS Nano*, **10**(11), pp. 9887–9898.

44. Lee, D. E., Na, J. H., Lee, S., Kang, C. M., Kim, H. N., Han, S. J., Kim, H., Choe, Y. S., Jung, K. H., Lee, K. C., Choi, K., Kwon, I. C., Jeong, S. Y., Lee, K.-H. and Kim, K. (2013). Facile method to radiolabel glycol chitosan nanoparticles with ^{64}Cu via copper-free click chemistry for microPET imaging, *Mol. Pharmaceutics*, **10**, pp. 2190–2198.

45. Shaffer, T. M., Harmsen, S., Khwaja, E., Kircher, M. F., Drain, C. M. and Grimm, J. (2016). Stable radiolabeling of sulfur-functionalized silica nanoparticles with copper-64, *Nano Lett.*, **16**, pp. 5601–5604.

46. Frigell, J., García, I., Gómez-Vallejo, V., Llop, J. and Penadés, S. (2014). ^{68}Ga-labeled gold glyconanoparticles for exploring blood–brain barrier

permeability: preparation, biodistribution studies, and improved brain uptake via neuropeptide conjugation, *J. Am. Chem. Soc.*, **136**, pp. 449–457.

47. Burke, B. P., Baghdadi, N., Clemente, G. S., Camus, N., Guillou, A., Kownacka, A. E., Domarkas, J., Halime, Z., Tripier, R. and Archibald, S. J. (2014). Final step gallium-^{68} radiolabeling of silica-coated iron oxide nanorods as potential PET/MR multimodal imaging agents, *Faraday Discuss.*, **175**, pp. 59–71.
48. Burke, B. P., Baghdadi, N., Kownacka, A. E., Nigam, S., Clemente, G. S., Al-Yassiry, M. M., Domarkas, J., Lorch, M., Pickles, M., Gibbs, P., Tripier, R., Cawthorne, C. and Archibald, S. J. (2015). Chelator free gallium-68 radiolabeling of silica coated iron oxide nanorods via surface interactions, *Nanoscale*, **7**, pp. 14889–14896.
49. Polyaka, A., Nagy, L. N., Mihaly, J., Görres, S., Wittneben, A., Leiter, I., Bankstahl, J. P., Sajti, L., Kellermayer, M., Zrínyi, M. and Ross, T. L. (2017). Preparation and ^{68}Ga-radiolabeling of porous zirconia nanoparticle platform for PET/CT-imaging guided drug delivery, *J. Pharm. Biomed. Anal.*, **137**, pp. 146–150.
50. Fazaeli, Y., Rahighi, R., Tayyebi, A. and Feizi, S. (2016). Synthesis, characterization and biological evaluation of a well dispersed suspension of gallium-68-labeled magnetic nanosheets of graphene oxide for *in vivo* coincidence imaging, *Radiochim. Acta*, **105**, pp. 65–73.
51. Karmani, L., Labar, D., Valembois, V., Bouchat, V., Nagaswaran, P. G., Bol, A., Gillart, J., Levêque, P., Bouzin, C., Bonifazi, D., Michiels, C., Ferone, O., Grégoire, V., Lucas, S., Borght, T. V. and Galleza, B. (2013). Antibody-functionalized nanoparticles for imaging cancer: influence of conjugation to gold nanoparticles on the biodistribution of ^{89}Zr-labeled cetuximab in mice, *Contrast Media Mol. Imaging*, **8**, pp. 402–408.
52. Boros, E., Bowen, A. M., Josephson, L., Vasdev, N. and Holland, J. P. (2015). Chelate-free metal ion binding and heat-induced radiolabeling of iron oxide nanoparticles, *Chem. Sci.*, **6**, pp. 225–236.
53. Chen, F., Goel, S., Valdovinos, H. F., Luo, H., Hernandez, R., Barnhart, T. E. and Cai, W. (2015). *In vivo* integrity and biological fate of chelator-free zirconium-89-labeled mesoporous silica nanoparticles, *ACS Nano*, **9**(8), pp. 7950–7959.
54. Li, N., Yu, Z., Pham, T. T., Blower, P. J. and Yan, R. (2017). A generic ^{89}Zr labeling method to quantify the *in vivo* pharmacokinetics of liposomal nanoparticles with positron emission tomography, *Int. J. Nanomed.*, **12**, pp. 3281–3294.

55. Felber, M. and Alberto, R. (2015). ^{99m}Tc radiolabeling of Fe_3O_4–Au core–shell and Au–Fe_3O_4 dumbbell-like nanoparticles, *Nanoscale*, **7**, pp. 6653–6660.

56. Sandiford, L., Phinikaridou, A., Protti, A., Meszaros, L. K., Cui, X., Yan, Y., Frodsham, G., Williamson, P. A., Gaddum, N., Botnar, R. M., Blower, P. J., Green, M. A. and de Rosales, R. T. M. (2013). Bisphosphonate-anchored PEGylation and radiolabeling of superparamagnetic iron oxide: long-circulating nanoparticles for *in vivo* multimodal (T1 MRI-SPECT) imaging, *ACS Nano*, **7**(1), pp. 500–512.

57. Misri, R., Meier, D., Yung, A. C., Kozlowski, P. and Häfeli, U. O. (2012). Development and evaluation of a dual-modality (MRI/SPECT) molecular imaging bioprobe, *Nanomed. Nanotechnol. Biol. Med.*, **8**, pp. 1007–1016.

58. Deng, S., Zhang, W., Zhang, B., Hong, R., Chen, Q., Dong, J., Chen, Y., Chen, Z. and Wu, Y. (2015). Radiolabeled cyclic arginine-glycine-aspartic (RGD)-conjugated iron oxide nanoparticles as single-photon emission computed tomography (SPECT) and magnetic resonance imaging (MRI) dual-modality agents for imaging of breast cancer, *J. Nanopart. Res.*, **17**, p. 19.

59. Chen, F., Ellison, P. A., Lewis, C. M., Hong, H., Zhang, Y., Shi, S., Hernandez, R., Meyer, M. E., Barnhart, T. E. and Cai, W. (2013). Chelator-free synthesis of a dual-modality PET/MRI agent, *Angew. Chem. Int. Ed.*, **125**, pp. 13561–13565.

60. Sharma, R., Xu, Y., Kim, S. W., Schueller, M. J., Alexoff, D., Smith, S. D., Wang, W. and Schlyer, D. (2013). Carbon-11 radiolabeling of iron-oxide nanoparticles for dual-modality PET/MR imaging, dual-modality imaging, using Magnetic Resonance Imaging (MRI) and Positron Emission, *Nanoscale*, **5**, pp. 7476–7483.

61. Truillet, C., Bouziotis, P., Tsoukalas, C., Brugière, J., Martini, M., Sancey, L., Brichart, T., Denat, F., Boschetti, F., Darbost, U., Bonnamour, I., Stellas, D., Anagnostopoulos, C. D., Koutoulidis, V., Moulopoulos, L. A., Perriat, P., Lux, F. and Tillement, O. (2015). Ultrasmall particles for Gd-MRI and ^{68}Ga-PET dual imaging, *Contrast Media Mol. Imaging*, **10**(4), pp. 309–319.

62. Bouziotis, P., Stellas, D., Thomas, E., Truillet, C., Tsoukalas, C., Lux, F., Tsotakos, T., Xanthopoulos, S., Paravatou-Petsotas, M., Gaitanis, A., Moulopoulos, L. I., Koutoulidis, V., Anagnostopoulos, C. D. and Tillement, O. (2017). ^{68}Ga-radiolabeled AGuIX nanoparticles as dual-modality imaging agent for PET/MRI guided radiation therapy, *Nanomedicine*, **12**(13), pp. 1561–1574.

63. Truillet, C., Thomas, E., Lux, F., Huynh, L. T., Tillement, O. and Evans, M. J. (2016). Synthesis and characterization of ^{89}Zr-labeled ultrasmall nanoparticles, *Mol. Pharmaceutics*, **13**(7), pp. 2596–2601.

64. Moon, S. H., Yang, B. Y., Kim, Y. J., Hong, M. K., Lee, Y. S., Lee, D. S., Chung, J. K. and Jeong, J. M. (2016). Development of a complementary PET/MR dual-modal imaging probe for targeting prostate-specific membrane antigen (PSMA), *Nanomed. Nanotechnol. Biol. Med.*, **12**, pp. 871–879.

65. Yang, B. Y., Moon, S. H., Seelam, S. R., Jeon, M. J., Lee, Y. S., Soo, D., Chung, L. J. K., Kim, Y. I. and Jeong, J. M. (2015). Development of a multimodal imaging probe by encapsulating iron oxide nanoparticles with functionalized amphiphiles for lymph node imaging, *Nanomedicine*, **10**(12), pp. 1899–1910.

66. Thorek, D. L. J., Ulmert, D., Diop, N. F. M., Lupu, M. E., Doran, M. G., Huang, R., Abou, D. S., Larson, S. M. and Grimm, J. (2014). Non-invasive mapping of deep-tissue lymph nodes in live animals using a multimodal PET/MRI nanoparticle, *Nat. Commun.*, **5**, p. 3097.

67. de Rosales, R. T. M., Tavare, R., Paul, R. L., Jauregui-Osoro, M., Protti, A., Glaria, A., Varma, G., Szanda, I. and Blower, P. J. (2011). Synthesis of ^{64}CuII–bis(dithiocarbamatebisphosphonate) and its conjugation with superparamagnetic iron oxide nanoparticles: *in vivo* evaluation as dual-modality PET–MRI agent, *Angew. Chem. Int. Ed.*, **50**, pp. 5509–5513.

68. Lamichhane, N., Dewkar, G. K., Sundaresan, G., Mahon R. N. and Zweit, J. (2017). [^{18}F]-fluorinated carboplatin and [^{111}In]-liposome for image-guided drug delivery, *Int. J. Mol. Sci.*, **18**, pp. e1079.

69. Banerjee, S. R., Foss, C. A., Horhota, A., Pullambhatla, M., McDonnell, K., Zale, S. and Pomper, M. G. (2017). An ^{111}In- and IRDye800CW-labeled PLA-PEG nanoparticle for imaging prostate-specific membrane antigen-expressing tissues, *Biomacromolecules*, **18**(1), pp. 201–209.

70. Yamaguchi, H., Tsuchimochi, M., Hayama, K., Kawase, T. and Tsubokawa, N. (2016). Dual-labeled near-infrared/^{99m}Tc imaging probes using PAMAM-coated silica nanoparticles for the imaging of HER2-expressing cancer cells, *Int. J. Mol. Sci.*, **17**, p. 1086.

71. Li, X., Xiong, Z., Xu, X., Luo, Y., Peng, C., Shen, M. and Shi, X. (2016). ^{99m}Tc-labeled multifunctional low generation dendrimer-entrapped gold nanoparticles for targeted SPECT/CT dual-mode imaging of tumors, *ACS Appl. Mater. Interfaces*, **8**(31), pp. 19883–19891.

72. Tang, Y., Zhang, C., Wang, J., Lin, X., Zhang, L., Yang, Y., Wang, Y., Zhang, Z., Bulte, J. W. M. and Yang, G. Y. (2015). MRI/SPECT/fluorescent tri-modal probe for evaluating the homing and therapeutic efficacy of

transplanted mesenchymal stem cells in a rat ischemic stroke model, *Adv. Funct. Mater.*, **25**(7), pp. 1024–1034.

73. Khan, M. K., Minc, L. D., Nigavekar, S. S., Kariapper, M. S., Nair, B. M., Schipper, M., Cook, A. C., Lesniak, W. G. and Balogh, L. P. (2008). Fabrication of {^{198}Au0} radioactive composite nanodevices and their use for nanobrachytherapy, *Nanomedicine*, **4**, pp. 57–69.

74. Chanda, N., Kan, P., Watkinson, L. D., Shukla, R., Zambre, A., Carmack, T., Engelbrecht, H., Lever, J., Katti, K., Fent, G., Casteel, S., Smith, J., Miller, W., Jurisson, S., Boote, E., Robertson, D., Cutler, C., Dobrovolskaia, M., Kannan, R. and Katti, K. (2010). Radioactive gold nanoparticles in cancer therapy: therapeutic efficacy studies of Ga-^{198}AuNP nanoconstruct in prostate tumor-bearing mice, *Nanomedicine*, **6**, pp. 201–209.

75. Shultz, M. D., Duchamp, J. C., Wilson, J., Shu, C., Ge, J. Zhang, J., Gibson, H., Fillmore, H., Hirsch, J., Dorn, H. and Fatouros, P. (2010). Encapsulation of a radiolabeled cluster inside a fullerene cage, $^{177}Lu_xLu_{(3-x)}N@C80$: an interleukin-13-conjugated radiolabeled metallofullerene platform, *J. Am. Chem. Soc.*, **132**, pp. 4980–4981.

76. Diener, M. D., Alford, J. M., Kennel, S. and Mirzadeh, S. (2007). 212Pb@C60 and its water-soluble derivatives: synthesis, stability, and suitability for radioimmunotherapy, *J. Am. Chem. Soc.*, **129**, pp. 5131–5138.

77. Bult, W., Varkevisser, R., Soulimani, F., Seevinck, P., Leeuw, H., Bakker, C., Luijten, P., van het Schip, A., Hennick, W. and Nijsen, F. (2010). Holmium nanoparticles: preparation and in vitro characterization of a new device for radioablation of solid malignancies, *Pharm. Res.*, **27**, pp. 2205–2212.

78. Bao, A., Goins, B., Klipper, R., Negrete, G., Mahindaratne, M. and Phillips, W. T. (2003). A novel liposome radiolabeling method using 99mTc-"SNS/S" complexes: in vitro and in vivo evaluation, *J. Pharm. Sci.*, **92**, pp. 1893–1904.

79. Shukla, R., Chanda, N., Zambre, A., Upendran, A., Katti, K., Kulkarni, R. R., Nune, S. K., Casteel, S. W., Smith, C. J., Vimal, J., Boote, E., Robertson, J. D., Kan, P., Engelbrecht, H., Watkinson, L. D., Carmack, T. L., Lever, J. R., Cutler, C. S., Caldwell, C., Kannan, R. and Katti, K. V. (2012). Laminin receptor specific therapeutic gold nanoparticles (^{198}AuNP-EGCg) show efficacy in treating prostate cancer, *Proc. Natl. Acad. Sci. U.S.A.*, **109**(31), pp. 12426–12431.

80. Jiménez-Mancilla, N., Ferro-Flores, G., Santos-Cuevas, C., Ocampo-García, B., Luna-Gutiérrez, M., Azorín-Vega, E., Isaac-Olivé, K., Camacho-

López, M. and Torres-García, E. (2013). Multifunctional targeted therapy system based on $^{99m}Tc/^{177}Lu$-labeled gold nanoparticles-Tat(49–57)-Lys3-bombesin internalized in nuclei of prostate cancer cells, *J. Label. Compd. Radiopharm.*, **56**, pp. 663–671.

81. Vilchis-Juárez, A., Ferro-Flores, G., Santos-Cuevas, C., Morales-Avila, E., Ocampo-García, B., Díaz-Nieto, L., Luna-Gutiérrez, M., Jiménez-Mancilla, N., Pedraza-López, M. and Gómez-Oliván, L. (2014). Molecular targeting radiotherapy with cyclo-RGDfK(C) peptides conjugated to ^{177}Lu-labeled gold nanoparticles in tumor-bearing mice, *J. Biomed. Nanotechnol.*, **10**(3), pp. 393–404.

82. Yook, S., Lu, Y., Jeong, J. J., Cai, Z., Tong, L., Alwarda, R., Pignol, J. P., Winnik, M. A. and Reilly, R. M. (2016). Stability and biodistribution of thiol-functionalized and ^{177}Lu-labeled metal chelating polymers (MCP) bound to gold nanoparticles, *Biomacromolecules*, **17**(4), pp. 1292–1302.

83. Yook, S., Cai, Z., Lu, Y., Winnik, M. A., Pignol, J. P. and Reilly, R. M. (2016). Intratumorally injected ^{177}Lu-labeled gold nanoparticles - gold nanoseed brachytherapy with application for neo-adjuvant treatment of locally advanced breast cancer (LABC), *J. Nucl. Med.*, **57**(6), pp. 936–942

84. Li, W., Liu, Z., Li, C., Li, N., Fang, L., Chang, J. and Tan, J. (2016). Radionuclide therapy using ^{131}I-labeled anti-epidermal growth factor receptor-targeted nanoparticles suppresses cancer cell growth caused by EGFR overexpression, *J. Cancer Res. Clin. Oncol.*, **142**, pp. 619–632.

85. Radovic, M., Vranjes-Djuric, S., Nikolic, N., Jankovic, D., Goya, G. F., Torres, T. E., Calatayud, M. P., Bruvera, I. J., Ibarra, M. R., Spasojevic, V., Jancare, B. and Antic, B. (2012). Development and evaluation of ^{90}Y-labeled albumin microspheres loaded with magnetite nanoparticles for possible applications in cancer therapy, *J. Mater. Chem.*, **22**, pp. 24017–24025.

86. McLaughlin, M. F., Woodward, J., Boll, R. A., Wall, J. S., Rondinone, A. J., Kennel, S. J., Mirzadeh, S. and Robertson, J. D. (2013). Gold coated lanthanide phosphate nanoparticles for targeted alpha generator radiotherapy, *PLoS One*, **8**(1), pp. e54531.

87. McLaughlin, M. F., Robertson, D., Pevsner, P. H., Wall, J. S., Mirzadeh, S. and Kennel, S. J. (2014). $LnPO_4$ nanoparticles doped with Ac-225 and sequestered daughters for targeted alpha therapy, *Cancer Biother. Radiopharm.*, **29**(1), pp. 34–41.

88. Lingappa, M., Song, H., Thompson, S., Bruchertseifer, F., Morgenstern, A. and Sgouros, G. (2010). Immunoliposomal delivery of ^{213}Bi for

α-emitter targeting of metastatic breast cancer, *Cancer Res.*, **70**(17), pp. 6815–6823.

89. Rojas, J. V., Woodward, J. D., Chen, N., Rondinone, A. J., Castano, C. H. and Mirzadeh, S. (2015). Synthesis and characterization of lanthanum phosphate nanoparticles as carriers for ^{223}Ra and ^{225}Ra for targeted alpha therapy, *Nucl. Med. Biol.*, **42**(7), pp. 614–620.

90. Chow, T. H., Lin, Y. Y., et al. (2008). Diagnostic and therapeutic evaluation of ^{111}Invinorelbine- liposomes in a human colorectal carcinoma HT-29/luc-bearing animal model, *Nucl. Med. Biol.*, **35**(5), pp. 623–634.

91. Liu, X., Nakamura, K., et al. (2010). Auger-mediated cytotoxicity of cancer cells in culture by an ^{125}I-antisense oligomer delivered as a three-component streptavidin nanoparticle, *J. Biomed. Nanotechnol.*, **6**(2), pp. 153–157.

92. Liu, X., Wang, Y., et al. (2009). Auger radiation-induced, antisense-mediated cytotoxicity of tumor cells using a 3-component streptavidin-delivery nanoparticle with ^{111}In, *J. Nucl. Med.*, **50**(4), pp. 582–590.

93. Reske, S. N., Deisenhofer, S., et al. (2007). ^{123}I-ITdU-mediated nanoirradiation of DNA efficiently induces cell kill in HL60 leukemia cells and in doxorubicin-, beta-, or gamma-radiation-resistant cell lines, *J. Nucl. Med.*, **48**(6), pp. 1000–1007.

94. Cai, Z., Chattopadhyay, N., Yang, K., Kwon, Y. L., Yook, S., Pignol, J. P. and Reilly, R. M. (2016). ^{111}In-labeled trastuzumab-modified gold nanoparticles are cytotoxic *in vitro* to HER2-positive breast cancer cells and arrest tumor growth *in vivo* in athymic mice after intratumoral injection, *Nucl. Med. Biol.*, **43**, pp. 818–826.

95. Song, L., Falzone, N. and Vallis, K. A. (2016). EGF-coated gold nanoparticles provide an efficient nano-scale delivery system for the molecular radiotherapy of EGFR-positive cancer, *Int. J. Radiat. Biol.*, **92**(11), pp. 716–723.

96. Gobbo, O. L., Sjaastad, K., Radomski, M. W., Volkov, Y. and Prina-Mello, A. (2015). Magnetic nanoparticles in cancer theranostics, *Theranostics*, **5**(11), pp. 1249–1263.

97. Chen, F., Ehlerding, E. B. and Cai, W. (2014). Theranostic nanoparticles, *J. Nucl. Med.*, **55**, pp. 1919–1922.

98. (a) Muthu, M. S., Leong, D. T., Mei, L. and Feng, S.-S. (2014). Nanotheranostics: application and further development of nanomedicine strategies for advanced theranostics, *Theranostics*, **4**, pp. 660–677. (b) Bouziotis, P., Psimadas, D., Tsotakos, T., Stamopoulos, D. Tsoukalas, C. (2013). Radiolabeled iron oxide nanoparticles as dual-

modality SPECT/MRI and PET/MRI agents, *Curr. Top. Med. Chem.*, **12**(23), pp. 2694–2702.

99. Nosrati, S., Shanehsazzadeh, S., Yousefnia, H., Gholami, A., Grüttner, C., Jalilian, A. R., Hosseini, R. H. and Lahooti, A. (2016). Biodistribution evaluation of ^{166}Ho–DTPA–SPION in normal rats, *J. Radioanal. Nucl. Chem.*, **307**, pp. 1559–1566.

100. Radovic, M., Calatayud, M. P., Goya, G. F., Ibarra, M. R., Antic, B., Spasojevic, V., Nikolic, N., Jankovic, D., Mirkovic, M. and Vranjes-Duric, S. (2015). Preparation and *in vivo* evaluation of multifunctional ^{90}Y-labeled magnetic nanoparticles designed for cancer therapy, *J. Biomed. Mater. Res. Part A*, **103**(1), pp. 126–134.

101. Cheng, Y., Zhu, J., Zhao, L., Xiong, Z., Tang, Y., Liu, C., Guo, L., Qiao, W., Shi, X. and Zhao, J. (2016). ^{131}I-labeled multifunctional dendrimers modified with BmK CT for targeted SPECT imaging and radiotherapy of gliomas, *Nanomedicine*, **11**(10), pp. 1253–1266.

102. Mendoza-Nava, H., Ferro-Flores, G., de María Ramírez, F., Ocampo-García, B., Santos-Cuevas, C., Aranda-Lara, L., Azorín-Vega, E., Morales-Avila, E. and Isaac-Olivé, K. (2016). ^{177}Lu-dendrimer conjugated to folate and bombesin with gold nanoparticles in the dendritic cavity: a potential theranostic radiopharmaceutical, *J. Nanomater.*, **2016**, Article ID 1039258 (11 pp.).

103. Zolata, H., Davani, F. A. and Afarideh, H. (2015). Synthesis, characterization and theranostic evaluation of Indium-111 labeled multifunctional superparamagnetic iron oxide nanoparticles, *Nucl. Med. Biol.*, **42**, pp. 164–170.

104. Farrag, N. S., El-Sabagh, H. A., Al-Mahallawi, A. M., Amin, A. M., AbdEl-Bary, A. and Mamdouh, W. (2017). Comparative study on radiolabeling and biodistribution of core-shell silver/polymeric nanoparticles-based theranostics for tumor targeting. *Int. J. Pharm.*, **521(**1–2), pp. 123–133.

105. Yang, X., Hong, H., Grailer, J. J., Rowland, I. J., Javadi, A., Hurley, S. A., Xiao, Y., Yang, Y., Zhang, Y., Nickles, R. J., Cai, W., Steeber, D. A. and Gong, S. (2011). cRGD-functionalized, DOX-conjugated, and ^{64}Cu-labeled superparamagnetic iron oxide nanoparticles for targeted anticancer drug delivery and PET/MR imaging, *Biomaterials*, **32**, pp. 4151–4160.

106. Wang, J., Zhao, H., Zhou, Z., Zhou, P., Yan, Y., Wang, M., Yang, H., Zhang, Y. and Yang, S. (2016). MR/SPECT imaging guided photothermal therapy of tumor-targeting Fe@Fe_3O_4 nanoparticles *in vivo* with low mononuclear phagocyte uptake, *ACS Appl. Mater. Interfaces*, **8**(31), pp. 19872–19882.

107. Tsiapa, I., Efthimiadou, E. K., Fragogeorgi, E., Loudos, G., Varvarigou, A. D., Bouziotis, P., Kordas, G. C., Mihailidis, D., Nikiforidis, G. C., Xanthopoulos, S., Psimadas, D., Paravatou-Petsotas, M., Palamaris, L., Hazle, J. D. and Kagadis, G. C. (2014). ^{99m}Tc-labeled aminosilane-coated iron oxide nanoparticles for molecular imaging of $\alpha_v\beta_3$ -mediated tumor expression and feasibility for hyperthermia treatment, *J. Colloid Interface Sci.*, **433**, pp. 163–175.

108. Gao, H., Liu, X., Tang, W., Niu, D., Zhou, B., Zhang, H., Liu, W., Gub, B., Zhou, X., Zheng, Y., Sun, Y., Jia, X. and Zhou, L. (2016). ^{99m}Tc-conjugated manganese-based mesoporous silica nanoparticles for SPECT, pH-responsive MRI and anti-cancer drug delivery, *Nanoscale*, **8**(47), pp. 19573–19580.

Chapter 11

In vivo Imaging as a Tool to Noninvasively Study Nanosystems

George Loudos and Maria Tina Rouchota
Technological Educational Institute of Athens
Athens, Attiki 15235, Greece
gloudos@teiath.gr; m.rouchota@upatras.gr

11.1 Introduction

In vivo imaging is continuously gaining interest as an efficient noninvasive technique of testing new biomolecules, drugs, and nanoparticles (NPs) in vivo. Over the past 30 years various physical principles describing interaction between radiation and matter have been explored, leading to a number of exciting methodologies that provide anatomic, functional, metabolic, and molecular information. Several techniques have been translated clinically, while all of them keep evolving in terms of improving performance and extending applications.

Nanotechnology is obviously a field that has benefitted a lot from in vivo imaging, although its use as a standard part of nanosystems evaluation is not established. One can argue that this delay is mainly

Drug Delivery Nanosystems: From Bioinspiration and Biomimetics to Clinical Applications
Edited by Costas Demetzos, Stergios Pispas, and Natassa Pippa

ISBN 978-981-4774-92-5 (Hardcover), 978-0-429-49054-5 (eBook)
www.panstanford.com

due to the multidisciplinary nature of nanomedicine; NPs are usually synthesized by chemists; in vivo applications are studied by biologists, and imaging is still led by groups of either medical physicists or engineers. However, over the past decade there have been various examples of using different imaging technologies for studying all types of NPs in different in vivo applications. As for other biomolecules, different imaging techniques aim to provide noninvasively answers to several questions that are raised when studying a new tracer. Some questions are:

- Do NPs reach the target for which they are designed?
- When are NPs in the highest concentration on the target?
- How long do they stay in blood circulation?
- Are they also concentrated in organs/tissues that are not targeted?
- Are they stable postinjection; do they form aggregates?
- What happens in the first few minutes postinjection?
- What is the optimal administration route?
- What is the optimal injected concentration?
- How shall we prepare the animals to maximize targeting?
- When is the best time for obtaining biodistribution points?

Definitely, the power of imaging modalities increases when NPs have physical properties that can enhance the imaging signals of one or more imaging modality. In this chapter the major in vivo imaging modalities, with emphasis on preclinical imaging, will be reviewed. Representative examples of performed studies will be given to demonstrate the added value of in vivo imaging in nanomedicine research.

Although part of the scientific community debates which modality is the best, the authors believe that each modality has its own advantages and disadvantages. Some of them are technical and some are related to cost and the availability of technology, and of course one should take into account that different modalities provide different nuggets of information. Thus, it is important that an end user be aware of all available technologies, understand the biological problem that needs to be solved, and decide on the proper technology or technologies to be used. Some basic characteristics of existing imaging modalities are given in Fig. 11.1.

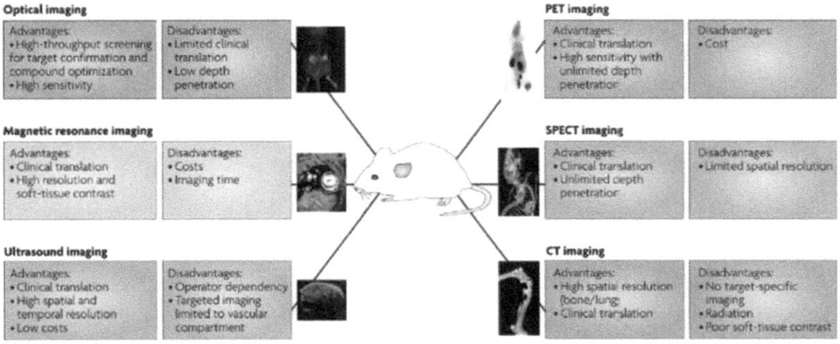

Figure 11.1 Pros and cons of main imaging technologies used in nanomedicine.

11.2 X-Ray Imaging

11.2.1 Basic Principles of X-ray and CT Imaging and Instrumentation

X-rays have been used in medicine as the basis of the first anatomical imaging technique, which continues to evolve up to now. It is based on the simple transmission of X-rays, which are emitted from a source (usually an X-ray tube) and are recorded from an analog or digital detector. As a result, an attenuation map of the object to be imaged is provided, which results in an image of gray values. In the simple X-ray imaging the resulting 2D image has no depth information and overlapping structures are projected in one plane. However, this technique provides a simple image of an animal or human interior and is considered as a trivial exam in many clinical applications. By rotating the object or the detector and applying reconstruction algorithms, one obtains tomographic images of high anatomical information, leading to computed tomography (CT) [1]. CT was invented by Hounsfield and today is a standard clinical tool in all hospitals worldwide. The power of CT imaging has been widely exploited in preclinical research. Downscaling of all necessary components and electronics has led to the development of micro-CT, which has superior performance compared to clinical systems and is now commercially available and optimized for small-animal imaging in preclinical research [2].

Modern micro-CT scanners offer superb cross-sectional images of soft-tissue and skeletal structures with submillimeter spatial resolution, subsecond temporal resolution, and good contrast. The spatial resolution and signal-to-noise ratio (SNR) of micro-CT depend on the operating characteristics of the X-ray tube, the pixel size of the detector, the distance of the examined object from the radiation source, the type of detector, and the focal spot size. Most micro-CT scanners use transmission targets with a focal spot size ranging from 1 to 10 μm, which is far smaller compared to clinical ones, allowing the reconstruction of images with a voxel size of 50 μm. The emitted fan beam or cone beam and the continuous spiral rotation of the X-ray source allow scanning of small objects in a single rotation, which is rather fast and eliminates motion artifacts [3].

11.2.2 Imaging of Gold Nanoparticles

Today CT imaging is usually a stand-alone anatomical technique or is combined with other molecular imaging techniques to provide the anatomical map of an animal or a human. However, the introduction of nanosystems, and mainly gold nanoparticles (GNPs), opened new prospects in its application in molecular imaging. GNPs have been actively studied over the past years as contrast agents in X-ray and CT imaging. GNPs are of particular interest in medical applications, mainly due to their unique optical and electronic properties, as well as their biological compatibility. The physicochemical properties of GNPs can be tuned by selecting their size and shape, as well as their surface functionalization. Details about their preparation and targeting can be found in several references [4]. Today a variety of different GNPs have been produced, including rods, wires, belts and combs, plates and prisms, polyhedra, cages and frames, caps, stars and flowers, and dendrites [5].

The solutions of GNPs show very intense absorption and different colors depending upon the size and shape of the NPs. Over the last decade GNPs have gained attention as an X-ray contrast agent since they exhibit a high X-ray attenuation coefficient compared with standard clinical contrast agents (barium sulfate and iodine), especially at the energy levels of clinical CT [6]. Moreover, they have a longer vascular retention time compared with iodine, due to their higher molecular weight, which increases the available imaging window. Since they are already tested at the clinical level, it is important for them to be designed so they meet the necessary requirements: delivery, nontoxicity, targeting, and contrast enhancement. Key properties include X-ray attenuation coefficient, colloidal stability in physiological media and during storage, vascular retention time, biodistribution, and cytotoxicity. Phantom studies have shown that the X-ray attenuation of GNPs increases linearly with mass concentration, indicating that the delivery of a high concentration of GNPs on the target will result in a high contrast [7].

Several applications of imaging GNPs have been reported, mostly focused on oncology, and some indicatives are given here. Nakagawa et al. [8] used NPs as a CT contrast agent to image tumors using an enhanced permeability and retention (EPR) effect. They showed that the localization of the GNPs in the tumor is affected by differences in particle size and was enhanced by the conjugation of a specific antibody against the tumor. Wang et al. [9] reported the use of folic acid–modified dendrimer-entrapped GNPs as nanoprobes for in vivo targeted CT imaging of human lung adenocarcinoma and successfully explored intravenous, intratumoral, and intraperitoneal administration of the particles. Kim et al. [10] labeled human mesenchymal stem cells with 40 nm citrate-stabilized GNPs and used CT imaging for different cell concentrations, showing that the number of labeled cells can be quantified in a way that is similar when radioactive or fluorine tracers are used. Chhour et al. [11] used GNPs to label monocytes located within plaques, allowing noninvasive CT imaging to be used as a tool to assess monocyte accumulation within plaques. In a very interesting study, Xu et al. [12] studied the interaction between renal clearable GNPs and the kidneys with normal function and unilateral ureteral obstruction. Their results show that the accumulation and clearance of renal clearable GNPs in normal and obstructed kidneys could be quantitatively and noninvasively evaluated with planar X-ray imaging at a contrast six times higher than that provided by iodine agents.

A typical image of commercially available GNPs is shown in Fig. 11.2.

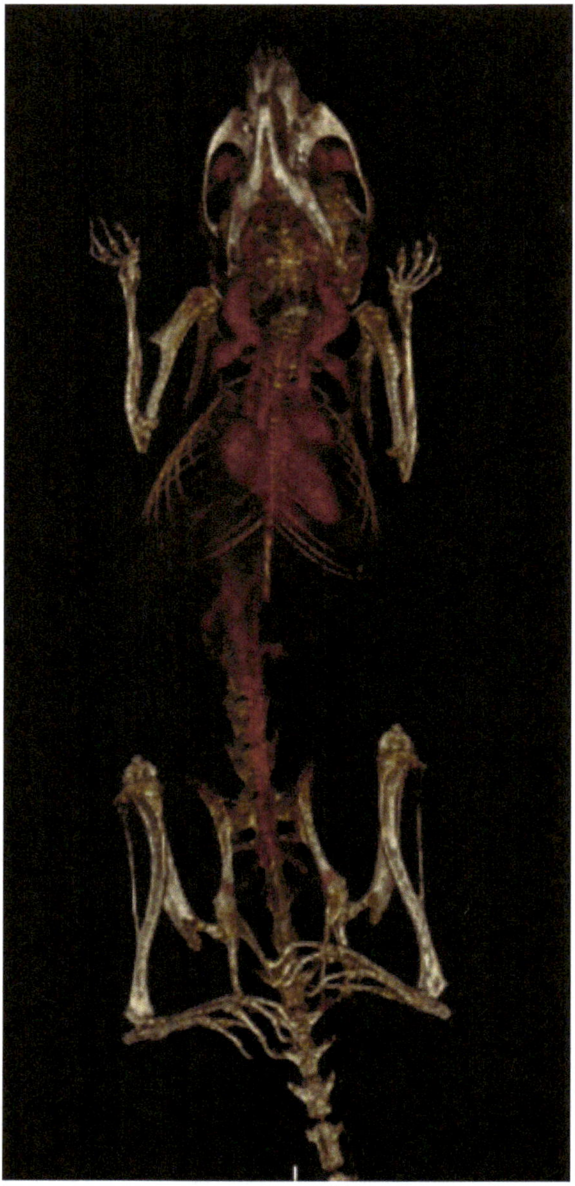

Figure 11.2 In vivo micro-CT of a mouse after injection with a commercial 15 nm X-ray contrast agent. Courtesy of BIOEMTECH, GR.

11.3 MRI

11.3.1 Basic Principles and Instrumentation

Magnetic resonance imaging (MRI) is a very powerful and versatile imaging modality with various clinical applications, ranging from anatomical to functional and molecular imaging. It exploits the magnetic properties of water hydrogen atoms, which are present in living organisms, when a strong static magnetic field, on the order of 0.5 to 9.4 tesla, is applied [13]. A series of repetitive radio frequency pulses and gradients excite the spins of hydrogen atoms, followed by Fourier space sampling to reconstruct multiplanar images of the organ(s) of interest. Different sophisticated MRI sequences have been developed, which extract rich information about anatomy, morphology, function, and metabolism.

Functional MRI allows imaging and anatomic identification of areas of the brain while the subject performs a specific task. Today dedicated micro-MRI systems provide noninvasive in vivo whole-body small-animal imaging with a high spatial resolution, around 100 μm for rodent studies, and excellent contrast for soft tissue differentiation [14]. Such systems are commercially available from various manufacturers and are a powerful tool in preclinical research, including the study of NPs, covering a wide range of applications, from oncology and brain research to cardiology and tissue engineering. Besides standard imaging, the principles of magnetic resonance are explored in other applications. The most common is magnetic resonance spectroscopy, which involves identification of the atomic spectra of regions of interest [14]. Finally, hyperpolarized MRI is a rapidly evolving technique that can dramatically increase the SNR in magnetic resonance [15] and will definitely have a strong impact on its applications, including nanomedicine.

11.3.2 Imaging of Magnetic Nanoparticles

Magnetic nanoparticles (MNPs) have attracted a lot of attention as MRI contrast agents. Iron oxide NPs (IONPs) and ferrite NPs shorten T2* relaxation times and have been successfully employed as T2

MRI contrast agents with improved properties. Extensive research has resulted in the development of T1 contrast agents, which bypass the drawbacks of iron oxide–negative T2 contrast agents. The use of MNPs as MRI contrast agents is an active but already mature field, which includes several applications at different and exciting domains besides oncology. While the recent trend is toward the use of MNPs for multimodal imaging, in this section examples of using only MRI are given. The recent literature is rich and some indicative examples are reported.

Schleich et al. used alternative strategies for targeting tumors: via the EPR effect and passive targeting, active targeting of $\alpha_v\beta_3$ integrin via arginine-glycine-aspartic (RGD) grafting, use of an external magnetic field a combination of the magnetic field and active targeting [16]. MRI successfully quantified and visualized the concentration of NPs in the tumors and the advantages of combining active and magnetic targeting. Yilmaz et al. [17] used IONPs and T2-/T2*-weighted MRI for noninvasive myocardial macrophage imaging. Although they did not observe significant enhancement of the myocardial (peri-)infarct zone using this imaging compared to conventional gadolinium-based necrosis/fibrosis imaging, the study was performed clinically, showing the potential of this approach. Cheng et al. [18] combined superparamagnetic iron oxide NPs (SPIONs) with curcumin, a natural compound that specifically binds to amyloid plaques, and used T2* MRI on mice to visualize amyloid plaques. Immunohistochemical examination of the mouse brains revealed that curcumin MNPs were colocalized with amyloid plaques, showing the potential of noninvasive diagnosis of Alzheimer's disease with MRI. Kim et al. [19] used MNPs to label bone-marrow-derived mesenchymal stromal cells and neural stem cells and then used a 3T MRI for imaging in vivo a cancer mouse model. The study showed that this approach should facilitate the translation of this agent to clinical trials for evaluation of trafficking of cells by MRI. Lee et al. [20] investigated the potential of limiting the aggravation of osteoporosis by reducing the activity of osteoclasts (OCs) through thermolysis, by culturing osteoblasts and OCs with IONPs. MRI was successfully used to visualize the accumulation of NPs in osteoporosis applications.

11.4 Ultrasound

11.4.1 Basic Principles and Instrumentation

Ultrasonography, or ultrasound (US), provides anatomical information about soft tissue structures by taking advantage of the differential transmission and reflection of US waves in the range of 5–20 MHz between adjacent tissue layers. The higher the delivered US frequency, the higher the tissue spatial resolution achieved, at the expense of higher attenuation by tissue, resulting in more superficial penetration [21].

Depending on probe wavelength and depth of the target organ, an US provides a fast, portable, and cost-efficient diagnostic image with a high frame rate, high resolution, high sensitivity, and sufficient contrast. Today, US imaging is a highly versatile real-time technique that can be useful in various applications, offering anatomical screening of organ disease and pathology on multiple anatomical planes.

On a preclinical level, high-frequency linear or curvilinear broadband transducers operating around 12–15 MHz are employed for solid organ and soft tissue imaging of small animals, like mice. US employs several real-time techniques, including M-Mode, which refers to 1D imaging of space over time; B-Mode, which is 2D imaging over time; 3D static or dynamic imaging; and color Doppler sonography, which provides hemodynamic information about heart and vessel blood flow on the basis of the Doppler frequency-shift phenomenon [22].

11.4.2 Imaging Nanobubbles

US contrast agents are gas-filled microbubbles (MBs) with diameters between 1 and 5 μm. Due to their size, MBs have optimal acoustic responses in the MHz range used for US imaging. In principle, multimodal US contrast agents entrap, attach, or adsorp other imaging agents, including NPs, in or on the shell of the MB in order to allow the exploitation of USs for NP imaging. In recent years, nanobubbles (NBs) with shells composed of polymers or phospholipids and gas, liquid, or solid cores have been applied in extravascular US imaging. A small particle size is a basic requirement for US contrast-enhanced agents that penetrate tumor blood vessel pores to allow for targeted imaging and therapy. However, compared to MBs, the nanoscale size of the particles used has the disadvantage of weakening the imaging ability of clinical diagnostic US.

Most reported applications of NBs focus on tumor imaging. Yin et al. [23] showed that lipid NBs with a size of ~435 nm were suitable for passive tumor targeting US imaging and suggested that the ultrasonic imaging ability was comparable to that of MBs. Yang et al. [24] developed uniform nanosized NBs of ~480 nm, which were conjugated antibody molecules with specific affinity to human epidermal growth factor receptor type 2 (HER2)-overexpressing tumors. These NBs presented good US enhancement, being a promising agent for efficient molecular imaging with potential application in early cancer quantitative diagnosis. Long et al. [25] have used oxygen NBs < 100 nm as a vehicle for site-specific oxygen delivery and simultaneously as a US contrast agent. In vivo studies showed that NBs can be used as a means for epigenetic regulation, US imaging, and cancer therapeutics, thus having a significant impact on new-age cancer treatment methods in oncology. Foroutan et al. [26] assessed the use of biodegradable P_2O_5–CaO–Na_2O phosphate-based glass nanospheres for labeling mesenchymal stem cells. Then US imaging was used and confirmed their promising use as contrast agents for this modality.

11.5 Scintigraphic and SPECT Imaging

11.5.1 Basic Principles and Instrumentation

Single-photon emission computed tomography (SPECT) imaging is based on the detection of gamma photons, emitted from radiotracers and injected in an animal or a human. The basic detector of a SPECT system is the Anger gamma camera [27], which includes all detector modules required to convert emitted photons to images. A collimator made by lead or tungsten is a grid of parallel holes (hexagonal or square), allows the detection of photons traveling parallel to its holes, and is the main limiting factor of a SPECT system's resolution and sensitivity. A scintillator converts all accepted photons to optical photons with energies of a few electron volts. The scintillator is coupled to a photomultiplier tube (PMT) by using an optical light guide and when optical photons strike the PMT's photocathode a number of photoelectrons are emitted. Inside the PMT those electrons are multiplied by a factor of 10^6 and an electron cloud hits the PMT's anode. This signal is collected, amplified, and processed to calculate the energy and position of each incident photon. Thus, a gamma camera works in a photon counting mode and provides planar images that have no depth information, similar to X-ray imaging. When the gamma camera is rotated around the object to be imaged, projection data are obtained and by using a proper reconstruction algorithm tomographic SPECT images are reconstructed [28].

The increased need for dedicated animal studies has pushed SPECT technology over the past 15 years. New collimator designs have drastically improved resolution and sensitivity, leading to systems with a submillimeter resolution. Significant advances have occurred in scintillator research, and several new materials can be used on a small scale, offering a high light output and a very good energy resolution. Position-sensitive PMT tubes were introduced by the end of the 1990s and are the detector of choice in most dedicated SPECT systems, since they offer a very high intrinsic resolution. Recent improvements in readout electronics have increased systems' sensitivity and mainly decreased their overall size and cost. Cadmium zinc telluride systems are an alternative to the combination of the scintillator-PMT modules, allowing direct photon detection with a significantly higher energy resolution. Over the past five years, the introduction of silicon photomultipliers (SiPMs), as a prominent alternative to PMTs, is being rapidly adopted in SPECT [29]. Today, micro-SPECT systems are available from several manufacturers and are usually combined with CT and/or positron emission tomography (PET).

11.5.2 Imaging Nanoparticles Labeled with Gamma Emitters

The use of gamma-emitting isotopes allows imaging NPs with high sensitivity compared to the previously mentioned techniques. Depending on the imaging system a spatial resolution of ~1 mm can provide accurate quantitative information of an NP's spatiotemporal biodistribution. By selecting isotopes of relatively long half-lives, it is possible to image various NPs for a period of 24 h (for ^{99m}Tc), up to several days when long-lived isotopes are used (i.e., ^{111}In). Furthermore, use of more than one radioisotope, emitting at different energies, is an advantage of SPECT, which allows simultaneous imaging of more than one NP at the same time or a combination of imaging an NP in parallel with a molecular mechanism of interest. While SPECT cannot provide fast 3D images, due to the need of multiple projections, scintigraphic imaging is a very efficient tool for fast screening of various NPs and can easily provide valuable information, especially during their synthesis and optimization steps.

An important consideration is that the labeling of NPs using radioisotopes needs special processing of the NPs and is not straightforward, as is the case for GNPs (with X-rays), MNPs (with MRI), and NBs (with US). Thus, it is important to perform all required stability and radiochemical quality control tests to ensure that labeling is stable and NPs maintain the same characteristics postlabeling; however, such procedures are in place for different biomolecules and can be tuned for application in nanomedicine. However, numerous publications have shown the advantages of this approach in different NP structures.

Although nuclear imaging of NPs is given in another chapter of this book, some indicative and challenging studies are reported here. This author group has used ^{99m}Tc labeling to image various types of nanosystems, including MNPs, liposomes, silver NPs, and polymer NPs. Recently, Fazaeli et al. [30] used graphene oxide (GO) sheets functionalized by aminopropylsilyl groups, labeled by ^{198,199}Au NP radioisotopes for fast in vivo targeting and SPECT imaging. Results showed that ^{198,199}Au@AF-GO provide excellent tumor targeting/imaging and are quickly washed out from the body, being potentially effective and promising nanomaterials in nanotechnology-based cancer diagnosis and therapy. GNPs were functionalized by Black et al. [31] with an MMP9-cleavable peptide and then radiolabeled with both ^{125}I and ^{111}In. The two isotopes allowed the formulation of two separate images during a single scan, enabling in vivo differentiation of tumors with differing MMP9 expression. Tseng et al. [32] used lipid calcium-phosphate NPs, labeled with ^{111}In and suitable for small interfering RNA delivery. Imaging studies showed preferential accumulation in the lymph nodes, which was significantly higher than liver and spleen accumulation in a 4T1 breast cancer lymph node metastasis model. Currently, SPECT is considered as a standard technology for studying NPs and more exciting applications include the combination of the technology with other imaging modalities, which take advantage of the unique NP properties and will be explained later in this chapter.

11.6 Coincidence and PET Imaging

11.6.1 Basic Principles and Instrumentation

PET imaging has several similarities with SPECT, since it includes radiotracer injection and photon detection. However, differences in the main physical principles affect detector design and potential applications. PET radiopharmaceuticals emit positrons instead of photons, which have variable kinetic energy [33]. Depending on this energy, a positron travels a short distance (up to a few millimeters) and when it hits an electron, both are annihilated, producing two antiparallel photons with energy equal to 511 keV. A PET detector should have at least two opposite detectors, while a full ring system maximizes the sensitivity of the technique. In conventional systems these photons are detected by using the same concept as that in the Anger camera, but a major difference is the absence of a collimator. The trajectory of the annihilation point is determined by the line that connects two photons, detected in a short time window (usually 4 to 20 ns). Then a reconstruction algorithm is applied to calculate the position of the annihilation point. PET performance is limited by the positron range, the photons' noncolinearity, scattering, attenuation, and random events, although advanced software tools compensate for them.

Evolution in PET usually starts from the preclinical level, and there are several examples of technological achievements that have been transferred to clinical application. Like SPECT, the combination of position-sensitive PMT tubes and pixelated scintillators leads to a significant improvement in resolution and sensitivity. Rapid evolution in electronics has allowed a significant improvement of temporal resolution on the order of a few picoseconds. This makes possible the calculation of the difference in the time of flight of detected photons. Like SPECT, several commercial micro-PET systems are available; in most cases they are coupled to CT, but the recent trend is their combination with MRI [34].

11.6.2 Imaging Nanoparticles Labeled with Positron Emitters

There are several advantages of using PET isotopes to radiolabel and image NPs. On the preclinical level, the spatial resolution in PET is slightly lower than that in SPECT, but still on the order of 1 mm, while PET sensitivity can be 100 times higher. Current PET systems have ring detectors, which in many cases can cover the entire body of a mouse in a single shot. In this way tomographic imaging is possible immediately after injection, allowing the performance of fast 3D dynamic studies and the use of novel tools, such as kinetic modeling and parametric imaging. Although on a clinical level ^{18}F-FDG and ^{18}F based tracers are used in the majority of applications, new isotopes gain interest. ^{66}Ga and ^{68}Ga, which can be made available by ^{68}Ge/^{68}Ga generators, can be easily coupled to many NPs and do not require a cyclotron. ^{64}Cu, ^{124}I, ^{81}Rb, and ^{89}Zr are being assessed by several research groups since they have long half-lives and they offer the possibility of studying NPs for a long period. Although several studies use PET for imaging various types of NPs, most of them use only PET as an imaging modality for obtaining images of NP biodistribution at different time points [35]. There is still a long way to fully exploiting the power of this technology, including the analysis of collected data and the use of new radioisotopes.

Some interesting examples are the work of Pérez-Medina et al. [36], who radiolabeled high-density lipid NPs with ^{89}Zr for PET imaging of tumor-associated macrophages. They showed that these ^{89}Zr-labeled NPs are specific for macrophages and can provide noninvasive quantitative information for macrophage PET imaging. Yang et al. [37] synthesized ^{64}Cu-doped Au nanocages as tracers for PET imaging. Results showed efficient passive accumulation in both 4T1 and patient-derived xenograft tumor models due to the EPR effect. Lee et al. [38] developed ^{124}I-labeled tannic acid GNPs for dendritic cell (DC) labeling and in vivo tracking of their migration with PET. This tracer was able to track the migration of

DCs to lymphoid organs even in extremely low concentrations. Stockhofe et al. [39] radiolabeled cross-linked micelles with ^{68}Ga as promising new PET imaging tracers. Sirianni et al. [40] used ^{18}F-4-fluorobenzylamine and a commercially available biotin derivate to label poly(lactic-*co*-glycolic acid) (PLGA) NPs. Then by applying PET imaging they measured the kinetics of delivering NPs of varying sizes to the rat brain, obtaining accurate information about NP distribution as a function of time, both during and after the infusion. Definitely, current research trend is a combination of PET with other anatomical or functional techniques for imaging NPs and benefit from their properties. The emphasis is on PET/MRI, as described later, although other interesting combinations are under active investigation.

11.7 Optical Imaging

11.7.1 Basic Principles and Instrumentation

Optical imaging methods use tracers that emit optical photons to image specific targets, without using radiation. Optical imaging can be divided into fluorescence imaging (FLI) and bioluminescence imaging (BLI) [41]. Bioluminescence is a normal process in animals like firefly that express an enzyme called luciferase, as a result of photochemical reactions. In BLI cells of interest have to be engineered first in order to express luciferase and then induced in the small animal. Injection of luciferine results in its oxidization by luciferase, and light is produced 10–12 min. after luciferin injection. This light signal is detected by a charge-coupled device (CCD) camera, and planar intensity images are produced. BLI is a highly sensitive technique, and only a few cells can provide sufficient signal. On the other hand in FLI the optical signal comes from a fluorescent molecule that can be either endogenous (collagen, hemoglobin, etc.) or injected (green fluorescent protein and other optical contrast agents). An external light source is used to excite the fluorophore, and a CCD detects the lower-energy emission light. Additional imaging components are filters that select excitation and emission wavelengths.

The main drawback of optical imaging is the strong absorption and scattering of optical photons, which travel only a few millimeters, thus limiting its application mostly to small animals [42]. However, near-infrared (NIR) fluorescence with emission wavelengths between 650 and 900 nm allows imaging at greater depths. Another challenge in optical imaging is tomographic imaging (fluorescence tomography), since scattering and attenuation vary according to the photons' wavelength and tissues through which they penetrate. In fluorescence tomography light coupling is performed using fibers in contact with the imaged object, or contact-free detection. The first mode limits flexibility. In the second mode model-based reconstruction methods have to be used, whose optimization is an open issue. Several commercial systems are available in the market that coupled with CT have good penetration as high-throughput preclinical screening tools.

11.7.2 Optical Imaging of Nanoparticles

The main benefit of using optical imaging in studying NPs is the lack of radiation and the relatively low cost of the technique. While it is possible to obtain very fast images, with increased throughput, a drawback is the low spatial resolution and absence of quantitative information. In addition, it is not possible to transfer this methodology to a clinical level in most cases due to the depth of absorption. However, this technology offers a robust screening tool, enabling repeated scanning of the same animal over a long period, and has been selected as a first in vivo step by many researchers. Although labeling NPs with fluorescent dyes is a standard way for their in vivo assessment [43] the recent challenge is the exploitation of novel NPs and materials that have interesting optical properties and can be used in in vivo imaging with no or minimum modification.

Quantum dots are among the first NPs whose optical properties attracted interest in in vivo imaging, with several reported examples [44]. Rampazzo et al. [45] studied luminescent silica NPs as contrast agents in optical imaging and optical sensing and for other high-sensitivity applications. Maldiney et al. [46] used NIR persistent luminescence NPs that are excited in vivo using highly penetrating low-energy red photons. Following their intravenous injection, it was possible to follow their biodistribution by simple whole-animal optical imaging, which opens new prospects for a variety of diagnosis applications. A very interesting application was the use of $NaGdF_4:Eu^{3+}$ NPs that are excited with X-rays and produce NIR light at 692 nm [47]. Gnach et al. [48] compared lanthanide-doped up-converting $NaYF_4$ and organic fluorophores for application in deep-tissue imaging, showing that NIR photoexcitation was favorable over conventional ultraviolet photoexcitation.

11.8 Multimodal Imaging

Each imaging modality has its own advantages and limitations, and the acquired information is actually complementary in-between them. The rationale behind multimodality imaging is to combine a low-sensitivity modality with high spatial resolution and tissue contrast (CT or MRI) with another low-resolution but high-sensitivity one. Commercially available systems for clinical practice and appropriately modified for preclinical small-animal research include PET-CT, SPECT-CT, PET-MRI, and even PET-CT-MRI. Recently new promising combinations of complementary modalities have entered the field.

11.8.1 PET/CT and SPECT/CT

The obvious combination of merging detailed X-ray anatomical imaging with the functional information of PET or SPECT was proposed in the late 1990s [49]. Sequential systems facilitating hardware fusion of scintigraphic and X-ray images provided accurate localization of the tracer's concentration in planar and tomographic mode. Using this concept, clinical PET/CT made a breakthrough in nuclear medicine market and almost eliminated standard PET scanners. SPECT/CT followed PET/CT and has now gained acceptance in medical community, and the same concept was transferred to small-animal imaging. There are two main advantages of merging anatomical with functional information. The first is the accurate localization of hot spots, which may be useful for inexperienced end users, and the second has to do with the use of anatomical information for attenuation correction [50], mostly in PET and then in SPECT. The true integration of these modalities in a single detector and the simultaneous acquisition of multimodal data remain a challenge.

Today almost all groups studying NPs with radioisotope techniques use combined SPECT/CT or PET/CT. Still, in this case we should not refer to multimodal NP imaging, since the CT information is used as an anatomic map and not to specifically image NPs, as in the case of Fig. 11.3, where calcium phosphate (CaP) nanoparticles are distributed into a normal mouse through the trachea and are located in the lungs.

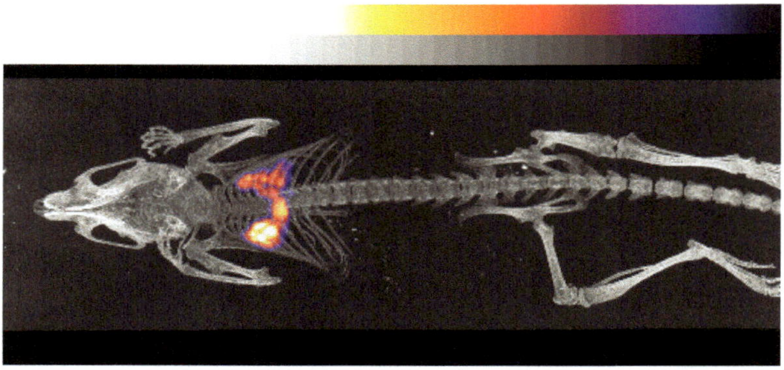

Figure 11.3 In vivo combined micro-SPECT/CT imaging of a mouse after injection of CaP nanoparticles radiolabeled with Tc99m through the trachea. Clear accumulation in the lungs is observed. Courtesy of BIOEMTECH, GR.

However, in the case of radiolabeled GNPs there are nice prospects of imaging the same tracer with both modalities and benefit from their complementarity. In this way CT can be used to image GNPs with a high resolution while PET or SPECT can add the quantitative information. The work of Li et al. [51] that combines SPECT and CT for targeting vulnerable atherosclerosis plaques supports this hypothesis. Furthermore, Xu et al. [52] used dendrimer-entrapped GNPs functionalized with an RGD peptide and labeled with ^{99m}Tc, delivering a promising nanoprobe for targeted SPECT/CT imaging of $\alpha_v\beta_3$ integrin–expressing tumors.

11.8.2 PET/MRI and SPECT/MRI

PET/MRI started as an engineering challenge, initially motivated by the success of PET/CT and the possible advantages that the replacement of CT with MRI would have [53]. PET/MRI is something more than replacing CT with MRI. Even if this was the only change, one can identify some important advantages; since MRI does not add an extra dose for the patient, it is possible to extend the PET applications in diagnostic cases were CT dosage seems useless and becomes the major preventing parameter, such as pediatric scans, brain imaging, and cardiac imaging. The second benefit is without a doubt the high soft tissue contrast, which is provided by MRI and besides tumor location can be valuable in both brain and cardiac imaging, where the soft tissue anatomy can be combined with PET functional information. Thirdly, PET requires data acquisition of a few minutes per bed position and this time can be exploited by the acquisition of different MRI sequences, thus resulting in a series of different images that will be diagnostically interpreted.

PET/MRI systems are needed to address several technical challenges. By the proper choice of avalanche photodiode detectors and other components and shielding of the associated electronics, it was possible to place a PET insert inside the MRI scanner and obtain simultaneously PET/MRI images during the early 2000s. However, the interest in PET/MRI technology increased exponentially following the introduction of SiPMs. Having the same advantages as PMTs (a supply voltage requirement of ~50 V, a very compact size, timing resolution down to 100 ps, and magnetic compatibility), it appears that SiPMs can be an ideal detector for whole-body PET/MRI. Slower but significant progress has been made toward SPECT/MRI, and current research is focused on smart geometries and collimator materials, aiming to provide simultaneous prototypes [54].

In terms of applications the real power of using PET/MRI for imaging NPs is in the fact that either PET tracers are used to label magnetic NPs or a combination of radioisotopes and MRI contrast agents are used simultaneously. The current status has been summarized in two very nice reviews, one from Tang et al. [55] and one from Lahooti et al. [56]. In most cases ^{68}Ga is used to label IONPs. Bouziotis et al. [57] used AGuIX NPs, which are ultrasmall NPs made of polysiloxane and surrounded by gadolinium chelates. Other examples are the use of ^{69}Ge-labeled IONPs [58], ^{64}Cu-labeled IONPs [59], and ^{89}Zr hyaluronan NPs [60].

11.8.3 Photoacoustic Imaging

Photoacoustic imaging (PAI) is a new modality that converts incident photons into US waves ultrasonically and overcomes the optical diffusion limit [61]. Thus, PAI combines the rich contrast of optical imaging with the high resolution and deep penetration of US imaging. With the rapid development of laser technology and US detection, PAI has enabled scalable visualization at levels from organelles to organs and has attracted tremendous attention over the past decade [62]. This new emerging, noninvasive, and nonionizing imaging technique can unveil different physiopathological processes and disease states in a wide range of biomedical applications. Photoacoustic molecular imaging is a promising technique for multiscalable biomedical applications and has tremendous potential in the emerging field of theranostics [61].

At the macroscopic level, photoacoustic computed tomography allows brain, organ, and whole-body imaging of creatures ranging from small animals to primates. Recently, PAI has received immense attention as a promising means of diagnostic and therapeutic monitoring. Although this technology is rather new, it has been rapidly adopted by nanomedicine community and different NP types have been studied in vivo. Xie et al. [63] studied the use of self-quenched semiconducting polymer NPs for amplified in vivo PAI. Sun et al. [64] developed PEGylated phosphorus NPs for combined PAI and photothermal cancer therapy. In a very promising study Miao et al. [65] used PA for semiconducting oligomer NPs for the in vivo imaging of pH in cancer mice models. Efforts to combine PAI with other modalities include combination with MRI, as reported by Sano et al. [66], or PAI with CT [67].

References

1. Hsieh, J. (2015). *Computed Tomography: Principles, Design, Artifacts, and Recent Advances*, 3rd edn., SPIE Press Book.
2. Badea, C. T., Drangova, M., Holdsworth, D. W. and Johnson, G. A. (2008). In vivo small-animal imaging using micro-CT and digital subtraction angiography, *Phys. Med. Biol.*, **53**, pp. 319–350.
3. Schambach, S. J., Bag, S., Schilling, L., et al. (2010). Application of micro-CT in small animal imaging, *Methods*, **50**, pp. 2–13.

4. Zeng, S., Yong, K. T., Roy, I., et al. (2011). A review on functionalized gold nanoparticles for biosensing applications, *Plasmonics*, **6**, p. 491.
5. Alex, S. and Tiwari, A. (2015). Functionalized gold nanoparticles: synthesis, properties and applications: a review, *J. Nanosc. Nanotech.*, **15**, pp. 1869–1894.
6. Hainfeld, J. F., Slatkin, D. N., Focella, T. M., et al. (2006). Gold nanoparticles: a new x-ray contrast agent, *Br. J. Radiol.*, **79**(939), pp. 248–253.
7. Galper, M. W., Saung, M. T., Fuster, V., et al. (2012). Effect of computed tomography scanning parameters on gold nanoparticle and iodine contrast, *Invest. Radiol.*, **47**(8), pp. 475–481.
8. Nakagawa, T., Gonda, K., Kamei, T., et al. (2016). X-ray computed tomography imaging of a tumor with high sensitivity using gold nanoparticles conjugated to a cancer-specific antibody via polyethylene glycol chains on their surface, *Sci. Technol. Adv. Mater.*, **17**, pp. 387–397.
9. Wang, H., Zheng, L., Peng, C., et. al. (2013). Folic acid-modified dendrimer-entrapped gold nanoparticles as nanoprobes for targeted CT imaging of human lung adenocarcinoma, *Biomaterials*, **34**(2), pp. 470–480.
10. Kim, T., Lee, N. D., Arifin, R., et al. (2017). In vivo micro-CT imaging of human mesenchymal stem cells labeled with gold-poly-l-lysine nanocomplexes, *Adv. Funct. Mater.*, **27**, p. 1604213.
11. Pratap, P., Sean, C. N. (2016). Labeling monocytes with gold nanoparticles to track their recruitment in atherosclerosis with computed tomography, *Biomaterials*, **87**, pp. 93–103.
12. Xu, J., Yu, M., Carter, P., et. al. (2017). In vivo x-ray imaging of transport of renal clearable gold nanoparticles in the kidneys, *Ang. Chem. Int.*, **56**(43), pp. 13356–13360.
13. Miraux, S., Massot, P., Ribot, E. J., et. al. (2008). 3D TrueFISP imaging of mouse brain at 4.7T and 9.4T, *J. Magn. Reson. Imaging*, **28**, pp. 497–503.
14. Beckmann, N., Kneuer, R., Gremlich, H.-U., et. al. (2007). In vivo mouse imaging and spectroscopy in drug discovery, *NMR Biomed.*, **20**, pp. 154–185.
15. Miloushev, V. Z., Keshari, K. R. and Holodny, A. I. (2016). Hyperpolarization MRI: preclinical models and potential applications in neuroradiology, *Top. Magn. Reson. Imaging*, **25**(1), pp. 31–37.

16. Schleich, N., Po, C., Jacobs, D., et al. (2014). Comparison of active, passive and magnetic targeting to tumors of multifunctional paclitaxel/SPIO-loaded nanoparticles for tumor imaging and therapy, *J. Control. Release*, **194**, pp. 82–91.

17. Yilmaz, A., Rösch, S., Klingel, K., et al. (2013). Magnetic resonance imaging (MRI) of inflamed myocardium using iron oxide nanoparticles in patients with acute myocardial infarction - preliminary results, *Int. J. Cardiol.*, **163**(2), pp. 175–182.

18. Cheng, K. K., Chan, P. S., Fan, S., et al. (2015). Curcumin-conjugated magnetic nanoparticles for detecting amyloid plaques in Alzheimer's disease mice using magnetic resonance imaging (MRI), *Biomaterials*, **44**, pp. 155–172.

19. Kim, S. J., Lewis, B., Steiner, M. S., et al. (2016). Superparamagnetic iron oxide nanoparticles for direct labeling of stem cells and in vivo MRI tracking, *Contr. Med. Mol. Imaging*, **11**(1), pp. 55–64.

20. Lee, M. S., Su, C. M., Yeh, J. C., et al. (2016). Synthesis of composite magnetic nanoparticles Fe_3O_4 with alendronate for osteoporosis treatment, *Int. J. Nanomed.*, **11**, pp. 4583–4594.

21. Voigt, J. U. (2009). Ultrasound molecular imaging, *Methods*, **48**, pp. 92–97.

22. Cheung, A. M., Brown, A. S., Hastie, L. A., et al. (2005). Three-dimensional ultrasound biomicroscopy for xenograft growth analysis, *Ultrasound Med. Biol.*, **31**, pp. 865–870.

23. Yin, T., Wang, P., Zheng, R., et al. (2012). Nanobubbles for enhanced ultrasound imaging of tumors, *Int. J. Nanomed.*, **7**, pp. 895–904.

24. Yang, H., Cai, W., Xu, L, et al. (2015). Nanobubble–affibody: novel ultrasound contrast agents for targeted molecular ultrasound imaging of tumor, *Biomaterials*, **37**, pp. 279–288.

25. Long, C. M., Bhandari, P. N. and Irudayaraj, J., (2016). Nanobubbles provide theranostic relief to cancer hypoxia, *The Summer Undergraduate Research Fellowship (SURF) Symposium*, Purdue University, Indiana, Paper 76.

26. Foroutan, F., Jokerst, J. V., Gambhir, S, S., et al. (2015). Sol–Gel synthesis and electrospraying of biodegradable $(P_2O_5)_{55}$–$(CaO)_{30}$–$(Na_2O)_{15}$ glass nanospheres as a transient contrast agent for ultrasound stem cell imaging, *ACS Nano*, **9**(2), pp. 1868–1877.

27. Anger, H. O., Powell, M. R., van Dyke, D. C., et al. (1967). Recent applications of the scintillation camera, *Strahlentherapie Sonderb.*, **65**, pp. 70–93.

28. O'Connor, M. K. and Kemp, B. J. (2006). Single-photon emission computed tomography/computed tomography: basic instrumentation and innovations, *Semin. Nucl. Med.*, **36**, pp. 258–266.

29. Kagadis, G., Loudos, G. and Katsanos, K. (2010). In vivo small animal imaging: current status and future prospects, *Med. Phys.*, **37**(12), pp. 6421–6441.

30. Fazaeli, Y., Akhavan, O., Rahighi, R., et al. (2014). In vivo SPECT imaging of tumors by 198,199Au-labeled graphene oxide nanostructures, *Mater. Sci. Eng. C*, **45**, pp. 196–204.

31. Black, K., Akers, W. J., Sudlow, G., et al. (2015). Dual-radiolabeled nanoparticle SPECT probes for bioimaging, *Nanoscale*, **7**, pp. 440–444.

32. Tseng, Y. C., Xu, Z., Guley, K., et al. (2014). Lipid–calcium phosphate nanoparticles for delivery to the lymphatic system and SPECT/CT imaging of lymph node metastases, *Biomaterials*, **35**(16), pp. 4688–4698.

33. Larobina, M., Brunetti, A. and Salvatore, M. (2006). Small animal PET: a review of commercially available imaging systems, *Curr. Med. Imaging Rev.*, **2**, pp. 187–192.

34. Catana, C., Wu, Y., Judenhofer, M. S., et al. (2006). Simultaneous acquisition of multislice PET and MR images: initial results with a MR-compatible PET scanner, *J. Nucl. Med.*, **47**, pp. 1963–1976.

35. Xing, Y., Zhao, J., Shi, X., et al. (2014). Recent development of radiolabeled nanoparticles for PET imaging, *Austin J. Nanomed. Nanotechnol.*, **2**(2), p. 1016.

36. Pérez-Medina, C., Tang, J., Abdel-Atti, D., et al. (2015). PET imaging of tumor-associated macrophages with 89Zr-labeled high-density lipoprotein nanoparticles, *J. Nucl. Med.*, **56**(8), pp. 1272–1277.

37. Yang, M., Huo, D., Gilroy, K. D., et al. (2017). Facile synthesis of ^{64}Cu-doped Au nanocages for positron emission tomography imaging, *ChemNanoMat*, **3**, pp. 44–50.

38. Lee, S. B., Lee, S. W., Jeong, S. Y., et al. (2017). Engineering of radioiodine-labeled gold core–shell nanoparticles as efficient nuclear medicine imaging agents for trafficking of dendritic cells, *ACS Appl. Mater. Interfaces*, **9**(10), pp. 8480–8489.

39. Stockhofe, K., Gimnich, M., Klinker, K., et al. (2016). Radiolabeling of cross-linked polymer micelles with 68Ga for PET-imaging, *J. Nucl. Med.*, **57**, p. 1082.

40. Sirianni, R. W., Zheng, M., Patel, T., et al. (2014). Radiolabeling of poly(lactic-co-glycolic acid) (PLGA) nanoparticles with biotinylated

F-18 prosthetic groups and imaging of their delivery to the brain with positron emission tomography, *Bioconjugate Chem.*, **25**(12), pp. 2157–2165.

41. Sadikot, R. T. and Blackwell, T. S. (2005). Bioluminescence imaging, *Proc. Am. Thorac. Soc.*, **2**, pp. 537–540.
42. Ntziachristos, V. (2006). Fluorescence molecular imaging, *Annu. Rev. Biomed. Eng.*, **8**, pp. 1–33.
43. Wolfbeis, O. S. (2015). An overview of nanoparticles commonly used in fluorescent bioimaging, *Chem. Soc. Rev.*, **44**, pp. 4743–4768.
44. Liab, J. and Zhu, J. J. (2013). Quantum dots for fluorescent biosensing and bio-imaging applications, *Analyst*, **138**, pp. 2506–2515.
45. Rampazzo, E., Prodi, L., Petrizza, L. and Zaccheroni, N. (2016). Luminescent silica nanoparticles featuring collective processes for optical imaging, *Top. Curr. Chem.*, **370**, pp. 1–28.
46. Maldiney, T., Bessière, A. and Seguin, J. (2014). The in vivo activation of persistent nanophosphors for optical imaging of vascularization, tumours and grafted cells, *Nat. Mater.*, **13**, pp. 418–426.
47. Sudheendra, L., Das, G. K., Li, C., et al. (2014). $NaGdF_4$:Eu_3+ nanoparticles for enhanced X-ray excited optical imaging, *Chem. Mater.*, **26** (5), pp. 1881–1888.
48. Gnach, A., Prorok, K., Misiak, M., et al. (2014). Up-converting $NaYF_4$:0.1%Tm_3+, 20%Yb_3+ nanoparticles as luminescent labels for deep-tissue optical imaging, *J. Rare Earths*, **32**(3), pp. 207–212.
49. Even-Sapir, E., Keidar, Z. and Bar-Shalom, R. (2009). Hybrid imaging SPECT/CT and PET/CT - improving the diagnostic accuracy of functional/metabolic and anatomic imaging, *Semin. Nucl. Med.*, **39**, pp. 264–275.
50. Zaidi, H. and Hasegawa, B. (2003). Determination of the attenuation map in emission tomography, *J. Nucl. Med.*, **44**, pp. 291–315.
51. Li, X., Wang, C., Tan, H., et al. (2016). Gold nanoparticles-based SPECT/CT imaging probe targeting for vulnerable atherosclerosis plaques, *Biomaterials*, **108**, pp. 71–80.
52. Xiaoying Xu, X., Zhao, L. and Li, X. (2017). Targeted tumor SPECT/CT dual mode imaging using multifunctional RGD-modified low generation dendrimer-entrapped gold nanoparticles, *Biomater. Sci.*, **5**, pp. 2393–2397.
53. Wehrl, H. F., Judenhofer, M. S., Wiehr, S. and Pichler, B. J. (2009). Pre-clinical PET/MR: technological advances and new perspectives in biomedical research, *Eur. J. Nucl. Med. Mol. Imaging*, **36**, pp. 56–68.

54. Hutton, B. F., Occhipinti, M., Kuehne, A., et al. (2018). Development of clinical simultaneous SPECT/MRI, *Br. J. Radiol.*, 91(1081), p. 20160690.
55. Tang, T., Garcia, J. and Louie, A. Y. (2017). PET/SPECT/MRI multimodal nanoparticles, *Des. Appl. Nanopart. Biomed. Imaging*, pp. 205–228.
56. Lahooti, A., Sarkar, S., Laurent, S. and Shanehsazzadeh, S. (2016). Dual nano-sized contrast agents in PET/MRI: a systematic review, *Contr. Med. Mol. Imaging*, **11**, pp. 428–447.
57. Bouziotis, P., Stellas, D. and Thomas, E., (2017). ^{68}Ga-radiolabeled AGuIX nanoparticles as dual-modality imaging agents for PET/MRI-guided radiation therapy, *Nanomedicine*, **12**(13), pp. 1561–1574.
58. Chakravarty, R., Valdovinos, H. F., Chen, F., et al. (2014). Intrinsically germanium-69-labeled iron oxide nanoparticles: synthesis and in-vivo dual-modality PET/MR imaging, *Adv. Mater.*, **26**(30), pp. 5119–5123.
59. Tu, C., Ng, T. S. C., Jacobs, R. E., et al. (2014). Multimodality PET/MRI agents targeted to activated macrophages, *J. Biol. Inorg. Chem.*, **19**, pp. 247–258.
60. Beldman, T. J., Senders, M. L., Alaarg, A., et al. (2017). Hyaluronan nanoparticles selectively target plaque-associated macrophages and improve plaque stability in atherosclerosis, *ACS Nano*, **11**(6), pp. 5785–5799.
61. Liu, Y., Nie, L. and Chen, X. (2016). Photoacoustic molecular imaging: from multiscale biomedical applications towards early-stage theranostics, *Trends in Biotechnol.*, **34**(5), pp. 420–433.
62. Wang, L. V. and Hu, S. (2012). Photoacoustic tomography: in vivo imaging from organelles to organs, *Science*, **335**, pp. 1458–1462.
63. Xie, C., Upputuri, P. K. and Zhen, X. (2017). Self-quenched semiconducting polymer nanoparticles for amplified in vivo photoacoustic imaging, *Biomaterials*, **119**, pp. 1–8.
64. Sun, C., Wen, L. and Zeng, J. (2016). One-pot solventless preparation of PEGylated black phosphorus nanoparticles for photoacoustic imaging and photothermal therapy of cancer, *Biomaterials*, **91**, pp. 81–89.
65. Miao, Q., Lyu, Y., Ding, D. and Pu, K. (2016). Photoacoustic imaging: semiconducting oligomer nanoparticles as an activatable photoacoustic probe with amplified brightness for in vivo imaging of pH, *Adv. Mater.*, **28**(19), pp. 3662–3668.
66. Sano, K. (2017). Development of molecular probes based on iron oxide nanoparticles for in vivo magnetic resonance/photoacoustic dual imaging of target molecules in tumors, *Yakugaku Zasshi*, **137**(1), pp. 55–60.

67. Cheheltani, R., Ezzibdeh, R. M., Chhour, P., et al. (2016). Tunable, biodegradable gold nanoparticles as contrast agents for computed tomography and photoacoustic imaging, *Biomaterials*, **102**, pp. 87–97.

Chapter 12

Nanotoxicity and Possible Health Risks

Elena Vlastou,[a] Efstathios P. Efstathopoulos,[a] and Maria Gazouli[a,b]
[a]*Department of Radiology, Medical School, National and Kapodistrian University of Athens, Rimini 1, Athens 12462, Greece*
[b]*Department of Basic Medical Science, Laboratory of Biology, School of Medicine, National and Kapodistrian, University of Athens, Michalakopoulou 176, Athens 11527, Greece*
mgazouli@med.uoa.gr

12.1 Introduction to Nanotoxicity

The giant steps toward nanosciences dictate the need to gain a broad knowledge about not only the beneficial but also the noxious properties of nanomaterials. Though there are remarkable advantages of nanoparticles (NPs) in medicine and industry, there are plenty of concerns that have been raised about their potential adverse effects in living organisms and on the ecosystems. Undoubtedly, it is critical to ensure that medical and industrial applications of NPs are made as safe as possible so that the balance is tilted in favor of the profits that society will earn. Nanotoxicology,

Drug Delivery Nanosystems: From Bioinspiration and Biomimetics to Clinical Applications
Edited by Costas Demetzos, Stergios Pispas, and Natassa Pippa

ISBN 978-981-4774-92-5 (Hardcover), 978-0-429-49054-5 (eBook)
www.panstanford.com

as a subfield of nanosciences, emphasizes detecting all the harmful consequences linked to NPs, along with the physical and chemical properties responsible for their toxicity, their interaction with biological systems, and the concentrations above which they threaten public health and the environment. It should be stated that the extent to which nanotoxicity affects organisms is also a matter of each one's genetic traits and so are the available weapons against it.

We should keep in mind that our interaction with NPs is an unavoidable phenomenon and has existed since we were born. NPs are present not only in the air we breathe but also in cosmetics, clothing, food, and water. Concerning air NPs, ultrafine dust is apparent in the atmosphere and in contrast to engineered NPs (ENPs), it has no advantageous properties. Airborne NPs owe their existence to vehicle emissions, industry applications, volcano explosions, and atmospheric pollution and are closely linked to severe respiratory and cardiac diseases [1, 2]. Health risk assessment though remains a challenging field due to the difficulty in measuring ENP concentration in the atmosphere. Moreover, NPs such as titanium oxide (TiO_2) and zinc oxide (ZnO) are used as ultraviolet (UV) filters in sunscreens and for water sterilization, so waste disposal and the use of sunscreens could be a potential source of water nanopollution [3]. Moreover, it has already been observed that silica (Si) and silver (Ag) NPs are widely used in fabrics as they enhance water and stain resistance. Lastly, the use of NPs in food packaging and NPs of vitamin E found in certain beverages indicate the strong presence of NPs in our daily nutrition habits too.

Nanotoxicology involves different aspects of science, from molecular biology to quantum physics and chemistry, and lays the foundations for eliminating all risks related to NP manufacturing and their applications. Several research studies have been conducted and published on NP toxicity, with various NPs of different properties, in cell lines, zebrafish, mice, and rats. The major obstacle associated with determining the hazardous impacts of NPs is the variety of parameters that are responsible for their adverse effects. It is widely known that the dosage, size, composition, aggregation, surface charge, structure, and chemistry and even the route of administration of the NPs and the duration of exposure to them are the main characteristics upon which nanotoxicity depends.

"You can't have one without the other" could definitely be the best quote to describe the strong connection between the beneficial and damaging effects that the same NP properties are responsible for.

12.2 Routes of Exposure

The existence of NPs in air, water, and food and their invasion in medicine reveal the possible ways for them to enter the human body. The skin, the respiratory system, and the gastrointestinal (GI) system are the main barriers that NPs override in their interaction with living organisms. In the case of NP delivery by an interstitial injection, the possible path of the NPs depends on dosage and nanomaterial properties. However, there is no doubt that in view of their small size, NPs can get easily transported to the systemic circulation and lymph system, leaching into any organ and tissue [4]. Particles smaller than 100 nm can cross cell membranes, while 40 nm and 30 nm particles are capable of penetrating into the cell nucleus and cross the blood-brain barrier (BBB), respectively [5]. The mechanisms that take place after NPs enter the human body and the potential damage caused will be analyzed later on.

12.2.1 Skin

Skin, which is the physical boundary between the organisms and the environment, is the first organ that NPs meet in their interaction with humans. The epidermis, the dermis, and the subcutaneous tissue are the three layers that build the skin anatomy. The stratum corneum, a keratinous membrane that forms the top sublayer of epidermis, consists of corneocytes and is the main barrier that secures organisms from any existing environmental threats. Dermal exposure to NPs could be achieved by application of drugs, sunscreens, creams, dry powder, sprays, or even clothing. Nanomaterial production is also a potential route of exposure for workers employed in this field. At first glance, sweat glands and hair follicles provide NPs the main path to enter human skin. However, it is under investigation whether and to what extent NPs could defeat the stratum corneum; enter the dermis and cause allergic effects, irritation, and toxicity to inner layers [6]; and enter the blood circulation. Obviously, under certain circumstances, such as sunburns, wounds, and acne, NPs gain access to the human body more easily. Kim et al. [7] have proved that quantum dots (QDs) could translocate from the dermis to lymph nodes and consequently enter the systemic vasculature, while Gontier et al. [8] reported a limited deposition of TiO_2 NPs in the stratum corneum. It is hypothesized that a TiO_2 NP coating hurts the skin and assists in their dispersion to the inner zones [9]. In general, various studies claim different levels of NP penetration in skin layers, from mediocre to deeper [1, 10–12], depending on the NPs' properties and dosage.

12.2.2 Respiratory Tract

Concerning the respiratory system, the deposition of inhaled NPs in lungs is the major topic of research in nanotoxicity. The three main areas that a respiratory system consists of are the nasopharyngeal, the tracheobronchial, and the alveolar. Lungs come in continuous contact with a mixture of airborne particles, but they also possess a series of defense structures that prevent infections and pathogenies. Especially the mucociliary system in the nasopharyngeal and tracheobronchial areas is responsible for catching inhaled particles and casting them out through the mouth.

However, when it comes to NPs, their small size makes it easier for them than for larger ones to overcome respiratory guards such as the bronchial epithelium and enter the systemic circulation or, subject to mucus clearance, translocate to the GI tract [13]. It is worth mentioning that patients with asthma or chronic obstructive pulmonary disease depict increased NP accumulation in lungs compared to the healthy population [14, 15]. According to the International Commission on Radiological Protection (1994), the majority of inhaled 1 nm NPs get accumulated in the nasopharyngeal region (90%), whereas the rest are mounted on the tracheobronchial one, leaving unharmed the alveolar region. NPs of 20 nm have shown the highest concentration in the alveolar region (50%), while only 15% is distributed in the nasopharyngeal and tracheobronchial regions [15, 16]. Lung cancer, asthma, bronchitis, and emphysema are some of the diseases linked to inhaled NPs.

It seems that NP absorption from lung regions is followed by their possible transfer to cell mitochondria, bone marrow, spleen, brain, nervous system, lymph node, and the heart [17]. It has been proved that olfactory nerves are the means for inhaled NPs to be transported to the olfactory bulb and the brain [18, 19]. NP accumulation in the nervous system could possibly result in Alzheimer s and Parkinson's diseases. Apart from various researchers [16, 17, 20, 21] the American Heart Association has also recently reported the direct correlation between airborne NP inhalation and cardiac diseases of mediocre to high severity.

12.2.3 Gastrointestinal Tract

NPs could enter into the GI tissues through oral exposure or nasal inhalation. Digested NPs from nanopolluted marine food, fruit, vegetables, water, or drug delivery could pass the layer of epithelium cells and the gastric mucosa to end in the stomach and surrounding tissues [17, 18, 22]. Especially for those employed in NP manufacture, hand to mouth is a common route for NPs in their digestive systems. In terms of biological functions, inhaled NPs that are cleared by the lung mucosa are subsequently absorbed by GI regions. It has been reported that the digestive gland cell membrane is harmed in the case of TiO_2 ingestion through oxidative stress induction [23]. Epithelium injuries, colon cancer, and Crohn's disease are related to GI absorption, while nanocopper particles have been found to inflict liver, spleen, and kidney damage in mice experiments [24].

12.3 NP Clearance

Biological clearance is the physical mechanism in charge of NP expulsion from the human body. The physicochemical characteristics, entry route, and region of accumulation of NPs define the series of procedures that occur after NPs interact with humans. NPs caught by the mucosa lining in the nasopharyngeal and tracheobronchial regions could be expelled through the mouth or be transported to the GI system. Particles located in the alveolar region are possibly trapped and destroyed by the alveolar macrophages through phagocytosis. This procedure constitutes clearance of one-third of the inhaled NPs and depends upon the macrophages' capability to recognize and attack the specific intruders [9, 25]. In case alveolar phagocytosis does not take place, soluble NPs are engulfed and expelled through the digestive system while nondegradable NPs may get transported to epithelial sites and pass into the circulatory system.

Once they enter systemic circulation, NPs are subject to opsonization and phagocytosis according to their properties and biodistribution. Besides, chemical dissolution involves soluble NPs' dilution in lipids or biological fluids. The products from this process are attached to proteins and other enzymes or end in the lymph system. Simultaneously, liver and splenic macrophages incorporate NPs gathered in the colon, bone marrow, liver, spleen, and lymph nodes to directly clear them from systemic circulation [17]. Finally, renal and hepatic clearance are the last mechanisms in NP eviction. The rectangular shape of the glomerular capillary wall, its negative charge, and its kidney filtration threshold (~5.5 nm) demonstrate NPs' characteristics that facilitate their penetration into kidneys [26]. Linear NPs, with sizes smaller than 5.5 nm, are easily filtered by the kidneys to end in urine, a method that prevents possible cytotoxicity compared to hepatic clearance [27]. The latter process occupies a complex liver network of hepatocytes and Kupffer and endothelial cells, which traps NPs through endocytosis to clear them through feces.

Understanding the nanoclearance mechanism is one of the key factors for combining NPs' high efficiency with minimized toxicity. With proper strategies and safe assumptions, nanotoxicology could propose great tools to manage NPs' malignant effects.

12.4 Factors Affecting Nanotoxicity

As mentioned before, the evaluation of NPs' adverse effects remains a great challenge for the scientific community due to the wealth of factors that nanotoxicity depends on. Size, surface area, dosing, shape, surface coating and charge, and bulk material are the basic parameters under investigation to assess the risk involved in NP usage. The cellular uptake, kinetics, and clearance of NPs are intensely affected by their physicochemical properties. The literature offers a huge variety of information about different studies in the specific area, some of which are briefly described below.

12.4.1 Size and Surface Area

The capacity of NPs to enter living organisms and interfere with cells and organs is highly associated with their size. NPs' size is considered to be the most critical feature that controls their distribution and clearance. Both beneficial and negative effects of ENPs follow from the fact that they are small enough to cross the human defense system and accumulate in particular areas of interest. It has been proven that decreasing NP size implies an increase in the surface area and a greater area-to-volume ratio per given mass. Consequently, the surface area contains more molecules of the bulk material, resulting in greater biological reactivity. Indeed, the greater toxicity induced by CuO and Ag NPs than their raw materials is experimentally confirmed [28, 29].

Various researchers claim that when inhaled ultrafine particles induce stronger deleterious effects than larger ones [30–32]. Similarly, the smallest inhaled NPs are mainly absorbed by the alveoli region and cause stronger pulmonary toxicity due to the difficulty in clearance compared to those accumulated in the upper airways [16, 33]. It has also been reported that there is quicker transport of injected NPs <50 nm to neighboring tissues in contrast to NPs >50 nm, while a comparison between 10 nm and 50 nm gold (Au) NPs agglomeration in human structures concluded that the tiniest have been found in all organs whereas 50 nm NPs have been concentrated in liver, spleen, and blood only [34]. Similarly, in experiments conducted on rats, 0.1% of 80 nm and 0.3%–0.5% of 15 nm iridium NPs immediately reached the rat's blood (within 1 min.) and was detected in liver [25] whereas TiO_2 NPs' size brought about toxicity variations in the rat's pulmonary system [26]. Experiments using Ag NPs that have been conducted in human lung cells [35], rats [36], and zebrafish [37] confirmed a size-dependent cytotoxicity.

An important conclusion derived from several experiments is that nanomaterial dosage should depend on NP surface area in terms of achieving the desirable results with eliminated health risk. Due to the strong connection between surface area and nanotoxicity, it has been assumed that a metric based on surface area should be established in order to ensure the safe administration of NPs [11, 33]. Hoet et al. reinforced this statement by reporting that a low dose of 20 nm TiO_2 particles induces greater toxicity than a high dose of 100 nm particles [38].

12.4.2 Shape

The impact of NPs' shape on their toxicity is a controversial subject. The difficulty researchers face is that alterations in NPs' shape are accompanied by changes in other properties so a straight shape-toxicity connection cannot be achieved. However, some studies where all NP properties but the shape have been kept stable have reported the impact of different NP shapes on various cells' uptake (cell lines, bacteria, zebrafish, plants, etc.) [39–43]. Gratton et al. discovered that cells are more accessible to rodlike NPs compared to cylindrical ones [44]. In the same direction, needlelike NPs [42, 45] have been found to evoke greater toxicity than other forms of NPs due to their easy access to cell membranes and tissues. Moreover, increased toxicity in lung epithelium cells has been identified in the case of ZnO nanorods compared to spherical ones [46]. However, the NP material and the characteristics of the biological system that interacts with the NPs may play a vital role in shape-dependent toxicity, so a more thorough look is needed into this field to come to a clear conclusion.

12.4.3 Surface Coating: Surface Charge

The precision and effectiveness of cell targeting are highly dependent on the NPs' biodegradability and solubility. Consequently, surface characteristics are among the most crucial NP properties that determine their interaction with biological systems and should be considered in NP applications. Several researchers [33, 38, 47–49] have shown the impact of an NP's surface coating and charge on toxicity. Hoet et al. have reported a strong correlation of a silica NP's toxicity with the concentration of surface radicals [38], while experiments on mice cell lines have concluded that uncoated Ag NPs induce less toxicity compared to those with an ammonium coating on their surface [50]. Generation of reactive oxygen species (ROS) too has been proved to be coating depended, as demonstrated by Shi et al., in experiments with copper NPs [51]. Surface charge has been proven to affect NP toxicity too. The main reason is the interaction of the negatively charged plasma membrane with positively charged NPs. In various experiments, positively charged NPs seem to lead to grander toxicity than negative or neutral stems [47–49, 52].

12.4.4 NP Material

Obviously, an NP material in terms of its chemical nature is a significant characteristic affecting each NP's toxicity. NP properties and effects are highly dependent on their bulk material, as shown in their toxic results analyzed in Section 12.6. Moreover, the comparative studies between different materials garner great interest and could be a good database for precise toxicity determination. Multiwalled carbon nanotubes (MWCNTs) appear less toxic compared to single-walled carbon nanotubes (SWCNTs) and carbon nanofibers [53]; SWCNTs are more toxic than carbon black particles, while carbon nanotubes (CNTs) containing nickel induce greater toxicity than quartz [54, 55]. Ag NP toxicity is higher than CeO_2 [56], whereas Stahl et al. note that silver NPs produce more harmful effects than gold ones in zebrafish [57]. Finally, the following NPs are classified from higher to lower toxicity according to a study by Wang et al. [58] in embryonic zebrafish: CuO > ZnO > CO_3O_4 > TiO_2. Similarly, the following NPs are classified from higher to lower toxicity in embryonic zebrafish by Lanone et al. [59]: CuO > ZnO > Al_2O_3 > Zr > W.

12.5 Mechanism of NP Toxicity

NPs, according to their characteristics and the cell cycle, penetrate into tissues, and subsequently there are specific procedures in action responsible for nanotoxicity. Let's assume that NPs pass through human "defense cells" (e.g., alveolar or splenic macrophages, pulmonary epithelium, and GI epithelium) without being trapped and destroyed. If they are not engulfed by a phagosome, which could prevent further nanochemical interaction, NPs, depending on their solubility, size, and chemical structure, could enter into the cell and get localized in different structures (nuclear membrane, cytoplasm, mitochondria, proteins, etc.). Phagocytosis is the main mechanism that offers NPs a cell access, while ion channels or plasma membrane pores have been found to favor the penetration of the tiniest NPs into cells [60].

ROS formation is the basic mechanism that causes nanotoxicity. ROS generation is a physiological/biological procedure resulting from oxygen metabolism; it can affect the homeostatic process, and it plays a vital part in cell signaling. Hydroxyl radicals ($^{\bullet}OH$), singlet oxygen ($^{1}O_2$), superoxide anions ($^{\bullet}O_2^{-}$), hydrogen peroxide (H_2O_2), and hypochlorous acid (HOCl) are the primary oxidative species, and they are created either in or outside the cell. They result from physical cell functions, such as inflammatory response and mitochondrial respiratory, or external factors, such as radiation, atmospheric pollution, tobacco, drugs, and ENPs. However, cells have their own weapons to defeat ROS generation. More specifically, antioxidant production is the main procedure that follows ROS appearance—an attempt to detoxify the oxidative species. A superoxide radical could be transformed into a reduced-activity peroxide radical by superoxide dismutase [61], a primary antioxidant of the cell defense mechanism [57]. Catalase is able to destroy the peroxide radical by converting it to water and molecular oxygen [62], while a secondary defense antioxidant, known as glutathione peroxidase, has been found to minimize the production of plenty of hydroperoxides [63].

Concerning NPs there are a variety of reasons leading to ROS creation. First of all, NP absorption by the cells activates macrophages and neutrophils, a procedure that accelerates ROS production [64]. In addition, metal NPs have been found to enhance $^{\bullet}OH$ and $^{\bullet}O_2^{-}$ creation through Fenton-type and Haber–Weiss reactions [65]. In various studies, surface-dependent oxidative stress exerts a major influence on ROS induction [65–67], while very small NPs have the ability to penetrate into mitochondria and cause directly oxidative stress [68].

ROS plethora within a cell though could cause unrepairable damage in cell function, DNA, lipids, and proteins. Besides, ROS are strongly connected to oxidative stress as a consequence of the cell's disability to eliminate oxidant effects. On a molecular basis, genotoxic effects arising from DNA strand breaks, lipid peroxidation, inflammation enhancement, and mitochondria perturbation and consequent cell death are among the most common impacts of oxidative stress. The expression of proinflammatory pathways, such as mitogen-activated protein kinase (MAPK) and nuclear factor

(NF-κB), and proinflammatory genes induced by the latter, such as TNF-α, IL-6, IL-7, and IL-8, indicate the direct correlation between NPs, oxidative stress, and inflammation.

Some of the diseases that are brought on by oxidative stress are Alzheimer's and Parkinson's disease, cancer, cardiovascular inflammation, and diabetes. The severity of NP toxicity on human health demonstrates the need for a deeper understanding of the exact mechanisms that take place in cell-NP interaction to finally come up with the most appropriate ways to limit the potential adverse effects.

12.6 NP Toxicity

12.6.1 Nonmetallic Material

12.6.1.1 Polymeric NPs

Polymeric NPs have widespread use as drug delivery systems for cancer treatment [69]. They seem to induce no inflammation, and they have been proven nontoxic among various applications. Khanna et al. report that there are no toxic effects of poly(lactic-*co*-glycolic acid) (PLGA) and polysachharide chitosan–based nanosystems [70], while Yildirimer et al. underline that a chitosan coating when applicable is a basic characteristic that minimizes toxicity [71].

12.6.1.2 Silica NPs

Apart from their presence in air, silica NPs are popular drug carriers and useful tools in diagnostic imaging. Depending on the administrated dosage, silica NPs have been found to induce ROS and oxidative stress [72, 73], whereas in experiments in lung cells [74] and keratinocyte cells [75], a dose-dependent toxicity has been discovered in cases where the NP concentration exceeded 50 mg/mL. In another experiment, the treatment of lung cancer cells with silica NPs activated various inflammatory cytokines [76]. Finally, Yildirimer et al. explain the inconsistent findings regarding generated liver toxicity as a result of silica NPs' size, coating, and route of administration effects [71].

12.6.1.3 Carbon NPs

The emerging applications of carbon NPs (CNPs) have attracted various researchers to evaluate carbon toxicity. Most of the studies highlight CNPs' strong harmful effects, especially in the case of inhalation route, despite the high complexity involved in their interaction with human tissues. SWCNTs and MWCNTs have been intensively investigated as they represent extremely revolutionary particles in biomedical engineering, drug delivery, gene therapies, etc. Greater toxicity has been noted in the case of SWCNT due to their larger surface area in comparison to MWCNT [77–79], while both of them have been observed to induce ROS and oxidative stress depending on their concentration [55, 80–83] and size [73, 84]. One minute has been proved enough for 3%–5% of the CNTs to be transported to the blood and be absorbed by the liver [85].

Lung cancer, asbestosis [86], and interstitial granuloma [55] seem to be possible effects of CNPs, while there are strong indications that ultrafine carbon particles are able to cross the BBB and translocate to the central nervous system (CNS) [87]. Several studies in the literature have reported lipid peroxidation [81, 88, 89], mitochondrial damage [78, 90], inflammation (with simultaneous activation of MAPK and NF-κB), and cell apoptosis [91–93]. Skin effects need to be investigated, as some studies have shown important cytotoxicity in keratinocytes [94, 95] combined with ROS formation and mitochondrial dysfunction [96], a fact that should raise worries about employees in a field involving CNP handling.

12.6.2 Metallic Material

12.6.2.1 Gold NPs

Gold NPs are the most appealing particles in targeted cancer therapy. Bulk gold is considered safe in biomedical applications, and combined with its manifold unique chemical properties, it seems an ideal material for the construction of safe NPs. Gold nanospheres of different sizes and cupping agents in keratinocytes [97], leukemia cell lines [98], and dendritic cell lines [99] have exhibited no cytotoxicity. Similarly, Patra et al. report no toxicity in baby hamsters' kidneys and human hepatocellular liver carcinoma cells [100], whereas Shukla et al. have discovered no activation of inflammatory markers after macrophage cells' exposure to Au NPs [101]. However, different outcomes have related the toxicity of Au NPs to their size [102, 103], dosage [71, 104], and even route of administration [105]. Furthermore, gold toxicity seems a matter of the kind of cell, as cytotoxicity has been induced in lung carcinoma cells in contrast to liver carcinoma cell lines, where no adverse effects have been noticed [100]. Wang et al. attributed the toxicity of gold nanorods to the stabilizing chemical cetyltrimethylammonium bromide coating [97]. The controversial results related to the potential hazards of Au NPs indicate the need for deep research prior to its first clinical applications. Experimental protocols, the biological system of interaction, and nanomaterial physicochemical properties should be well standardized so one can extract trustworthy results concerning the safety and biocompatibility of gold NPs.

12.6.2.2 Silver NPs

Silver NPs' antibacterial properties have attracted the interest of medicine and clothing industries. Silver nanomaterials are found in wound dressings and clothing, so human skin is directly exposed to Ag NPs' possible harmful effects. Gray-blue skin and liver discoloration, widely known as argyria, have been detected as a result of exposure to Ag NPs [106–108]. Oxidative stress, reduced mitochondrial function, genotoxicity, and cell apoptosis in animal tissues [88]; human skin carcinoma [109]; and leukemia [110] are among the crucial side effects of exposure to silver. Neuronal degeneration in rat models [111] and noxious changes in the synaptic function of zebrafish embryos [112] have been also reported, whereas accumulation in the liver depending on Ag NPs' shape and size has been proved to lead to mitochondrial dysfunction and increased ROS creation [71, 113]. Besides, it is the different extents of toxicity that lead to questions by many research groups. For instance, in mouse cells and fibroblasts, uncoated silver NPs cause milder effects than coated [114], while Haase et al. report higher cytotoxicity in the case of peptide-coated compared to citrate-coated 20 nm Ag NPs [115]. From experiments in keratinocytes, uncoated Ag NPs have been found to be more toxic than carbon-coated particles [116], while another study reveals that 100 mg/mL of silver nitrate in solution has been proven toxic compared to silver nanospheres and nanoprisms, which have produced no toxic effects [15].

12.6.2.3 Metal oxide NPs

Metal oxide NPs have various applications in both industrial and medical fields. Titanium dioxide NPs, found in sunscreens and clothing, seem responsible for ROS in BEAS-2B cells [117] and for a significant expansion of oxidative stress in mice fibroblast cells at dosages above 60 μg/mL [118]. In addition to producing ROS and surface coating-dependent cytotoxicity [71, 118–120], TiO_2 NPs 5–200 nm in size have been found to affect a rodent's immune system, liver, spleen, lipids, and myocardium [26, 73]. Generally, it seems that TiO_2 particles induce cell type-dependent toxicity [121] and at the same time, experiments in volunteers have shown prompt TiO_2 absorption by human hair follicles [122] and mice lung inflammation generated by 2–5 nm particles [123]. In experiments conducted with TiO_2 and ZnO, DNA damage have been attributed to both NPs, while cell malfunction has also been reported in the case of ZnO particles [124, 125].

Similar to TiO_2, ZnO NPs lead to cytotoxicity and cell death [126], demonstrated in various mammalian cell lines [73] such as bronchial epithelium and phagocytic cells [127] through ROS generation. Brunner et al. tested ZnO in human mesothelioma and rodent fibroblast cells. It ultimately lead to cell death in concentrations higher than 49 mg/mL [128]. Alterations in human hepatocytes, embryonic kidney cells [129], and mice liver enzymes [130] have also been reported in different studies.

Concerning iron oxide NPs, apart from inflammation they have depicted surface coating-dependent toxicity in one study where chitosan- and dextran-coated particles of different concentrations and sizes were tested [131]. ROS production, lipid peroxidation, and DNA damage have been also correlated to these NPs [73, 126], while after inhalation they are assumed to get transported to lungs, liver, and spleen and cross the BBB [132]. Concerning superparamagnetic NPs, parallel with their tremendous potential in CNS imaging, they are linked to great cytotoxicity and neuronal damage, depending on their coating, size, and concentration. Therefore, the scientific community should focus on detailed human neurological toxicity estimation.

12.6.3 Quantum Dots

QDs are widely exploited in medicine and electronics industries due to their manifold physicochemical properties. Detection of cancerous cells, biomedical imaging, drug delivery, CNS mapping, and cell labeling are among applications employing QDs. It has been reported that QD toxicity is strongly connected with experimental conditions and each QD's particular properties, which vary a lot from one QD to another [15, 133–135], resulting in a lack of agreement between different published results. However, any toxic effect found is assumed to originate from the release of metal ions from the QD core caused by UV light irradiation and oxidative environments. In the case of cell lines exposed to cadmium (Cd)-based QDs, evidence confirms that Cd ion liberation results in cytotoxicity and ROS generation [133, 136–138]. Surface coating appears to be another critical factor affecting QD toxicity [15, 71, 137]. For instance, a mercaptoundecanoic acid coating has been proved significantly more toxic [137, 139] than polyethylene glycol (PEG) and polymaleic anhydride octadecene (QD-PC) coatings. It has been also noticed that irradiation of ZnS-coated CdSe QDs does not produce any ROS [140], while only spleen, kidney, and liver accumulation, with no noxious effects, has been reported from experiments in Sprague–Dawley mice [141]. QDs with a carboxylic acid coating have been detected in the upper stratum corneum layers of rats and mice [135, 142], while intraperitoneal CdSe and ZnSe injection in mice brought about brain transportation without causing any functional damage [143]. Overall, precise in vivo and in vitro protocols in stable environmental conditions, using adequate and appropriate QD coating to limit ion leaching, would be suggested for a reliable assessment of QD toxicity.

12.7 Nanotoxicity in the Environment

Nanosized particles' presence in ecosystems dates back to the early years of the earth's creation. As mentioned before, forest fires, volcano eruptions, soil erosion, and desert dust storms are among the natural NP sources, while minerals and bacteria could be also considered as environmental nanostructures. Burned wood in fireplaces, gases emitted from diesel engines, and nanowaste from industrial applications belong to the sources of unintentional NP delivery into the environment. Environmental remediation and wastewater treatment plants are additional factors that contribute to nanoecotoxicity because of the metal oxides and iron NPs that are commonly involved. Obviously, the huge increase in NP use over the last decades justifies the growing scientific worries regarding environmental nanotoxicity. It should be emphasized that airborne NPs and nanomaterials in liquids and the soil are more likely to undergo environmental dispersion [144].

Air, water, and soil directly interact with a variety of NPs, a phenomenon that possibly results in harmful effects in living organisms and plants and the NPs ending up in humans through inhalation or the food chain. Unfortunately, the expansion in NP applications does not go hand in hand with the estimation of ecological hazards. The heterogeneity of NP characteristics; the possible transformation, agglomeration, or alteration in surface properties; and the strong influence of the environmental conditions (sunlight, UV radiation) on the NPs' behavior outline the uncertainty in their fate once they are released in the environment, hence the complexity involved in nanoecotoxicity assessment.

12.7.1 NPs in Air

Natural and man-made NPs apparent in air have exhibited a significant impact on the environmental burden. Vehicle emissions, cigarette smoke, meteorite dust, and stationary combustion sources together with ENPs handling and conditioning constitute the basis of air nanocontamination. Further interaction between emitted NPs and existing air impurities creates daughter particles with properties dissimilar to the parental ones [145]; thus, the environmental damage is hard to quantitatively determine.

Apart from dissolution and aggregation, in terms of our ecosystem's defense weapons, environmental hydroxyl radicals could be compared to human macrophages as they are in charge of breaking down organic pollutants. Yet, contact between NPs and the free hydroxyl radicals brings about a significant decrease in these ecoguards, limiting the degradation of atmospheric pollutants. This phenomenon increases the greenhouse gases obtainable in the atmosphere—the major kind of gases guilty of leading to ozone layer depletion [146].

Glacier melting may also be linked to the impact of NPs on the global climate. Black carbon is incorporated in glaciers, leading to an increase in heat absorption by the glaciers and finally resulting in glacier melting. Brown clouds that are made of black CNPs and fuel combustion products encompass high amounts of ozone, which may pose a high risk to agriculture. Additionally, the increased exposure to this atmosphere might increase the risk of exposure to pathogenic microorganisms. The health impact of exposure to this brown cloud is an increase in diseases (i.e., cardiovascular, pulmonary, bacterial diseases) as well as chronic respiratory problems [146].

12.7.2 NPs in Water

Water pollution is an additional consequence of the widespread application of NPs over the preceding years. NPs apparent in the atmosphere could translocate to the sea, rivers, and oceans through rain, wind, or storms. However, discharge of wastewater containing medical and industrial NPs and their further disposal in surface water is the main origin of water nanocontamination. In terms of nature and concentration, NPs existing in wastewater interact with particles that participate in wastewater treatment processes. Wastewater treatment degradation could be a possible result of these interactions, leading to incomplete waste disinfection and consequently severe water pollution [145]. It is remarkable that NPs used in wastewater treatment might concurrently result in water contamination, a fact that should trouble scientists in terms of the safe concentration levels of NPs in any relevant application. Finally, the presence of nanomaterials in consumer products such as paints, sunscreens, creams, and cosmetics, along with NPs used in environmental remediation, seems an important cause of water contamination.

Apart from humans, aquatic species could be directly affected by water nanopollution. *Daphnia magna* toxicity and mortality caused by TiO_2 [9, 147, 148] and C60 NPs [148, 149] could possibly lead to a major disruption in the aquatic food chain. Zebrafish that are directly fed by *Daphnia magna* may be indirectly exposed to these NPs in addition to direct straight contact and interaction with them. Zebrafish molting and offspring production setback has been reported in the case of three weeks of exposure to C60 NPs [150]. Short-term exposure to TiO_2 seems nontoxic for adult zebrafish [9, 151], while long-term exposure appears toxic for its gills, liver, and brain. Two weeks of exposure to TiO_2 NPs has caused an important decrease in zebrafish egg production [152].

A plethora of experiments have demonstrated the toxic effects of calcium oxide, copper oxide, magnesium oxide, and silver NPs on both embryo and adult zebrafish [151, 153, 154]. Furthermore, ZnO NPs may cause oxidative stress on zebrafish gill and intestine [155] and DNA damage in its embryos [156]. Finally, controversial outcomes have been published regarding the effects of different types of silica NPs on embryonic zebrafish [157, 158], indicating the difficulty in getting consistent results, even when trying to determine nanotoxicity in aquatic organisms when experimental protocols differ from one study to another.

12.7.3 NPs in Soil

Soil-NP interaction remains a complex issue for the scientific community. The numerous differences in soil structure in terms of chemical substances, minerals, humidity, bacteria, and other microorganisms portray the huge difficulty in soil toxicity determination. Most of the experiments have been conducted with higher-than-real concentrations of untouched NPs in artificial instead of sandy soil samples [159], creating sufficient uncertainties in toxicity measurements.

Undoubtedly, fertilizers, pesticides, airstreams, and wastewater treatment plant sludge offer NPs the potential to penetrate into soil; interact with the variety of organic and inorganic soil substances; and induce toxicity in bacteria, eukaryotic organisms, and plants. Naturally occurring NPs existing in soil, for example, metal hydroxides and clay minerals, probably are the least toxic NPs for bacteria and protozoa [160], in contrast to man-made NPs, such as TiO_2 and fullerenes. In particular, TiO_2 NPs have an important impact on bacteria cell viability due to ROS formation and subsequent oxidative stress [161]. Similarly, C60 fullerenes have caused a notable reduction in soil bacteria population [162], while a 48 h exposure to silver NPs has proved to induce toxicity in bacterium colonies too [163].

Several different types of earthworms have been tested in terms of nanotoxicity. Copper NPs at a concentration below 65 mg per kg of soil have not exhibited any noxious impact, while no genetic effect has been reported in the case of gold NPs for concentrations below 50 mg per kg of soil. On the other hand, reproductive harm has occurred due to higher gold NP concentrations [164] and in the case of copper and TiO_2 concentrations of 1000 mg per kg of soil [165]. Depending on their concentration [166], coating, and size [167] silver NPs have decreased earthworms' growth rate whereas ZnO and CeO NPs may raise survival issues in earthworms too [9].

12.7.4 NP Effects in Plants

Plants could possibly be affected by airborne or soil NPs in different ways. To begin with, nanosized leaf pores, stomata, and roots are the main entrances for NPs existing in air and soil into plants. CNTs seem to enter cell membranes [168] and interact with the root surface [169]. Various studies recently reviewed the impact of NPs of different materials, sizes, and concentrations on different plant cells, from soybean and tobacco to fruit and vegetables [167, 146]. It seems that all nanophysicochemical properties play a vital role in the influence of NPs on plants, while the toxic effects induced are comparable to those in mammals, fish, and cell lines. DNA damage, ROS generation, and cell viability are among the results, but seed germination and root elongation rates could also depict potential nanotoxicity. Besides, NP accumulation in leaves could be related to a reduction in the photosynthesis phenomenon, resulting in a decrease in plant growth rate [146].

It is a highly debatable topic whether the noticed effects are a result of NP presence alone. The concentration of unidentified NPs in air and soil, along with the probable changes in the NPs' nature as they come in contact with air pollutants and soil substances, poses a great challenge for the scientific community in determining plant nanotoxicity. However, from nanotoxicological point of view, plant species important for human nutrition should attract researchers' attention as they characterize the foundation of the food chains that ensure the earth's survival.

References

1. Forbe, T., García, M. and Gonzalez, E. (2011). Potencial risks of nanoparticles, *Ciênc. Tecnol. Aliment.*, **4**, pp. 835–842.
2. Handy, R. D. and Shaw, B. J. (2007). Toxic effects of nanoparticles and nanomaterials: Implications for public health, risk assessment and the public perception of nanotechnology, *Health Risk Soc.*, **9**(2), pp. 125–144.
3. Ward, J. E. and Kach, D. J. (2009). Marine aggregates facilitate ingestion of nanoparticles by suspension-feeding bivalves, *Mar. Environ. Res.*, **68**(3), pp. 137–142.
4. Radomski, A., Jurasz, P., Alonso-Escolano, D., Drews, M., Morandi, M., Malinski, T. and Radomski, M. W. (2005). Nanoparticle-induced platelet aggregation and vascular thrombosis, *Br. J. Pharmacol.*, **146**(6), pp. 882–893.
5. Oberdörster, G., Elder, A. and Rinderknecht, A. (2009). Nanoparticles and the brain: cause for concern?, *J. Nanosci. Nanotechnol.*, **9**(8), pp. 4996–5007.
6. Holsapple, M. P., Farland, W. H., Landry, T. D. Monteiro-Riviere, N. A., Carter, J. M., Walker, N. J. and Thomas, K. V. (2005). Research strategies for safety evaluation of nanomaterials, Part II: Toxicological and safety evaluation of nanomaterials, current challenges and data needs, *Toxicol. Sci.*, **88**(1), pp. 12–17.
7. Kim, S., Lim, Y. T., Soltesz, E. G., De Grand, A. M., Lee, J., Nakayama, A., Parker, J. A., Mihaljevic, T., Laurence, R. G., Dor, D. M., Cohn, L. H., Bawendi, M. G. and Frangioni, J. V. (2004). Near-infrared fluorescent type ii quantum dots for sentinel lymph node mapping, *Nat. Biotechnol.*, **22**(1), pp. 93–97.
8. Gontier, E., Ynsa, M. D., Biro, T., Hunyadi, J., Kiss, B., Gaspar, K., Pinheiro, T., Silva, J. N., Filipe, P., Stachura, J., Dabros, W., Reinert, T., Butz, T., Moretto, P. and Surleve-Bazeille, J. E. (2008). Is there penetration of titania nanoparticles in sunscreens through skin? A comparative electron and ion microscopy study, *Nanotoxicology*, **2**(4), pp. 218–231.
9. Sajid, M., Ilyas, M., Basheer, C., Tariq, M., Daud, M., Baig, N. and Shehzad, F. (2015). Impact of nanoparticles on human and environment: review of toxicity factors, exposures, control strategies, and future prospects, *Environ. Sci. Pollut. Res. Int.*, **22**(6), pp. 4122–4143.
10. Hagens, W. I., Oomen, A. G., de Jong, W. H., Cassee, F. R. and Sips, A. J. (2007). What do we (need to) know about the kinetic properties of

nanoparticles in the body? *Regul. Toxicol. Pharmacol.*, **49**(3), pp. 217–229.

11. Oberdörster, G., Oberdörster, E. and Oberdörster, J. (2005). Nanotoxicology: an emerging discipline evolving from studies of ultrafine particles, *Environ. Health Perspect.*, **113**(7), pp. 823–839.
12. Tinkle, S. S., Antonini, J. M., Rich, B. A., Roberts, J. R., Salmen, R., DePree, K. and Adkins, E. J. (2003). Skin as a route of exposure and sensitization in chronic beryllium disease, *Environ. Health Perspect.*, **111**(9), pp. 1202–1208.
13. Fröhlich, E. and Roblegg, E. (2012). Models for oral uptake of nanoparticles in consumer products, *Toxicology*, **291**(1–3), pp. 10–17.
14. Kreyling, W. G., Semmler-Behnke, M. and Moller, W. (2006). Ultrafine particle-lung interactions: does size matter?, *J. Aerosol. Med.*, **19**(1), pp. 74–83.
15. Ray, P. C., Yu, H. and Fu, P. P. (2009). Toxicity and environmental risks of nanomaterials: challenges and future needs, *J. Environ. Sci. Health C*, **27**(1), pp. 1–35.
16. Zhao, Y., Wang, B., Feng, W. and Bai, C. (2012). Nanotoxicology: toxicological and biological activities of nanomaterials, in *Encyclopedia of Life Support Systems (EOLSS)*, Oxford, UK.
17. Arora, S., Rajwade, J. M. and Paknikar, K. M. (2012). Nanotoxicology and in vitro studies: the need of the hour, *Toxicol. Appl. Pharmacol.*, **258**, pp. 151–165.
18. Janrao, K. K., Gadhave, M. V., Banerjee, S. K. and Gaikwad, D. D. (2014). Nanoparticle induced nanotoxicity: an overview, *Asian J. Biomed. Pharm. Sci.*, **4**(32), pp. 1–7.
19. Oberdörster, G., Sharp, Z., Atudorei, V., Elder, A., Gelein, R., Lunts, A., Kreyling, W. and Cox, C. (2002). Extrapulmonary translocation of ultrafine carbon particle following whole-body inhalation exposure of rats, *J. Toxicol. Environ. Health A*, **65**, pp. 1531–1543.
20. Nurkiewicz, T. R., Porter, D. W., Barger, M., Millecchia, L., Rao, K. M., Marvar, P. J., Hubbs, A. F., Castranova, V. and Boegehold, M. A. (2006). Systemic microvascular dysfunction and inflammation after pulmonary particulate matter exposure, *Environ. Health Perspect.*, **114**(3), pp. 412–419.
21. Bu, Q., Yan, G., Deng, P., Peng, F., Lin, H., Xu, Y., Cao, Z., Zhou, T., Xue, A., Wang, Y., Cen, X. and Zhao, Y. L. (2010). NMR-based metabonomic study of the sub-acute toxicity of titanium dioxide nanoparticles in rats after oral administration, *Nanotechnology*, **21**(12), p. 125105.

22. Bergin, I. L. and Witzmann, F. A. (2013). Nanoparticle toxicity by the gastrointestinal route: evidence and knowledge gaps, *Int. J. Biomed. Nanosci. Nanotechnol.*, **3**(1–2), doi: 10.1504/IJBNN.2013.054515.

23. Valant, J., Drobne, D. and Novak, S. (2012). Effect of ingested titanium dioxide nanoparticles on the digestive gland cell membrane of terrestrial isopods, *Chemosphere*, **87**(1), pp. 19–25.

24. Curtis, J., Greenberg, M., Kester, J., Phillips, S. and Krieger, G. (2006). Nanotechnology and nanotoxicology: a primer for clinicians, *Toxicol. Rev.*, **25**(4), pp. 245–260.

25. Kreyling, W. G., Semmler, M., Erbe, F., Mayer, P., Takenaka, S., Schulz, H., Oberdörster, G. and Ziesenis, A. (2002). Translocation of ultrafine insoluble iridium particles from lung epithelium to extrapulmonary organs is size dependent but very low, *J. Toxicol. Environ. Health A*, **65**(20), pp. 1513–1530.

26. Liu, R., Zhang, X., Pu, Y., Yin, L., Li, Y., Zhang, X., Liang, G., Li, X. and Zhang, J. (2010). Small-sized titanium dioxide nanoparticles mediate immune toxicity in rat pulmonary alveolar macrophages in vivo, *J. Nanosci. Nanotechnol.*, **10**(8), pp. 5161–5169.

27. Longmire, M., Choyke, P. L. and Kobayashi, H. (2008). Clearance properties of nano-sized particles and molecules as imaging agents: considerations and caveats, *Nanomedicine (Lond)*, **3**(5), pp. 703–717.

28. Batchelor-McAuley, C., Tschulik, K., Neumann, C. C., Laborda, E. and Compton, R. G. (2014). Why are silver nanoparticles more toxic than bulk silver? Towards understanding the dissolution and toxicity of silver nanoparticles, *Int. J. Electrochem. Sci*, **9**, pp. 1132–1138.

29. Mortimer, M., Kasemets, K. and Kahru, A. (2010). Toxicity of ZnO and CuO nanoparticles to ciliated protozoa tetrahymena thermophila, *Toxicology*, **269**(2–3), pp. 182–189.

30. Braakhuis, H. M., Gosens, I., Krystek, P., Boere, J. A., Cassee, F. R., Fokkens, P. H., Post, J. A., van Loveren, H. and Park, M. V. (2014). Particle size dependent deposition and pulmonary inflammation after short-term inhalation of silver nanoparticles, *Part. Fibre Toxicol.*, **11**(1), p. 49.

31. Donaldson, K. and Stone, V. (2003). Current hypotheses on the mechanisms of toxicity of ultrafine particles, *Ann. Ist. Super. Sanita.*, **39**(3), pp. 405–410.

32. Renwick, L. C., Brown, D., Clouter, A. and Donaldson, K. (2004). Increased inflammation and altered macrophage chemotactic responses caused by two ultrafine particle types, *Occup. Environ. Med.*, **61**(5), pp. 442–447.

33. Shin, S., Song, I. and Um, S. (2015). Role of physicochemical properties in nanoparticle toxicity, *Nanomaterials*, **5**(3), p. 1351.

34. De Jong, W. H., Hagens, W. I., Krystek, P., Burger, M. C., Sips, A. J. and Geertsma, R. E. (2008). Particle size-dependent organ distribution of gold nanoparticles after intravenous administration, *Biomaterials*, **29**(12), pp. 1912–1919.

35. Gliga, A. R., Skoglund, S., Wallinder, I. O., Fadeel, B. and Karlsson, H. L. (2014). Size-dependent cytotoxicity of silver nanoparticles in human lung cells: the role of cellular uptake, agglomeration and ag release, *Part. Fibre Toxicol.*, **11**, p. 11.

36. Lankveld, D. P., Oomen, A. G., Krystek, P., Neigh, A., Troost-de Jong, A., Noorlander, C. W., Van Eijkeren, J. C., Geertsma, R. E. and De Jong, W. H. (2010). The kinetics of the tissue distribution of silver nanoparticles of different sizes, *Biomaterials*, **31**(32), pp. 8350–8361.

37. Chen, Z., Meng, H., Xing, G., Chen, C., Zhao, Y., Jia, G., Wang, T., Yuan, H., Ye, C., Zhao, F., Chai, Z., Zhu, C., Fang, X., Ma, B. and Wan, L. (2006). Acute toxicological effects of copper nanoparticles in vivo, *Toxicol. Lett.*, **163**(2), pp. 109–120.

38. Hoet, P. H., Brüske-Hohlfeld, I. and Salata, O. V. (2004). Nanoparticles known and unknown health risks, *J. Nanobiotechnol.*, **2**(1), p. 12.

39. Agarwal, R., Singh, V., Jurney, P., Shi, L., Sreenivasan, S. V. and Roy, K. (2013). Mammalian cells preferentially internalize hydrogel nanodiscs over nanorods and use shape-specific uptake mechanisms, *Proc. Natl. Acad. Sci. U.S.A.*, **110**(43), pp. 17247–17252.

40. Gorka, D. E., Osterberg, J. S., Gwin, C. A., Colman, B. P., Meyer, J. N., Bernhardt, E. S., Gunsch, C. K., DiGulio, R. T. and Liu, J. (2015). Reducing environmental toxicity of silver nanoparticles through shape control, *Environ. Sci. Technol.*, **49**(16), pp. 10093–10098.

41. Ispas, C., Andreescu, D., Patel, A., Goia, D. V., Andreescu, S. and Wallace, K. N. (2009). Toxicity and developmental defects of different sizes and shape nickel nanoparticles in zebrafish, *Environ. Sci. Technol.*, **43**(16), pp. 6349–6356.

42. Nagai, H., Okazaki, Y., Chew, S. H., Misawa, N., Yamashita, Y., Akatsuka, S., Ishihara, T., Yamashita, K., Yoshikawa, Y., Yasui, H., Jiang, L., Ohara, H., Takahashi, T., Ichihara, G., Kostarelos, K., Miyata, Y., Shinohara, H. and Toyokuni, S. (2011). Diameter and rigidity of multiwalled carbon nanotubes are critical factors in mesothelial injury and carcinogenesis, *Proc. Natl. Acad. Sci. U.S.A.*, **108**(49), pp. E1330–E1338.

43. Tucker, A. K. and Hernandez, R. (2011). Absence of enhanced diffusion in the dynamics of a thick needle through three-dimensional fixed spherical scatterers, *J. Phys. Chem. B*, **115**(15), pp. 4412–4418.

44. Gratton, S. E., Ropp, P. A., Pohlhaus, P. D., Luft, J. C., Madden, V. J., Napier, M. E. and DeSimone, J. M. (2008). The effect of particle design on cellular internalization pathways, *Proc. Natl. Acad. Sci. U.S.A.*, **105**(33), pp. 11613–11618.

45. Barua, S., Yoo, J. W., Kolhar, P., Wakankar, A., Gokarn, Y. R. and Mitragotri, S. (2013). Particle shape enhances specificity of antibody-displaying nanoparticles, *Proc. Natl. Acad. Sci. U.S.A.*, **110**(9), pp. 3270–3275.

46. Hsiao, I. L. and Huang, Y. J. (2011). Effects of various physicochemical characteristics on the toxicities of ZnO and TiO nanoparticles toward human lung epithelial cells, *Sci. Total Environ.*, **409**(7), pp. 1219–1228.

47. Feng, Z. V., Gunsolus, I. L., Qiu, T. A., Hurley, K. R., Nyberg, L. H., Frew, H., Johnson, K. P., Vartanian, A. M., Jacob, L. M., Lohse, S. E., Torelli, M. D., Hamers, R. J., Murphy, C. J. and Haynes, C. L. (2015). Impacts of gold nanoparticle charge and ligand type on surface binding and toxicity to gram-negative and gram-positive bacteria, *Chem. Sci.*, **6**(9), pp. 5186–5196.

48. Fröhlich, E. (2012). The role of surface charge in cellular uptake and cytotoxicity of medical nanoparticles, *Int. J. Nanomed.*, **7**, pp. 5577–5591.

49. Jiang, J., Oberdörster, G. and Biswas, P. (2009). Characterization of size, surface charge, and agglomeration state of nanoparticle dispersions for toxicological studies, *J. Nanopart. Res.*, **11**(1), pp. 77–89.

50. Suresh, A. K., Pelletier, D. A., Wang, W., Moon, J.-W., Gu, B., Mortensen, N. P., Allison, D. P., Joy, D. C., Phelps, T. J. and Doktycz, M. J. (2010). Silver nanocrystallites: biofabrication using *Shewanella oneidensis*, and an evaluation of their comparative toxicity on gram-negative and gram-positive bacteria, *Environ. Sci. Technol.*, **44**(13), pp. 5210–5215.

51. Shi, H., Magaye, R., Castranova, V. and Zhao, J. (2013). Titanium dioxide nanoparticles: a review of current toxicological data, *Part. Fibre Toxicol.*, **10**, p. 15.

52. Seiffert, J., Hussain, F., Wiegman, C., Li, F., Bey, L., Baker, W., Porter, A., Ryan, M. P., Chang, Y., Gow, A., Zhang, J., Zhu, J., Tetley, T. D. and Chung, K. F. (2015). Pulmonary toxicity of instilled silver nanoparticles: influence of size, coating and rat strain, *PLoS One*, **10**(3), p. e0119726.

53. Magrez, A., Kasas, S., Salicio, V., Pasquier, N., Seo, J. W., Celio, M., Catsicas, S., Schwaller, B. and Forro, L. (2006). Cellular toxicity of carbon-based nanomaterials, *Nano Lett.*, **6**(6), pp. 1121–1125.

54. Lam, C. W., James, J. T., McCluskey, R. and Hunter, R. L. (2004). Pulmonary toxicity of single-wall carbon nanotubes in mice 7 and 90 days after intratracheal instillation, *Toxicol. Sci.*, **77**, pp. 126–134.

55. Smart, S. K., Cassady, A. I., Lu, G. Q. and Martin, D. J. (2006). The biocompatibility of carbon nanotubes, *Carbon*, **44**(6), pp. 1034–1047.

56. Gaiser, B. K., Fernandes, T. F., Jepson, M. A., Lead, J. R., Tyler, C. R., Baalousha, M., Biswas, A., Britton, G. J., Cole, P. A., Johnston, B. D., Ju-Nam, Y., Rosenkranz, P., Scown, T. M. and Stone, V. (2012). Interspecies comparisons on the uptake and toxicity of silver and cerium dioxide nanoparticles, *Environ. Toxicol. Chem.*, **31**(1), pp. 144–154.

57. Stahl, W., Junghans, A., de Boer, B., Driomina, E. S., Briviba, K. and Sies, H. (1998). Carotenoid mixtures protect multilamellar liposomes against oxidative damage: synergistic effects of lycopene and lutein, *FEBS Lett.*, **427**(2), pp. 305–308.

58. Wang, Y., Aker, W. G., Hwang, H. M., Yedjou, C. G., Yu, H. and Tchounwou, P. B. (2011). A study of the mechanism of in vitro cytotoxicity of metal oxide nanoparticles using catfish primary hepatocytes and human HepG2 cells, *Sci. Total Environ.*, **409**(22), pp. 4753–4762.

59. Lanone, S., Rogerieux, F., Geys, J., Dupont, A., Maillot-Marechal, E., Boczkowski, J., Lacroix, G. and Hoet, P. (2009). Comparative toxicity of 24 manufactured nanoparticles in human alveolar epithelial and macrophage cell lines, *Part. Fibre Toxicol.*, **6**, p. 14.

60. Porter, A. E., Muller, K., Skepper, J., Midgley, P. and Welland, M. (2006). Uptake of C60 by human monocyte macrophages, its localization and implications for toxicity: studied by high resolution electron microscopy and electron tomography, *Acta Biomater.*, **2**(4), pp. 409–419.

61. Fridovich, I. (1995). Superoxide radical and superoxide dismutases, *Annu. Rev. Biochem.*, **64**, pp. 97–112.

62. Mates, J. M. and Sanchez-Jimenez, F. (1999). Antioxidant enzymes and their implications in pathophysiologic processes, *Front. Biosci.*, **4**, pp. 339–345.

63. Jornot, L., Petersen, H. and Junod, A. F. (1998). Hydrogen peroxide-induced DNA damage is independent of nuclear calcium but dependent on redox-active ions, *Biochem. J.*, **335**(Pt 1), pp. 85–94.

64. Risom, L., Moller, P. and Loft, S. (2005). Oxidative stress-induced DNA damage by particulate air pollution, *Mutat. Res.*, **592**(1–2), pp. 119–137.

65. Petersen, E. J. and Nelson, B. C. (2010). Mechanisms and measurements of nanomaterial-induced oxidative damage to DNA, *Anal. Bioanal. Chem.*, **398**(2), pp. 613–650.

66. Donaldson, K. and Tran, C. L. (2002). Inflammation caused by particles and fibers, *Inhalation Toxicol.*, **14**(1), pp. 5–27.

67. Rani, V. and Yadav, U. C. S. (2014). *Free Radical in Human Health and Disease*, Springer, New Delhi, India.

68. Sioutas, C., Delfino, R. J. and Singh, M. (2005). Exposure assessment for atmospheric ultrafine particles (UFPs) and implications in epidemiologic research, *Environ. Health Perspect.*, **113**(8), pp. 947–955.

69. Parveen, S. and Sahoo, S. K. (2008). Polymeric nanoparticles for cancer therapy, *J. Drug Target.*, **16**(2), pp. 108–123.

70. Khanna, P., Ong, C., Bay, B. and Baeg, G. (2015). Nanotoxicity: an interplay of oxidative stress, inflammation and cell death, *Nanomaterials*, **5**(3), p. 1163.

71. Yildirimer, L., Thanh, N. T. K., Loizidou, M. and Seifalian, A. M. (2011). Toxicological considerations of clinically applicable nanoparticles, *Nano Today*, **6**, pp. 585–607.

72. Akhtar, M. J., Ahamed, M., Kumar, S., Siddiqui, H., Patil, G., Ashquin, M. and Ahmad, I. (2010). Nanotoxicity of pure silica mediated through oxidant generation rather than glutathione depletion in human lung epithelial cells, *Toxicology*, **276**(2), pp. 95–102.

73. Bahadar, H., Faheem, M., Kamal, N. and Mohammad, A. (2016). Toxicity of nanoparticles and an overview of current experimental models, *Iran. Biomed. J.*, **20**(1), pp. 1–11.

74. Lison, D., Thomassen, L. C., Rabolli, V., Gonzalez, L., Napierska, D., Seo, J. W., Kirsch-Volders, M., Hoet, P., Kirschhock, C. E. and Martens, J. A. (2008). Nominal and effective dosimetry of silica nanoparticles in cytotoxicity assays, *Toxicol. Sci.*, **104**(1), pp. 155–162.

75. Park, E. J., Yi, J., Kim, Y., Choi, K. and Park, K. (2010). Silver nanoparticles induce cytotoxicity by a trojan-horse type mechanism, *Toxicol. in Vitro*, **24**(3), pp. 872–878.

76. Cho, M., Cho, W. S., Choi, M., Kim, S. J., Han, B. S., Kim, S. H., Kim, H. O., Sheen, Y. Y. and Jeong, J. (2009). The impact of size on tissue distribution and elimination by single intravenous injection of silica nanoparticles, *Toxicol. Lett.*, **189**(3), pp. 177–183.

77. Firme III, C. P. and Bandaru, P. R. (2010). Toxicity issues in the application of carbon nanotubes to biological systems, *Nanomed. Nanotechnol. Biol. Med.*, **6**(2), pp. 245–256.

78. Ghanbary, F., Naserzadeh, P., Seydi, E., Ghasemi, A., Joghataei, M. T., Ashtari, K. and Akbari, M. (2017). Mitochondrial oxidative stress and dysfunction induced by single- and multi-wall carbon nanotubes: a comparative study, *J. Biomed. Mater. Res. A*, **105**(7), pp. 2047–2055.

79. Tian, F., Cui, D., Schwarz, H., Estrada, G. G. and Kobayashi, H. (2006). Cytotoxicity of single-wall carbon nanotubes on human fibroblasts, *Toxicol. in Vitro*, **20**(7), pp. 1202–1212.

80. He, X., Young, S. H., Schwegler-Berry, D., Chisholm, W. P., Fernback, J. E. and Ma, Q. (2011). Multiwalled carbon nanotubes induce a fibrogenic response by stimulating reactive oxygen species production, activating nf-kappab signaling, and promoting fibroblast-to-myofibroblast transformation, *Chem. Res. Toxicol.*, **24**(12), pp. 2237–2248.

81. Manke, A., Wang, L. and Rojanasakul, Y. (2013). Mechanisms of nanoparticle-induced oxidative stress and toxicity, *BioMed Res. Int.*, **2013**, Article ID 942916 (15 pp.).

82. Mitchell, L. A., Gao, J., Wal, R. V., Gigliotti, A., Burchiel, S. W. and McDonald, J. D. (2007). Pulmonary and systemic immune response to inhaled multiwalled carbon nanotubes, *Toxicol. Sci.*, **100**(1), pp. 203–214.

83. Wang, J., Sun, P., Bao, Y., Liu, J. and An, L. (2011). Cytotoxicity of single-walled carbon nanotubes on PC12 cells, *Toxicol. in Vitro*, **25**(1), pp. 242–250.

84. Herzog, E., Casey, A., Lyng, F. M., Chambers, G., Byrne, H. J. and Davoren, M. (2007). A new approach to the toxicity testing of carbon-based nanomaterials--the clonogenic assay, *Toxicol. Lett.*, **174**(1–3), pp. 49–60.

85. Nemmar, A., Vanbilloen, H., Hoylaerts, M. F., Hoet, P. H., Verbruggen, A. and Nemery, B. (2001). Passage of intratracheally instilled ultrafine particles from the lung into the systemic circulation in hamster, *Am. J. Respir. Crit. Care Med.*, **164**(9), pp. 1665–1668.

86. Jia, G., Wang, H., Yan, L., Wang, X., Pei, R., Yan, T., Zhao, Y. and Guo, X. (2005). Cytotoxicity of carbon nanomaterials: single-wall nanotube, multi-wall nanotube, and fullerene, *Environ. Sci. Technol.*, **39**(5), pp. 1378–1383.

87. Silva, V. M., Corson, N., Elder, A. and Oberdorster, G. (2005). The rat ear vein model for investigating in vivo thrombogenicity of ultrafine particles (UFP), *Toxicol. Sci.*, **85**(2), pp. 983–989.

88. Kim, S. and Ryu, D. Y. (2013). Silver nanoparticle-induced oxidative stress, genotoxicity and apoptosis in cultured cells and animal tissues, *J. Appl. Toxicol.*, **33**(2), pp. 78–89.

89. Monserrat, J. M., Seixas, A. L., Ferreira-Cravo, M., Burguer-Mendonca, M., Garcia, S. C., Kaufmann, C. G. Jr. and Ventura-Lima, J. (2017). Interference of single walled carbon nanotubes (SWCNT) in the measurement of lipid peroxidation in aquatic organisms through tbars assay, *Ecotoxicol. Environ. Saf.*, **140**, pp. 103–108.

90. Chen, T., Zang, J., Wang, H., Nie, H., Wang, X., Shen, Z., Tang, S., Yang, J. and Jia, G. (2012). Water-soluble taurine-functionalized multi-walled carbon nanotubes induce less damage to mitochondria of raw 264.7 cells, *J. Nanosci. Nanotechnol.*, **12**(10), pp. 8008–8016.

91. Bonner, J. C. (2007). Lung fibrotic responses to particle exposure, *Toxicol. Pathol.*, **35**(1), pp. 148–153.

92. Crouzier, D., Follot, S., Gentilhomme, E., Flahaut, E., Arnaud, R., Dabouis, V., Castellarin, C. and Debouzy, J. C. (2010). Carbon nanotubes induce inflammation but decrease the production of reactive oxygen species in lung, *Toxicology*, **272**(1–3), pp. 39–45.

93. Muller, J., Huaux, F., Moreau, N., Misson, P., Heilier, J.-F., Delos, M., Arras, M., Fonseca, A., Nagy, J. B. and Lison, D. (2005). Respiratory toxicity of multi-wall carbon nanotubes, *Toxicol. Appl. Pharmacol.*, **207**(3), pp. 221–231.

94. Ding, L., Stilwell, J., Zhang, T., Elboudwarej, O., Jiang, H., Selegue, J. P., Cooke, P. A., Gray, J. W. and Chen, F. F. (2005). Molecular characterization of the cytotoxic mechanism of multiwall carbon nanotubes and nano-onions on human skin fibroblast, *Nano Lett.*, **5**(12), pp. 2448–2464.

95. Maynard, A. D., Baron, P. A., Foley, M., Shvedova, A. A., Kisin, E. R. and Castranova, V. (2004). Exposure to carbon nanotube material: aerosol release during the handling of unrefined single walled carbon nanotube material, *J. Toxicol. Environ. Health A*, **67**, pp. 87–107.

96. Shvedova, A., Castranova, V., Kisin, E., Schwegler-Berry, D., Murray, A., Gandelsman, V., Maynard, A. and Baron, P. (2003). Exposure to carbon nanotube material: assessment of nanotube cytotoxicity using human keratinocyte cells, *J. Toxicol. Environ. Health A*, **66**(20), pp. 1909–1926.

97. Wang, S., Lu, W., Tovmachenko, O., Rai, U. S., Yu, H. and Ray, P. C. (2008). Challenge in understanding size and shape dependent toxicity of gold nanomaterials in human skin keratinocytes, *Chem. Phys. Lett.*, **463**(1–3), pp. 145–149.

98. Connor, E. E., Mwamuka, J., Gole, A., Murphy, C. J. and Wyatt, M. D. (2005). Gold nanoparticles are taken up by human cells but do not cause acute cytotoxicity, *Small*, **1**(3), pp. 325–327.

99. Villiers, C., Freitas, H., Couderc, R., Villiers, M.-B. and Marche, P. (2010). Analysis of the toxicity of gold nano particles on the immune system: effect on dendritic cell functions, *J. Nanopart. Res.*, **12**(1), pp. 55–60.

100. Patra, H. K., Banerjee, S., Chaudhuri, U., Lahiri, P. and Dasgupta, A. K. (2007). Cell selective response to gold nanoparticles, *Nanomedicine*, **3**(2), pp. 111–119.

101. Shukla, R., Bansal, V., Chaudhary, M., Basu, A., Bhonde, R. R. and Sastry, M. (2005). Biocompatibility of gold nanoparticles and their endocytotic fate inside the cellular compartment: a microscopic overview, *Langmuir*, **21**(23), pp. 10644–10654.

102. Chen, Y. S., Hung, Y. C., Liau, I. and Huang, G. S. (2009). Assessment of the in vivo toxicity of gold nanoparticles, *Nanoscale Res. Lett.*, **4**(8), pp. 858–864.

103. Sonavane, G., Tomoda, K. and Makino, K. (2008). Biodistribution of colloidal gold nanoparticles after intravenous administration: effect of particle size, *Colloids Surf. B*, **66**(2), pp. 274–280.

104. Goodman, C. M., McCusker, C. D., Yilmaz, T. and Rotello, V. M. (2004). Toxicity of gold nanoparticles functionalized with cationic and anionic side chains, *Bioconjugate Chem.*, **15**(4), pp. 897–900.

105. Lipka, J., Semmler-Behnke, M., Sperling, R. A., Wenk, A., Takenaka, S., Schleh, C., Kissel, T., Parak, W. J. and Kreyling, W. G. (2010). Biodistribution of peg-modified gold nanoparticles following intratracheal instillation and intravenous injection, *Biomaterials*, **31**(25), pp. 6574–6581.

106. Fung, M. C. and Bowen, D. L. (1996). Silver products for medical indications: risk-benefit assessment, *J. Toxicol. Clin. Toxicol.*, **34**(1), pp. 119–126.

107. Panyala, N. R., Peña-Méndez, E. M. and Havel, J. (2008). Silver or silver nanoparticles: a hazardous threat to the environment and human health, *J. Appl. Biomed.*, **6**(3), pp. 117–129.

108. White, J. M., Powell, A. M., Brady, K. and Russell-Jones, R. (2003). Severe generalized argyria secondary to ingestion of colloidal silver protein, *Clin. Exp. Dermatol.*, **28**(3), pp. 254–256.

109. Poon, V. K. and Burd, A. (2004). In vitro cytotoxity of silver: implication for clinical wound care, *Burns*, **30**(2), pp. 140–147.

110. Foldbjerg, R., Olesen, P., Hougaard, M., Dang, D. A., Hoffmann, H. J. and Autrup, H. (2009). PVP-coated silver nanoparticles and silver ions induce reactive oxygen species, apoptosis and necrosis in THP-1 monocytes, *Toxicol. Lett.*, **190**(2), pp. 156–162.

111. Tang, J., Xiong, L., Wang, S., Wang, J., Liu, L., Li, J., Yuan, F. and Xi, T. (2009). Distribution, translocation and accumulation of silver nanoparticles in rats, *J. Nanosci. Nanotechnol.*, **9**(8), pp. 4924–4932.

112. Powers, C. M., Levin, E. D., Seidler, F. J. and Slotkin, T. A. (2011). Silver exposure in developing zebrafish produces persistent synaptic and behavioral changes, *Neurotoxicol. Teratol.*, **33**(2), pp. 329–332.

113. Teodoro, J. S., Simoes, A. M., Duarte, F. V., Rolo, A. P., Murdoch, R. C., Hussain, S. M. and Palmeira, C. M. (2011). Assessment of the toxicity of silver nanoparticles in vitro: a mitochondrial perspective, *Toxicol. in Vitro*, **25**(3), pp. 664–670.

114. Ahamed, M., Alsalhi, M. S. and Siddiqui, M. K. (2010). Silver nanoparticle applications and human health, *Clin. Chim. Acta*, **411**, pp. 1841–1848.

115. Haase, A., Tentschert, J., Jungnickel, H., Graf, P., Mantion, A., Draude, F., Plendl, J., Goetz, M. E., Galla, S., Mašić, A., Thuenemann, A. F., Taubert, A., Arlinghaus, H. F. and Luch, A. (2011). Toxicity of silver nanoparticles in human macrophages: uptake, intracellular distribution and cellular responses, *J. Phys. Conf. Ser.*, **304**(1).

116. Samberg, M. E., Oldenburg, S. J. and Monteiro-Riviere, N. A. (2010). Evaluation of silver nanoparticle toxicity in skin in vivo and keratinocytes in vitro, *Environ. Health Perspect.*, **118**(3), pp. 407–413.

117. Park, E. J., Yi, J., Chung, K. H., Ryu, D. Y., Choi, J. and Park, K. (2008). Oxidative stress and apoptosis induced by titanium dioxide nanoparticles in cultured BEAS-2B cells, *Toxicol. Lett.*, **180**(3), pp. 222–229.

118. Jin, C. Y., Zhu, B. S., Wang, X. F. and Lu, Q. H. (2008). Cytotoxicity of titanium dioxide nanoparticles in mouse fibroblast cells, *Chem. Res. Toxicol.*, **21**(9), pp. 1871–1877.

119. Chiang, H. M., Xia, Q., Zou, X., Wang, C., Wang, S., Miller, B. J., Howard, P. C., Yin, J. J., Beland, F. A., Yu, H. and Fu, P. P. (2012). Nanoscale ZnO induces cytotoxicity and DNA damage in human cell lines and rat primary neuronal cells, *J. Nanosci. Nanotechnol.*, **12**(3), pp. 2126–2135.

120. Wang, C. C., Wang, S., Xia, Q., He, W., Yin, J. J., Fu, P. P. and Li, J. H. (2013). Phototoxicity of zinc oxide nanoparticles in hacat keratinocytes-generation of oxidative DNA damage during uva and visible light irradiation, *J. Nanosci. Nanotechnol.*, **13**(6), pp. 3880–3888.

121. Pan, Z., Lee, W., Slutsky, L., Clark, R. A., Pernodet, N and Rafailovich, M. H. (2009). Adverse effects of titanium dioxide nanoparticles on human dermal fibroblasts and how to protect cells, *Small*, **5**(4), pp. 511–520.

122. Lademann, J., Weigmann, H., Rickmeyer, C., Barthelmes, H., Schaefer, H., Mueller, G. and Sterry, W. (1999). Penetration of titanium dioxide microparticles in a sunscreen formulation into the horny layer and the follicular orifice, *Skin Pharmacol. Appl. Skin Physiol.*, **12**, pp. 247–256.

123. Grassian, V. H., O'Shaughnessy, P. T., Adamcakova-Dodd, A., Pettibone, J. M. and Thorne, P. S. (2007. Inhalation exposure study of titanium dioxide nanoparticles with a primary particle size of 2 to 5 nm, *Environ. Health Perspect.*, **115**(3), pp. 397–402.

124. Karlsson, H. L., Cronholm, P., Gustafsson, J. and Moller, L. (2008). Copper oxide nanoparticles are highly toxic: a comparison between metal oxide nanoparticles and carbon nanotubes, *Chem. Res. Toxicol.*, **21**(9), pp. 1726–1732.

125. Osman, I. F., Baumgartner, A., Cemeli, E., Fletcher, J. N. and Anderson, D. (2010). Genotoxicity and cytotoxicity of zinc oxide and titanium dioxide in hep-2 cells, *Nanomedicine (Lond)*, **5**(8), pp. 1193–1203.

126. Fu, P. P., Xia, Q., Hwang, H. M., Ray, P. C. and Yu, H. (2014). Mechanisms of nanotoxicity: generation of reactive oxygen species, *J. Food Drug Anal.*, **22**, pp. 64–75.

127. Xia, T., Kovochich, M., Liong, M., Madler, L., Gilbert, B., Shi, H., Yeh, J. I., Zink, J. I. and Nel, A. E. (2008). Comparison of the mechanism of toxicity of zinc oxide and cerium oxide nanoparticles based on dissolution and oxidative stress properties, *ACS Nano*, **2**(10), pp. 2121–2134.

128. Brunner, T. J., Wick, P., Manser, P., Spohn, P., Grass, R. N., Limbach, L. K., Bruinink, A. and Stark, W. J. (2006). In vitro cytotoxicity of oxide nanoparticles: comparison to asbestos, silica, and the effect of particle solubility, *Environ. Sci. Technol.*, **40**(14), pp. 4374–4381.

129. Guan, R., Kang, T., Lu, F., Zhang, Z., Shen, H. and Liu, M. (2012). Cytotoxicity, oxidative stress, and genotoxicity in human hepatocyte and embryonic kidney cells exposed to ZnO nanoparticles, *Nanoscale Res. Lett.*, **7**(1), p. 602.

130. Sharma, V., Singh, P., Pandey, A. K. and Dhawan, A. (2012). Induction of oxidative stress, DNA damage and apoptosis in mouse liver after sub-acute oral exposure to zinc oxide nanoparticles, *Mutat. Res.*, **745**(1–2), pp. 84–91.

131. Zhu, M. T., Feng, W. Y., Wang, B., Wang, T. C., Gu, Y. Q., Wang, M., Wang, Y., Ouyang, H., Zhao, Y. L. and Chai, Z. F. (2008). Comparative study of

pulmonary responses to nano- and submicron-sized ferric oxide in rats, *Toxicology*, **247**, pp. 278–284.

132. Liu, G., Gao, J., Ai, H. and Chen, X. (2013). Applications and potential toxicity of magnetic iron oxide nanoparticles, *Small*, **9**(9–10), pp. 1533–1545.

133. Derfus, A. M., Chan, W. C. W. and Bhatia, S. N. (2004). Probing the cytotoxicity of semiconductor quantum dots, *Nano Lett.*, **4**(1), pp. 11–18.

134. Tsoi, K. M., Dai, Q., Alman, B. A. and Chan, W. C. (2013). Are quantum dots toxic? Exploring the discrepancy between cell culture and animal studies, *Acc. Chem. Res.*, **46**(3), pp. 662–671.

135. Zhang, L. W., Yu, W. W., Colvin, V. L. and Monteiro-Riviere, N. A. (2008). Biological interactions of quantum dot nanoparticles in skin and in human epidermal keratinocytes, *Toxicol. Appl. Pharmacol.*, **228**(2), pp. 200–211.

136. Chen, N., He, Y., Su, Y., Li, X., Huang, Q., Wang, H., Zhang, X., Tai, R. and Fan, C. (2012). The cytotoxicity of cadmium-based quantum dots, *Biomaterials*, **33**(5), pp. 1238–1244.

137. Galeone, A., Vecchio, G., Malvindi, M. A., Brunetti, V., Cingolani, R. and Pompa, P. P. (2012). In vivo assessment of CdSe-ZnS quantum dots: coating dependent bioaccumulation and genotoxicity, *Nanoscale*, **4**(20), pp. 6401–6407.

138. Li, K. G., Chen, J. T., Bai, S. S., Wen, X., Song, S. Y., Yu, Q., Li, J. and Wang, Y. Q. (2009). Intracellular oxidative stress and cadmium ions release induce cytotoxicity of unmodified cadmium sulfide quantum dots, *Toxicol. in Vitro*, **23**(6), pp. 1007–1013.

139. Hoshino, A., Hanaki, K., Suzuki, K. and Yamamoto, K. (2004). Applications of t-lymphoma labeled with fluorescent quantum dots to cell tracing markers in mouse body, *Biochem. Biophys. Res. Commun.*, **314**(1), pp. 46–53.

140. Ipe, B. I., Lehnig, M. and Niemeyer, C. M. (2005). On the generation of free radical species from quantum dots, *Small*, **1**(7), pp. 706–709.

141. Hauck, T. S., Anderson, R. E., Fischer, H. C., Newbigging, S. and Chan, W. C. (2010). In vivo quantum-dot toxicity assessment, *Small*, **6**(1), pp. 138–144.

142. Mortensen, L. J., Oberdorster, G., Pentland, A. P. and Delouise, L. A. (2008). In vivo skin penetration of quantum dot nanoparticles in the murine model: the effect of UVR, *Nano Lett.*, **8**(9), pp. 2779–2787.

143. Kato, S., Itoh, K., Yaoi, T., Tozawa, T., Yoshikawa, Y., Yasui, H., Kanamura, N., Hoshino, A., Manabe, N., Yamamoto, K. and Fushiki, S. (2010). Organ distribution of quantum dots after intraperitoneal administration, with special reference to area-specific distribution in the brain, *Nanotechnology*, **21**(33), p. 335103.

144. Boldrin, A., Hansen, S. F., Baun, A., Hartmann, N. I. B. and Astrup, T. F. (2014). Environmental exposure assessment framework for nanoparticles in solid waste, *J. Nanopart. Res.*, **16**(6), p. 2394.

145. Ingole, S., Gupta, A., Pugh, K. and Kurwadkar, S. (2015). Nanoparticles in the environment: occurrence, distribution, and risks, *J. Hazard. Toxic Radioact. Waste*, **19**(3).

146. Smita, S., Gupta, S. K., Bartonova, A., Dusinska, M., Gutleb, A. C. and Rahman, Q. (2012). Nanoparticles in the environment: assessment using the causal diagram approach, *Environ. Health*, **11**(Suppl 1), pp. S13–S13.

147. Bundschuh, M., Seitz, F., Rosenfeldt, R. R. and Schulz, R. (2012). Titanium dioxide nanoparticles increase sensitivity in the next generation of the water flea daphnia magna, *PLoS One*, **7**(11), pp. e48956.

148. Lovern, S. B. and Klaper, R. (2006). Daphnia magna mortality when exposed to titanium dioxide and fullerene (C60) nanoparticles, *Environ. Toxicol. Chem.*, **25**(4), pp. 1132–1137.

149. Zhu, S., Oberdörster, E. and Haasch, M. L. (2006). Toxicity of an engineered nanoparticle (fullerene, C60) in two aquatic species, daphnia and fathead minnow, *Mar. Environ. Res.*, **62**, pp. S5–S9.

150. Oberdörster, E., Zhu, S., Blickley, T. M., McClellan-Green, P. and Haasch, M. L. (2006). Ecotoxicology of carbon-based engineered nanoparticles: effects of fullerene (C60) on aquatic organisms, *Carbon*, **44**(6), pp. 1112–1120.

151. Kovrižnych, J. A., Sotníková, R., Zeljenková, D., Rollerová, E., Szabová, E. and Wimmerová, S. (2013). Acute toxicity of 31 different nanoparticles to zebrafish (danio rerio) tested in adulthood and in early life stages – comparative study, *Interdiscip. Toxicol.*, **6**(2), pp. 67–73.

152. Wang, J., Zhu, X., Zhang, X., Zhao, Z., Liu, H., George, R., Wilson-Rawls, J., Chang, Y. and Chen, Y. (2011). Disruption of zebrafish (danio rerio) reproduction upon chronic exposure to TiO_2 nanoparticles, *Chemosphere*, **83**(4), pp. 461–467.

153. Griffitt, R. J., Weil, R., Hyndman, K. A., Denslow, N. D., Powers, K., Taylor, D. and Barber, D. S. (2007). Exposure to copper nanoparticles causes

gill injury and acute lethality in zebrafish (danio rerio), *Environ. Sci. Technol.*, **41**(23), pp. 8178–8186.

154. Morgan, T. P. and Wood, C. M. (2004). A relationship between gill silver accumulation and acute silver toxicity in the freshwater rainbow trout: support for the acute silver biotic ligand model, *Environ. Toxicol. Chem.*, **23**(5), pp. 1261–1267.

155. Xiong, D. W., Fang, T., Chen, X. D., Sima, X. F. and Zhu, W. T. (2010). Oxidative stress effects and damage of nanoscale TiO_2 and ZnO on zebrafish, *Huan Jing Ke Xue*, **31**(5), pp. 1320–1327.

156. Zhao, X., Wang, S., Wu, Y., You, H. and Lv, L. (2013). Acute ZnO nanoparticles exposure induces developmental toxicity, oxidative stress and DNA damage in embryo-larval zebrafish, *Aquat. Toxicol.*, **136–137**, pp. 49–59.

157. Duan, J., Yu, Y., Shi, H., Tian, L., Guo, C., Huang, P., Zhou, X., Peng, S. and Sun, Z. (2013). Toxic effects of silica nanoparticles on zebrafish embryos and larvae, *PLoS One*, **8**(9), p. e74606.

158. Fent, K., Weisbrod, C. J., Wirth-Heller, A. and Pieles, U. (2010). Assessment of uptake and toxicity of fluorescent silica nanoparticles in zebrafish (danio rerio) early life stages, *Aquat. Toxicol.*, **100**(2), pp. 218–228.

159. Cornelis, G., Hund-Rinke, K., Kuhlbusch, T., van den Brink, N. and Nickel, C. (2014). Fate and bioavailability of engineered nanoparticles in soils: a review, *Crit. Rev. Environ. Sci. Technol.*, **44**(24), pp. 2720–2764.

160. Theng, B. K. G. and Yuan, G. (2008). Nanoparticles in the soil environment, *Elements*, **4**, p. 395.

161. Dalai, S., Pakrashi, S., Kumar, R. S. S., Chandrasekaran, N. and Mukherjee, A. (2012). A comparative cytotoxicity study of TiO_2 nanoparticles under light and dark conditions at low exposure concentrations, *Toxicol. Res.*, **1**(2), pp. 116–130.

162. Johansen, A. (2008). Effects of C60 fullerene nanoparticles on soil bacteria and protozoans, *Environ. Toxicol. Chem.*, **27**, p. 1895.

163. Fajardo, C. (2014). Impact of ag and Al_2O_3 nanoparticles on soil organisms: in vitro and soil experiments, *Sci. Total Environ.*, **46**(17), pp. 254–261.

164. Unrine, J. M., Tsyusko, O. V., Hunyadi, S. E., Judy, J. D. and Bertsch, P. M. (2010). Effects of particle size on chemical speciation and bioavailability of copper to earthworms (eisenia fetida) exposed to copper nanoparticles, *J. Environ. Qual.*, **39**(6), pp. 1942–1953.

165. Heckmann, L. H., Hovgaard, M. B., Sutherland, D. S., Autrup, H., Besenbacher, F. and Scott-Fordsmand, J. J. (2011). Limit-test toxicity screening of selected inorganic nanoparticles to the earthworm eisenia fetida, *Ecotoxicology*, **20**(1), pp. 226–233.

166. van der Ploeg, M. J., Handy, R. D., Waalewijn-Kool, P. L., van den Berg, J. H., Herrera Rivera, Z. E., Bovenschen, J., Molleman, B., Baveco, J. M., Tromp, P., Peters, R. J., Koopmans, G. F., Rietjens, I. M. and van den Brink, N. W. (2014). Effects of silver nanoparticles (nm-300k) on lumbricus rubellus earthworms and particle characterization in relevant test matrices including soil, *Environ. Toxicol. Chem.*, **33**(4), pp. 743–752.

167. Maurer-Jones, M. A., Gunsolus, I. L., Murphy, C. J. and Haynes, C. L. (2013). Toxicity of engineered nanoparticles in the environment, *Anal. Chem.*, **85**(6), pp. 3036–3049.

168. Serag, M. F., Kaji, N., Gaillard, C., Okamoto, Y., Terasaka, K., Jabasini, M., Tokeshi, M., Mizukami, H., Bianco, A. and Baba, Y. (2011). Trafficking and subcellular localization of multiwalled carbon nanotubes in plant cells, *ACS Nano*, **5**(1), pp. 493–499.

169. Canas, J. E., Long, M., Nations, S., Vadan, R., Dai, L., Luo, M., Ambikapathi, R., Lee, E. H. and Olszyk, D. (2008). Effects of functionalized and nonfunctionalized single-walled carbon nanotubes on root elongation of select crop species, *Environ. Toxicol. Chem.*, **27**(9), pp. 1922–1931.

Index